Breast Imaging

Editors

CHRISTOPHER E. COMSTOCK
CECILIA L. MERCADO

RADIOLOGIC CLINICS
OF NORTH AMERICA

www.radiologic.theclinics.com

Consulting Editor
FRANK H. MILLER

May 2014 • Volume 52 • Number 3

ELSEVIER

1600 John F. Kennedy Boulevard • Suite 1800 • Philadelphia, Pennsylvania, 19103-2899

http://www.theclinics.com

RADIOLOGIC CLINICS OF NORTH AMERICA Volume 52, Number 3
May 2014 ISSN 0033-8389, ISBN 13: 978-0-323-26126-5

Editor: John Vassallo (j.vassallo@elsevier.com)
Developmental Editor: Donald Mumford

Radiologic Clinics of North America (ISSN 0033-8389) is published bimonthly by Elsevier Inc., 360 Park Avenue South, New York, NY 10010-1710. Months of issue are January, March, May, July, September, and November. Periodicals postage paid at New York, NY and additional mailing offices. Subscription prices are USD 460 per year for US individuals, USD 709 per year for US institutions, USD 220 per year for US students and residents, USD 535 per year for Canadian individuals, USD 905 per year for Canadian institutions, USD 660 per year for international individuals, USD 905 per year for international institutions, and USD 315 per year for Canadian and foreign students/residents. To receive student and resident rate, orders must be accompanied by name of affiliated institution, date of term and the signature of program/residency coordinatior on institution letterhead. Orders will be billed at individual rate until proof of status is received. Foreign air speed delivery is included in all *Clinics* subscription prices. All prices are subject to change without notice. **POSTMASTER:** Send address changes to *Radiologic Clinics of North America*, Elsevier Health Sciences Division, Subscription Customer Service, 3251 Riverport Lane, Maryland Heights, MO63043. **Customer Service: Telephone: 1-800-654-2452** (U.S. and Canada); **1-314-447-8871** (outside U.S. and Canada). **Fax: 1-314-447-8029. E-mail: journalscustomerservice-usa@ elsevier.com** (for print support); **journalsonlinesupport-usa@elsevier.com** (for online support).

Reprints. For copies of 100 or more of articles in this publication, please contact the Commercial Reprints Department, Elsevier Inc., 360 Park Avenue South, New York, New York 10010-1710. Tel.: +1-212-633-3874; Fax: +1-212-633-3820; E-mail: reprints@elsevier.com.

Radiologic Clinics of North America also published in Greek Paschalidis Medical Publications, Athens, Greece.

Radiologic Clinics of North America is covered in *MEDLINE/PubMed (Index Medicus), EMBASE/Excerpta Medica, Current Contents/Life Sciences, Current Contents/Clinical Medicine, RSNA Index to Imaging Literature, BIOSIS, Science Citation Index,* and *ISI/BIOMED*.

Printed in the United States of America.

Contributors

CONSULTING EDITOR

FRANK H. MILLER, MD
Professor of Radiology; Chief, Body
Imaging Section and Fellowship Program
and GI Radiology; Medical Director MRI,
Department of Radiology, Feinberg School
of Medicine, Northwestern University,
Chicago, Illinois

EDITORS

CHRISTOPHER E. COMSTOCK, MD
Associate Professor of Radiology,
Department of Radiology, Memorial
Sloan Kettering Cancer Center, New York,
New York

CECILIA L. MERCADO, MD
Associate Residency Program Director,
Assistant Professor of Radiology, Department
of Radiology, New York University School of
Medicine, NYU Cancer Institute, New York
University Langone Medical Center, New York,
New York

AUTHORS

CHRISTOPHER E. COMSTOCK, MD
Associate Professor of Radiology,
Department of Radiology, Memorial
Sloan Kettering Cancer Center, New York,
New York

EMILY F. CONANT, MD
Professor, Department of Radiology,
Perelman School of Medicine at the University
of Pennsylvania, Philadelphia, Pennsylvania

STEPHEN A. FEIG, MD
Fong and Jean Tsai Professor of Women's
Imaging; Director of Breast Imaging,
Department of Radiological Sciences,
University of California Irvine Medical Center,
Orange, California

RICHARD HA, MD
Assistant Professor of Clinical Radiology,
Columbia University Medical Center,
New York, New York

R. EDWARD HENDRICK, PhD, FACR
Clinical Professor, Department of
Radiology, School of Medicine, University
of Colorado–Denver, Aurora,
Colorado

MAXINE JOCHELSON, MD
Department of Radiology, Memorial
Sloan-Kettering Cancer Center;
Associate Professor of Clinical Radiology,
Weill Cornell Medical College, New York,
New York

STUART S. KAPLAN, MD, FACR
Section Chief, Breast Imaging, Comprehensive
Cancer Center; Vice Chairman, Department
of Radiology, Mount Sinai Medical Center,
Miami Beach, Florida

JAMES G. MAINPRIZE, PhD
Sunnybrook Research Institute, Toronto,
Ontario, Canada

ELLEN B. MENDELSON, MD, FACR
Professor of Radiology; Section Chief,
Department of Radiology, Lynn Sage
Comprehensive Breast Center, Feinberg
School of Medicine, Northwestern Memorial
Hospital–Prentice 4, Northwestern University,
Chicago, Illinois

CECILIA L. MERCADO, MD
Associate Residency Program Director,
Assistant Professor of Radiology, Department
of Radiology, New York University School of
Medicine, NYU Cancer Institute, New York
University Langone Medical Center, New York,
New York

GINGER M. MERRY, MD, MPH
Breast Imaging Radiologist, Colorado
Permanente Medical Group, Denver, Colorado;
Department of Radiology, Lynn Sage
Comprehensive Breast Center, Feinberg
School of Medicine, Northwestern Memorial
Hospital–Prentice 4, Northwestern University,
Chicago, Illinois

MICHAEL S. MIDDLETON, MD, PhD
Assistant Clinical Professor of Radiology,
Department of Radiology, University of
California San Diego School of Medicine, San
Diego, California

LINDA MOY, MD
Assistant Professor of Radiology, Department
of Radiology, New York University School of
Medicine, New York, New York

SARAH PALESTRANT, MD, MPhil
Department of Radiology, New York
University School of Medicine, New York,
New York

JANICE S. SUNG, MD
Assistant Attending, Department of Radiology,
Memorial Sloan-Kettering Cancer Center,
New York, New York

MARTIN J. YAFFE, PhD
Department of Medical Biophysics;
Sunnybrook Research Institute, Toronto,
Ontario, Canada

Contents

Numerous clinical studies have confirmed that screening women age 40 years and older reduces breast cancer mortality by 30% to 50%. Several factors including faster breast cancer growth rates and lower breast cancer incidence among younger women, as well as shorter life expectancy and more comorbid conditions among older women, should also be considered in screening guidelines. Annual screening beginning at age 40 years and continuing with no upper age limit, as long as a woman has a life expectancy of at least 5 years and no significant comorbid conditions, is currently recommended.

The updated American College of Radiology (ACR) Breast Imaging Reporting and Data System (BI-RADS) has been newly released. This article summarizes the changes and updates that have been made to BI-RADS. The goal of the revised edition continues to be the same: to improve clarification in image interpretation, maintain reporting standardization, and simplify the monitoring of outcomes. The new BI-RADS also introduces new terminology to provide a more universal lexicon across all 3 imaging modalities.

Digital breast tomosynthesis is an extension of digital mammography that produces quasi three-dimensional reconstructed images from a set of low-dose x-ray projections acquired over a limited angular range. The quality of the reconstructed image and the dose to the breast are dependent on the angular range and number of projections, the dose used per projection, and detector resolution and noise characteristics. This article discusses various aspects of tomosynthesis optimization.

Digital breast tomosynthesis is rapidly being implemented in breast imaging clinics across the world as early clinical data demonstrate that this innovative technology may address some of the long-standing limitations of conventional mammography. This article reviews the recent clinical data supporting digital breast tomosynthesis implementation, the basics of digital breast tomosynthesis image interpretation using case-based illustrations, and potential issues to consider as this new technology is integrated into daily clinical use.

images. When reading the examination, the radiologist should approach the images from both a global and focused perspective, synthesizing findings into a report that includes a management plan. This article reviews a systematic and organized approach to breast MR imaging interpretation.

An enhancing focus is a commonly encountered type of lesion on breast magnetic resonance (MR) imaging. No set criteria for appropriate management are available. Often management of these lesions depends on the interpreting radiologist, with varying recommendations for biopsy, short-term follow-up, or routine surveillance. This article reviews published studies in order to develop a strategy for the management of enhancing foci identified on breast MR imaging.

This article describes the rationale and indications for breast implant–related magnetic resonance (MR) imaging, alone or in combination with breast cancer–related MR imaging. Basic silicone chemistry, implant styles, and normal appearances of breast implants are described. The various presentations of breast implant rupture are described, and a 4-point staging scheme for intracapsular rupture is reviewed. Finally, a discussion of what the reviewing physician needs to know is presented, both before breast implant MR examinations are requested and afterward, when results are reported.

Mammography is the only technology documented to reduce breast cancer mortality. Its sensitivity, however, is 75% to 80% at best and reduced to 30% to 50% in women with dense breasts. MR imaging is a sensitive modality for the detection of breast cancer but cannot be used in all patients. Its sensitivity is due in large part to its ability to detect enhancement of tumor vascularity so cancers can be detected before a mass is present. Contrast-enhanced dual-energy mammography uses the same capability of vascular enhancement and has been demonstrated to be more sensitive than routine mammography.

PROGRAM OBJECTIVE

The objective of the *Radiologic Clinics of North America* is to keep practicing radiologists and radiology residents up to date with current clinical practice in radiology by providing timely articles reviewing the state of the art in patient care.

TARGET AUDIENCE

Practicing radiologists, radiology residents, and other health care professionals who provide patient care utilizing radiologic findings.

LEARNING OBJECTIVES

Upon completion of this activity, participants will be able to:

1. Discuss the approach to breast magnetic resonance imaging interpretation.
2. Review the evidence related to screening mammography benefit controversies.
3. Explain magnetic resonance evaluation of breast implants.

ACCREDITATION

The Elsevier Office of Continuing Medical Education (EOCME) is accredited by the Accreditation Council for Continuing Medical Education (ACCME) to provide continuing medical education for physicians.

The EOCME designates this enduring material for a maximum of 15 *AMA PRA Category 1 Credit*(s)™. Physicians should claim only the credit commensurate with the extent of their participation in the activity.

All other health care professionals requesting continuing education credit for this enduring material will be issued a certificate of participation.

DISCLOSURE OF CONFLICTS OF INTEREST

The EOCME assesses conflict of interest with its instructors, faculty, planners, and other individuals who are in a position to control the content of CME activities. All relevant conflicts of interest that are identified are thoroughly vetted by EOCME for fair balance, scientific objectivity, and patient care recommendations. EOCME is committed to providing its learners with CME activities that promote improvements or quality in healthcare and not a specific proprietary business or a commercial interest.

The planning committee, staff, authors and editors listed below have identified no financial relationships or relationships to products or devices they or their spouse/life partner have with commercial interest related to the content of this CME activity:
Christopher E. Comstock, MD; Stephen A. Feig, MD; Richard Ha, MD; Kristen Helm; Brynne Hunter; Maxine Jochelson, MD; Stuart S. Kaplan, MD, FACR; Jill McNair; Cecilia L. Mercado, MD; Ginger M. Merry, MD, MPH; Frank H. Miller, MD; Linda Moy, MD; Sarah Palestrant, MD, MPhil; Karthikeyan Subramaniam; Janice S. Sung, MD; John Vassallo.

The planning committee, staff, authors and editors listed below have identified financial relationships or relationships to products or devices they or their spouse/life partner have with commercial interest related to the content of this CME activity:
Emily F. Conant, MD is on speakers bureau and is a consultant/advisor for Hologic, Inc.; is on speakers bureau and has a research grant from National Institutes of Health/National Cancer Institute population-based research.

R. Edward Hendrick, PhD, FACR is a consultant/advisor for GE Healthcare.

James G. Mainprize, PhD has a research grant from GE Healthcare.

Ellen B. Mendelson, MD, FACR is a consultant/advisor for Philips N.V., Quantason LLC, Delphinus Medical Technologies, Hologic, Inc. and Siemens Corporation.

Michael S. Middleton, MD, PhD is a consultant/advisor for Allergan, Inc.

Martin J. Yaffe, MSc, PhD has a research grant from GE Healthcare.

UNAPPROVED/OFF-LABEL USE DISCLOSURE

The EOCME requires CME faculty to disclose to the participants:

1. When products or procedures being discussed are off-label, unlabelled, experimental, and/or investigational (not US Food and Drug Administration (FDA) approved); and
2. Any limitations on the information presented, such as data that are preliminary or that represent ongoing research, interim analyses, and/or unsupported opinions. Faculty may discuss information about pharmaceutical agents that is outside of FDA-approved labelling. This information is intended solely for CME and is not intended to promote off-label use of these medications. If you have any questions, contact the medical affairs department of the manufacturer for the most recent prescribing information.

TO ENROLL

To enroll in the *Radiologic Clinics of North America* Continuing Medical Education program, call customer service at 1-800-654-2452 or sign up online at http://www.theclinics.com/home/cme. The CME program is available to subscribers for an additional annual fee of USD $315.

METHOD OF PARTICIPATION

In order to claim credit, participants must complete the following:

1. Complete enrolment as indicated above.
2. Read the activity.
3. Complete the CME Test and Evaluation. Participants must achieve a score of 70% on the test. All CME Tests and Evaluations must be completed online.

CME INQUIRIES/SPECIAL NEEDS

For all CME inquiries or special needs, please contact elsevierCME@elsevier.com.

RADIOLOGIC CLINICS OF NORTH AMERICA

Preface

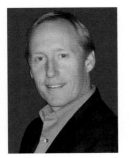 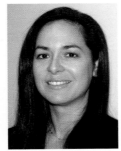

Christopher E. Comstock, MD   Cecilia L. Mercado, MD

Editors

The field of breast imaging has undergone tremendous growth in recent years. In addition to mammography, ultrasound, and MRI, new technologies including tomosynthesis and contrast-enhanced digital mammography have emerged to improve the sensitivity and specificity of breast cancer detection. In addition, recent state breast density notification legislation has led to the proliferation of the use of ultrasound for breast cancer screening in women with dense breasts.

This issue of the *Radiologic Clinics of North America* begins by reaffirming the importance of breast imaging and early cancer detection. The first article reviews the most current studies regarding screening mammography and presents strong evidence that screening mammography reduces mortality from breast cancer. The issue also provides an update on the newly released Breast Imaging Reporting and Data System (BI-RADS) Atlas, which has undergone a significant revision after 11 years. One of the articles discusses some key changes that have been made to BI-RADS and also reviews the new terminology that has been introduced to the breast imaging lexicon.

Several articles focus on magnetic resonance (MR) imaging of the breast. Topics include how to perform high-quality breast MR imaging, useful guidelines on breast MR interpretation to improve diagnostic accuracy, and techniques to optimize MR interventional procedures. The management of enhancing foci on breast MR is also discussed. As recommended by the FDA, breast MRI is also routinely used to evaluate for rupture of silicone implants. Valuable information on the interpretation and evaluation of breast implants on MR imaging is provided.

Ultrasound has emerged as the most common modality for supplemental screening in women with dense breasts. Factors to consider to optimize image quality on ultrasound are reviewed. This edition provides updated information on screening breast ultrasonography and offers guidelines for the implementation of a screening breast ultrasound program. Digital breast tomosynthesis (DBT) is rapidly being adopted by many practices and will likely become the standard mammographic screening technique. Two articles review the basic technical aspects and clinical implementation of DBT. Automated whole breast ultrasound and contrast-enhanced mammography are two additional new technologies that are expected to play an increasing role in supplemental screening for breast carcinoma as breast density notification laws become more widespread.

We trust that this issue will be a valuable resource to practicing radiologists as well as radiologists just completing their training. Many thanks to the contributors, who have generously shared their time, knowledge, and expertise in the field of breast imaging.

Christopher E. Comstock, MD
Department of Radiology
Memorial Sloan Kettering Cancer Center
300 East 66th Street
New York, NY 10065, USA

Cecilia L. Mercado, MD
Department of Radiology
New York University School of Medicine
NYU Cancer Institute
New York University Langone Medical Center
560 First Avenue
New York, NY 10016, USA

E-mail addresses:
ComstocC@mskcc.org (C.E. Comstock)
Cecilia.Mercado@nyumc.org (C.L. Mercado)

radiologic.theclinics.com

Radiol Clin N Am 52 (2014) xi
http://dx.doi.org/10.1016/j.rcl.2014.02.014
0033-8389/14/$ – see front matter © 2014 Published by Elsevier Inc.

Screening Mammography Benefit Controversies
Sorting the Evidence

Stephen A. Feig, MD

KEYWORDS

- Screening • Mammography • Benefit • Controversies

KEY POINTS

- Numerous clinical studies have confirmed that screening women age 40 years and older reduces breast cancer mortality by 30% to 50%.
- Several factors including faster breast cancer growth rates and lower breast cancer incidence among younger women, as well as shorter life expectancy and more comorbid conditions among older women, should also be considered in screening guidelines.
- Annual screening beginning at age 40 years and continuing with no upper age limit, as long as a woman has a life expectancy of at least 5 years and no significant comorbid conditions, is currently recommended by the American Cancer Society, the American College of Radiology, and the Society of Breast Imaging.

Screening mammography by virtue of its ability to substantially reduce death rates from the most common type of malignancy among women and the second leading cause of their death from cancer represents one of the major medical achievements of our time. Yet, unlike other medical advancements, the value of screening women age 40 years and older did not become apparent until after many years of clinical trials which began in the 1960s. Lengthy observational follow-up was required, because breast cancer is a chronic disease. During subsequent decades, there have been numerous improvements in technology, beginning with the replacement of direct exposure film mammography by film/screen mammography, the more recent conversion to digital mammography, and the current clinical evaluation of digital tomosynthesis. There have also been improvements in performance of mammography, such as better breast compression paddles and automatic exposure devices, mammographic grids, use of the mediolateral oblique (MLO) view instead of the straight mediolateral view. Some advances, such as use of 2-view screening (craniocaudal and MLO), instead of a single MLO view alone, screening at an annual rate rather than semiannual intervals, and double reading by 2 radiologists, have still not been universally accepted because of concerns regarding cost-effectiveness.

Screening controversies began in 1975 and continue. Some issues are legitimate, but most have been artificially contrived. No other medical test has been more thoroughly scrutinized and debated over the past 40 years. Keeping informed on these complex issues has been challenging for all physicians, including breast imagers. The public especially deserves empathy, because their information is channeled through the nonmedical media. Thus, the purpose of this article is to assess our current knowledge of screening benefits. Comprehensive reviews of adverse consequences and costs of screening may be found in the author's previous articles in the *Radiologic Clinics of North America*.[1,2]

Department of Radiological Sciences, University of California Irvine Medical Center, 101 City Drive South, Orange, CA 92869-3298, USA
E-mail address: sfeig@uci.edu

Radiol Clin N Am 52 (2014) 455–480
http://dx.doi.org/10.1016/j.rcl.2014.02.009
0033-8389/14/$ – see front matter © 2014 Elsevier Inc. All rights reserved.

RANDOMIZED TRIALS HAVE PROVEN THAT EARLY DETECTION REDUCES BREAST CANCER DEATH RATES

The ability of widespread screening to detect breast cancers at smaller size and earlier stage than encountered in the general population was first established at the Breast Cancer Detection Demonstration Project (BCDDP), a program that screened 280,000 women throughout the United States with both mammography and physical examination from 1973 to 1981, sponsored by the American Cancer Society (ACS) and National Cancer Institute. In this program, 39% (1375) of the 3548 cancers were found by mammography alone, 7% (257) by clinical examination alone, and 51% (1805) by both mammography and clinical examination.[3] The 20-year relative survival rates at the BCDDP were 80.5% (overall), 85% for cancers detected by mammography alone, 82% for cancers detected by physical examination alone, and 74% for cancers detected by both mammography and physical examination.[4] These rates can be compared with the contemporaneous 20-year survival rate of 53% among US women who were largely not being screened.[5] Although these results were promising, there are several reasons why improved survival rates among such women who volunteer to be screened do not necessarily establish benefit from screening. They include selection bias, lead time bias, length bias, and interval cancers.[6] Thus, differences in survival rates may be influenced by factors other than the screening process itself.

Selection bias refers to the possibility that women who volunteer for screening differ from those who do not volunteer in ways that may alter the outcome of their disease, such as health status and behavioral factors. Therefore, survival rates in screened and nonscreened women may be influenced by factors other than the screening process itself.

Lead time bias implies that screening may affect the date of detection but not necessarily the date of death from breast cancer. Let us suppose that a woman who has never been screened finds her breast cancer serendipitously in 2009. She dies from her disease 5 years later, in 2014. If this same woman had been screened, her cancer might have been detected by mammography in the year 2005. Although small, the cancer detected in this woman by mammography might have dissemination beyond the breast. Despite screening, the woman dies from her disease in the year 2014. Because of screening, she is said to have survived for 9 years instead of 5 years. Therefore, the seemingly 4-year improvement in survival may not be real.

Length-biased sampling postulates that cancers detected at screening contain a disproportionate number of less aggressive cancers. Their growth rates are so slow that in the absence of screening, they might never reach sufficient size to surface clinically. Even if undetected, such indolent cancers might never result in death.

Possibly, the favorable survival rates for screen-detected cancers might be negated by lower survival rates for faster-growing interval cancers, which are undetected by mammography and surface clinically between screenings.

Considering these potential biases, benefit from screening cannot be proved by observation of improved survival rates. Rather, such proof requires prospective comparison of breast cancer death rates among a study group of women offered screening and a control group of women not offered screening in a randomized clinical trial (RCT).[6] Apart from the offer to be screened, these groups should not differ in any other substantial way. Therefore, a statistically significant difference in breast cancer deaths between the groups on follow-up represents incontrovertible proof of benefit from the screening. Observation of lower mortality for the screened group in a well-designed and well-conducted RCT is not affected by selection bias, lead time bias, length bias, or interval cancers.

RESULTS OF RCTS

Seven population-based trials of breast cancer screening by mammography alone or in combination with physical examination have been conducted. They are as follows: (1) the Health Insurance Plan of Greater New York (HIP) trial,[7] (2) the Swedish Two-County trial consisting of Kopparberg and Ostergotland counties,[8–10] (3) the Malmö (Sweden) Mammographic Screening trial,[11–15] (4) the Stockholm (Sweden) trial,[14–17] (5) the Gothenburg (Sweden) Breast Screening trial,[14,15,18–20] (6) the Edinburgh (Scotland) trial,[21,22] and (7) the UK Age trial.[23] In a population-based RCT, study and control groups are randomly selected from a predefined population. There has also been 1 non–population-based RCT, the National Breast Screening Study of Canada (NBSSC).[24–26] In a non–population-based RCT, study and control groups are randomly selected from women who volunteer to participate.

Protocols and results for women of all ages at entry into these 8 RCTs are shown in **Table 1**. Mortality reduction is equal to 1 minus the relative risk (RR) of dying from breast cancer in the study group women versus the control group. The HIP trial, the

Table 1
Randomized trials of mammography screening: protocols and results

Trial (y)	Age at Entry (y)	Number of Views	Frequency of Mammography (mo)	Rounds (n)	CBE	Follow-Up (y)	Relative Risk (95% Confidence Interval)	Mortality Reduction (%)
HIP trial (1963–1969)	40–64	2	12	4	Annual	18	0.78 (0.61–0.97)	22
Malmö, Sweden (1976–1986)	46–69	1–2	18–24	5	None	20	0.78 (0.65–0.95)	22
Two-County Swedish (1979–1988)	40–74	1	23–33	4	None	30	0.68 (0.54–0.80)	32
Edinburgh, Scotland (1979–1988)	45–64	1–2	24	4	Annual	14	0.78 (0.62–0.97)	22
NBSSC (1980–1987) NBSSC-1	40–49	2	12	5	None	13	0.97 (0.78–1.33)	0.3
NBSSC-2	50–59	2	12	5	Yes	13	1.02 (0.78–1.33)	–2
Stockholm, Sweden (1981–1988)	40–64	1	28	2	None	16	0.90 (0.63–1.28)	10
Gothenburg, Sweden (1982–1988)	40–59	2	18	4	None	14	0.79 (0.58–1.08)	21
UK Age trial (1991–2005)	39–41	1–2	12	8	None	10	0.83 (0.66–1.04)	17

Data from Refs. 7,9,11,12,17,19,20,22,23,25,26

first RCT ever conducted, found a 22% reduction in breast cancer deaths (RR = 0.78).[7]

The Two-County Swedish trial was the first to show a statistically significant benefit from screening by mammography alone. The latest 30-year follow-up for this trial found a 32% reduction in breast cancer deaths among women aged 40 to 74 years at entry.[9] In the Edinburgh trial, screening by annual physical examination and biennial mammography resulted in a statistically significant 22% decrease in breast cancer deaths among women aged 45 to 64 years at entry.[21,22]

The Gothenburg Breast Screening trial had a 21% reduction in deaths from breast cancer among women aged 40 to 59 years at entry into screening, a finding that had marginal statistical significance.[14,15,18–20] The Malmö Mammographic Screening trial found a significant 22% reduction in breast cancer deaths among women who began screening between ages 45 and 60 years.[11–15] The Stockholm trial described a nonsignificant 10% reduction in breast cancer deaths among women screened between 40 and 60 years of age, which was not statistically significant.[14–17]

Combined results from a 15.8-year follow-up of women aged 38 to 75 years at entry into 4 Swedish trials (Malmö, Ostergotland, Stockholm, and Gothenburg) showed a statistically significant 21% reduction (confidence interval = 0.70–0.89) in breast cancer mortality with screening.[14,15]

NBSSC failed to show any benefit for mammography screening in women aged 50 to 59 years.[24,25] In that trial, women undergoing annual mammography and physical examination were compared with those being screened by physical examination alone. Possible explanations for the variance between NBSSC results and those of the 7 other randomized trials include poor technical quality of mammography improper study design, and control group contamination with advanced cancers.[27–36]

Of the 8 randomized screening trials, 7 showed evidence of benefit from screening.[37] Breast cancer mortality reduction was statistically significant in each of 4 trials (HIP, Swedish Two-County, and Edinburgh) and in combined results from the Stockholm, Malmö, Ostergotland, and Gothenburg trials, and marginally significant in the Gothenburg trial. Only 1 trial, the NBSSC, found no evidence of benefit.

Origins of the Controversy Regarding Women Aged 40 to 49 Years

Initial reports from the HIP trial found a difference in breast cancer death rates between study and control groups for women 50 years of age and older at entry that was apparent by year 4.[7] However, a difference for women aged 40 to 49 years did not emerge until 7 to 8 years of follow-up. By 18 years of follow-up, the reduction in breast cancer deaths among study women aged 40 to 49 years at entry was 23%, the same as that for women aged 50 to 64 years at entry. Yet, even by that time, benefit for younger women was still not statistically significant according to the original investigators.[7] This lack of statistical significance was a consequence of the smaller number of younger women enrolled and the lower breast cancer incidence. Nevertheless, the apparent lack of statistically significant benefit led to controversy regarding screening of women in their 40s.[37–39]

However, the HIP trial was designed to determine the efficacy of screening a single group of all women aged 40 to 65 years rather than the efficacy of screening separate age groups. Attempts to subdivide the study group reduced statistical power. The observation that results for younger women lacked statistical significance was often cited in the subsequent screening debate. The fact that the data for women aged 50 to 59 years as well as 60 years and older at entry, when analyzed separately, also lacked statistical significance was largely ignored.[7,40] Subsequently, Chu and colleagues,[41] using a different method of analysis, found statistically significant mortality reductions of 24% for women aged 40 to 49 years and 21% for those aged 50 to 64 years at entry into the HIP trial. Despite the report by Chu and colleagues, some observers were still not convinced that screening would benefit women in their 40s for several reasons. First, the reduction in the breast cancer death rates in the trials for younger women did not appear until several years after appearance of the reduction for women older than 50 years. Second, results for younger women were not statistically significant for any other individual trial until 1997.

The controversy intensified in 1992, with publication of the 7-year follow-up report from the NBSSC.[24] This study found no evidence of benefit among women aged 40 to 49 years who were offered 5 annual screenings by mammography and physical examination. There are several explanations for these disappointing results. First, the technical quality of mammography was poor.[27–29] During most of the trial, more than 50% of the mammograms were poor or completely unacceptable by an independent expert panel, even as assessed by the standards of the day. Second, there are indications that the randomization process through which women were assigned to study and control groups was undermined.[30–35]

All women were given a physical examination before randomization to the study trial. This protocol may have allowed preferential allocation of women with palpable masses (later-stage breast cancers) to the study group.[29–36] As a likely consequence, an excess of late-stage breast cancers and breast cancer deaths was found in the study group compared with the control group throughout the trial.

Mortality Reduction Among Women Screened in Their 40s

Beginning in 1993, several successive meta-analyses of combined data for multiple RCTs were performed to accrue more women-years of follow-up than possible from any 1 RCT alone. However, the earliest meta-analyses, published in 1993 and 1995, suggested little if any benefit from screening women younger than 50 years.[42–44]

Subsequent meta-analyses published by Smart and colleagues[45] in 1995 and the Falun Meeting Committee[46] in 1996 included later follow-up data. These studies showed a statistically significant mortality reduction of 24%, for women aged 40 to 49 years at entry into the 7 population-based RCTs (Table 2). They also found a 15% to 16% mortality reduction, which barely missed statistical significance when the NBSSC, a non–population-based RCT, was also included. A meta-analysis of these trials, published by Hendrick and colleagues[47] in 1997, found statistically significant mortality reductions among women invited to undergo screening in their 40s: 18% for all 8 RCTs and 29% for the 5 Swedish RCTs (see Table 2). Thus, with increasing length of follow-up, successive meta-analyses have shown progressively greater and statistically significant mortality reductions for women who began

screening between 40 and 49 years of age. Regardless of whether NBSSC results are included or excluded, meta-analyses for screening women aged 40 to 49 years show statistically significant benefit. Subsequently, 2 other individual RCTs besides the HIP were each able to show benefit for women aged 40 to 49 years (Table 3). Bjurstam and colleagues[18–20] reported a statistically significant 45% mortality reduction for women aged 39 to 49 years at randomization in the Gothenburg trial. Andersson and Janzon[13] reported a statistically significant 35% breast cancer mortality reduction for women in the Malmö trial who began screening mammography at age 45 to 49 years. A randomized trial of women aged 39 to 41 years at entry in the UK study showed a statistically nonsignificant 17% mortality reduction for those invited and 24% mortality reduction for those screened.[13] Deficiencies that restricted results in the study included use of 1 rather than 2 mammographic views on incidence screens, which the investigators knew missed 20% to 25% of cancers, failure to biopsy clustered calcifications (causing them to miss additional small cancers), low recall rates and insufficient women-years of follow-up, a low 68% compliance rate, considerable contamination of the unscreened control population with private facilities offering mammograms, and mortality follow-up limited to 10 years.[48,49] Later analysis is likely to show more benefit. We also now have data from many service screening studies, showing statistically significant mortality reduction from screening women aged 40 to 49 years, equal to that found for screening older women. For example, in Ostergotland and Dalarma counties in Sweden, Tabar and colleagues[50] found breast cancer mortality reductions of 48% for women aged 40 to 49 years and 44% for all women aged 40 to 69 years. No such decline was seen in the 30-year to 39-year age group, in which none was offered screening. In British Columbia, Coldman and colleagues[51] found that breast cancer deaths were reduced 39% among women aged 40 to 49 years versus 40% for all women aged 40 to 79 years. In the 2 northern Swedish counties of Vasternorrland and Norrbotten, breast cancer deaths were reduced 35% to 38% for women aged 40 to 49 years versus 30% for all women aged 40 to 74 years.

Screening Women 75 Years of Age and Older

The question of mammographic screening for elderly women is clinically relevant, because there are more than 10 million women aged 75 years and older in the United States. The average life expectancy for women at age 75 years is 13 years.[52]

Table 2
Meta-analyses of RCTs of mammography showing statistically significant mortality reduction for women aged 40 to 49 years

Trials	Follow-Up (y)	Mortality Reduction (%)
All 8 trials[a]	10.5–18.0	15
7 trials[b]	7.0–18.0	24
5 Swedish trials[c]	11.4–15.2	29

[a] HIP, 5 Swedish trials, Edinburgh trial. UK Age trial and NBSSC-1.
[b] All trials except NBSSC-1.
[c] Malmö Mammographic Screening trial; Swedish Two-County trial, Kopparberg and Ostergotland; Stockholm trial; and Gothenburg Breast Screening trial.
Data from Refs.[45–47]

Table 3
Follow-up of RCTs of mammography showing statistically significant breast cancer mortality reduction for women aged 40 to 49 years

Trial (y)	Age at Entry (y)	Number of Views	Frequency of Mammography (mo)	Clinical Breast Examination	Follow-Up (y)	Mortality Reduction (%)
HIP (1963–1969)	40–49	2	12	Annual	18.0	24
Malmö Mammographic Screening Program (1976–1990)	45–49	1–2	18–24	None	12.7	36
Gothenburg Breast Screening trial (1982–1988)	39–49	2	18	None	12.0	45

Data from Refs.[13,18,41]

Women with good general health have a longer than average life expectancy. Thus, it is reasonable to expect that elderly women might benefit from screening.[53] Reduction in breast cancer mortality among women aged 50 years and older becomes apparent within 4 years of entry into RCTs. Therefore, for many older women with screening-detected breast cancer, death from another illness does not occur before they experience the benefit from screening.[54]

Benefit from screening women 75 years older has not been proved, because this age group was not included in any RCT.[55] Nevertheless, there is no biological reason why early detection should not be effective for these women. The detection sensitivity of mammography is higher in elderly women because of their generally more fatty breast composition.[56,57] However, because of the lower life expectancy in older women, there is a potential for diagnosis of tumors that would not have given rise to symptoms during their remaining lifetime. In addition, screening is warranted only if the woman is suitable for appropriate therapy in the event of a cancer diagnosis. Taking these considerations, especially comorbidity issues, it seems reasonable that screening mammography should be performed in women aged 75 years having generally good health and life expectancy of 5 years or longer.[58,59]

Why Do Randomized Trials Underestimate the Benefit from Screening?

There are at least 6 reasons why results from all the early RCTs have underestimated the benefit to an individual woman undergoing screening with current advanced mammography technology:

- Mammographic image quality below current standards

- Use of only 1 mammographic view per breast in some RCTs
- Noncompliance of some study group women
- Contamination of the control group
- Excessively long screening intervals (more than annual)
- Inadequate number of screening rounds

First, there have been many technical improvements in mammographic technique since the early 1980s, when these trials were conducted. These innovations in mammographic equipment, screen-film systems, and processing as well as replacement of analog (film) mammography by digital mammography allow images to have better sharpness, exposure, and contrast.[60–65] Better image quality facilitates early detection of breast cancer.[62–65]

Second, women in the RCTs were mostly screened with 1 view per breast. The current standard, 2 views per breast examination has been shown to detect 3% to 20% more cancers than found using an MLO view alone.[66–71] Of the 7 population-based RCTs, only the HIP trial[7] used 2 views on all examinations. For example, the Gothenburg trial[18] used 2-view mammography at the first screen and either single view or 2 views at subsequent screens, depending on breast density. The Malmö trial[11] used 2 views in the first 2 screenings but only an MLO view alone on all subsequent screenings, except in patients with dense breasts. The Edinburgh trial[21] used 2-view screening on the initial screening but only 1 view on all subsequent screenings. The Stockholm and Swedish Two-County trials[8,16] used a single MLO view in all screenings.

Two fundamental reasons why RCTs underestimate the benefit from screening are as follows: (1) not all study group women accept the invitation to be screened (noncompliance); and (2) some control group women obtained mammography screening outside the trial (contamination). Yet, to avoid selection bias, an RCT must compare the breast cancer death rate among all study group women, both screened and nonscreened, with that among all control group women, including those who are screened on their own initiative. Thus, both noncompliance of some study women and contamination of control group women reduce the calculated benefit from RCTs.

Among the RCTs, the noncompliance rate ranged from 10% to 39%.[72] Studies performed on data from the individual trials have estimated that if all women in the study group had attended each screening round, there would have been an additional reduction in breast cancer deaths. Data from the Gothenburg, Malmö, and Swedish Two-County trials as well as the NBSSC indicate that the rate of control group contamination ranged from 13% to 25%.[72]

Randomized trials might have also underestimated the potential benefit of screening, because screening intervals were too long.[73] Aside from the HIP trial, screening intervals in RCTs have been longer than the annual intervals now recommended. For example, women in the Swedish Two-County trial were screened every 24 to 33 months,[8] and those in the Edinburgh trial every 24 months.[21] Numerous studies suggest that greater benefit should result from annual screening, especially for women aged 40 to 49 years, in whom breast cancer growth rates seem to be faster.[74–77] From a tumor growth rate model, Michaelson and colleagues[78] calculated that annual screening would result in a 51% reduction in the rate of distant metastatic disease compared with a 22% reduction at a screening interval of 2 years.

It has been estimated that the use of annual screening in the Swedish Two-County trial could have resulted in an additional 18% mortality reduction for women aged 40 to 49 years at entry, who were screened every 2 years, and an additional 12% mortality reduction for women aged 50 to 59 years at entry, who were screened every 33 months.[79] For women aged 39 to 49 years at entry into the Gothenburg trial, who were screened every 18 months, it has been estimated that annual screening could have resulted in an additional 20% mortality reduction.[80]

Several investigators have used mathematical models of RCT data to calculate the benefit to an average woman who is screened every year and for whom results are not affected by noncompliance and contamination.[46,74,80,81] For example, from an observed 45% reduction in breast cancer mortality among women aged 39 to 49 years offered screening every 18 months in the Gothenburg trial, Feig calculated that the mortality reduction could have been as high as 65% with annual screening at the observed 80% compliance rate and as high as 75% at a 100% compliance rate.[80]

The fact that the results of some trials were based on a short screening period and small numbers of screening rounds represents a sixth reason why such trials may underestimate the potential benefits of screening. Most trials do not achieve the highest steady state of benefit until after 8 to 11 years of follow-up.[82] Short trial durations substantially underestimate the mortality reduction that would be achieved with continued annual screening from ages 40 to 80 years, inclusive.

Validity of RCT Results: the Gotzsche and Olsen Controversy

From results from RCTs conducted over the past quarter of a century and involving more than 500,000 women, consensus has been reached in the medical community in favor of screening mammography.

In the face of such near-unanimous agreement about the value of screening mammography, 2 studies made the seemingly incredible claim that none of the trials provided any convincing evidence that screening prevents breast cancer deaths.[83,84] In these studies, Gotzsche and Olsen, asserted that only 2 of the 8 screening trials (the Malmö Mammographic Screening trial and the NBSSC) were valid and that neither of these trials found evidence of benefit. The studies, published in 2000 and 2001, were highly publicized because of the sensational nature of their claim, which questioned the widely held belief in the efficacy of early detection through mammography screening.

The only 2 points of which Gotzsche and Olsen and all other observers agree are as follows: (1) that the NBSSC failed to find benefit for screening in women aged 50 to 70 years with mammography and clinical examination versus clinical examination alone,[24,25] and (2) the NBSSC found no benefit for mammographic screening of women aged 40 to 49 years.[26] However, at this point, advocates of screening part ways with Gotzsche and Olsen, because their explanations for the negative NBSSC results are vastly different. It is difficult to understand how Gotzsche and Olsen could view the NBSSC as the paradigm of a well-conducted study for several reasons. First, independent reviews found that the technical quality of mammography in the NBSSC was poor, even when measured by the standards of the 1980s, when the trial was conducted.[27–29] Second, performance of clinical breast examination before randomization of trial subjects may have allowed channeling of symptomatic women into the study group.[29–36] The finding of an excess of advanced cancers in the study group aged 40 to 49 years was not shown in any of the other 7 trials and suggests that randomization at NBSSC was not performed blindly.

Third, NBSSC was not a population-based trial. Rather, participants were self-selected volunteers. Because self-selected women are more likely to be symptomatic, adequate randomization of such subjects is more problematic, especially when clinical examination has already been performed. Self-selected asymptomatic women may have higher survival rates than randomly selected asymptomatic women. Thus, benefit may be harder to show in a trial with such subjects than in a population-based trial. Contrary to the judgment of Gotzsche and Olsen, almost any of these problems to trial design and implementation could render the NBSSC incapable of providing meaningful results.

The statement by Gotzsche and Olsen that the Malmö trial showed no evidence of benefit is more difficult to understand. Gotzsche and Olsen considered only an early report of a small but insignificant 5% mortality reduction among women aged 45 to 70 years.[12] These investigators ignored later reports of breast cancer mortality reductions of 19% for women aged 45 to 70 years, 26% for women aged 55 to 70 years, and 36% for women aged 45 to 50 years at entry into the Malmö trial.[13] Moreover, several months after publication of the second Olsen and Gotzsche study, Miettinen and colleagues reported using 3-year moving averages of RR estimates to estimate that the true mortality reduction from the Malmö trial was 55% for women aged 55 to 69 years and 60% for women aged 45 to 57 years at entry into screening.[82]

Gotzsche and Olsen also claimed to have identified age differences of 1 to 5 months between study and control groups in the HIP and Edinburgh trials and all Swedish trials aside from the Malmö trial. The writers suggested that the observed reduction in breast cancer death rates was caused by these age differences rather than by the screening process itself. Gotzsche and Olsen were unaware that when the screening trials used cluster randomization rather than individual randomization, such small age differences were not unexpected, in some cases biased the studies against screening, and were in any case fully accounted for in analyses, leaving the conclusion of a significant mortality reduction unchanged.[85–87]

Screening trials and therapeutic trials are different in nature and may be different in design. In therapeutic trials, all participants have disease. The main variables are treatment versus no treatment and dose regimen. Study and control groups are small. Individual randomization is required, and small age differences are significant to the study. In screening mammography trials, there is low disease prevalence, so large study and control groups are necessary. For this reason, individual randomization may not be necessary. Individual randomization may not be practical, and cluster randomization is usually necessary.[87]

The age difference between the 2 groups that Gotzsche and Olsen purported to have discovered in the Swedish Two-County trial had been previously acknowledged by Tabar and colleagues[88] in 1989. After adjustment for age, mortality was only minimally different: 31% versus 30% for women aged 40 to 70 years in the Swedish Two-County trial and 45% instead of 46% for women aged 39 to 49 years in the Gothenburg trial.[86] Thus, there was no way that these small differences in age could have altered the overall conclusion that mammography screening results in a substantial reduction in deaths from breast cancer.

In another criticism, Gotzsche and Olsen suggested that assignment of the cause of death among women in the Swedish screening trials might have been inaccurate. Accurate assignment of cause of death is critical to proper assessment of trial results. Death in a woman with breast cancer may be either causally related or unrelated to her malignancy. Because screening trials compare deaths caused by breast cancer in women in study groups and control groups, attribution of the cause of death must be performed in a consistent and unbiased manner. However, the criticism by Gotzsche and Olsen was baseless. The methods had been previously described in detail by Nystrom and colleagues.[89] The process consisted of independent blind evaluation by 4 physicians and resulted in unanimous agreement in a remarkable 93% of cases.[14,15,89]

Gotzsche and Olsen also observed that no statistically significant decrease in death rates from all causes combined had yet been shown in any of the Swedish trials. These investigators interpreted this observation to mean that any benefit from reduction in breast cancer deaths would be countered by increased deaths from other causes. This incorrect conclusion disregarded the fact that breast cancer accounts for only about 5% of total mortality. Thus, even the largest individual trial would be unlikely to show any statistically significant decrease in all-cause mortality. On this issue, Gotzsche and Olsen were again proved wrong.

After publication of the second Olsen and Gotzsche study, Nystrom and colleagues[14,15] were able to find a 2% decrease in all-cause mortality among study group women in 5 Swedish trials combined. In addition, Tabar and colleagues[90] observed a significant 19% reduction in deaths from all causes among breast cancer cases in the group invited to screening in the Swedish Two-County trial. Thus, the Gotzsche and Olsen conjecture regarding all-cause mortality was incorrect.

To further their thesis that data from the Swedish Two-County trial were unreliable. Gotzsche and Olsen asserted that the reported study group size was different in the articles by Tabar and colleagues. In response to the criticism, Duffy and Tabar acknowledged that the study population size did differ among their published reports. Tabar and colleagues had previously noted that these differences were caused by progressive identification and exclusion of women diagnosed with breast cancer before the trial began. This is an acceptable and commendable practice. The irony of this unjustified criticism is that Tabar and colleagues were faulted for practicing good science.

In their studies, Gotzsche and Olsen also reiterated the conclusion of a study by Sjonell and Stahle,[91] which claimed that widespread service screening in Sweden had not affected breast cancer mortality in the population. The basic mistake made by Sjonell and Stahle in this claim was that they had measured death rates too early after screening was started. Decreased mortality from screening should not be expected until 5 to 8 years after the start of screening. They had mistakenly begun to tally breast cancer deaths before the beginning of the service screening programs that they were attempting to assess. In addition, their calculations did not consider the increase in breast cancer incidence over time.

Although the report by Gotzsche and Olsen received considerable publicity in the US media, no medical organization or government changed its screening policy from their conclusions. After review of the Gotzsche and Olsen studies, 11 leading medical organizations (American Academy of Family Physicians, ACS, American Congress of Obstetricians and Gynecologists, American College of Physicians, American College of Preventive Medicine, American Medical Association, American Society of Internal Medicine, Cancer Research Foundation of America, National Medical Association, Oncology Nursing Society, and the Society of Gynecologic Oncologists) reaffirmed their support of screening in a full-page advertisement published in the New York Times on January 31, 2002.[87] Also,

the NCI and the United States Preventive Services Task Force (USPSTF) concluded that despite Gotzsche and Olsen's contentions, the results from RCTs of screening were still valid. In addition, the Swedish National Board of Health and Welfare, the Danish National Board of Health, the Health Council of the Netherlands, the European Institute of Oncology, and the World Health Organization dismissed Gotzsche and Olsen's arguments and concluded that the evidence for benefit of screening for breast cancer was convincing.[92–96]

SERVICE SCREENING STUDIES

After the success of the Swedish randomized trials, organized service screening mammography became routine in nearly all Swedish counties by the 1990s. Unlike randomized trials, which are conducted primarily as clinical research studies, service screening is performed mainly as a public health initiative. Nevertheless, results from service screening projects have provided strong confirmation that screening mammography is effective in reducing mortality from breast cancer.[97] Data from service screening can be analyzed using 3 different methods: incidence-based mortality (IBM) studies, case-control studies, and trend studies.[98]

IBM Studies

IBM studies compare breast cancer mortality among women who were screened as well as the larger group of women who were offered screening and may or may not have agreed to be screened with breast cancer mortality expected in the absence of screening, which may be estimated in 1 of 3 ways:

1. Mortality in a cohort of women not yet invited to screening
2. Historical mortality data from the same region as well as from both historical and current data from a region
3. Historical data from the same region and if necessary adjusted for change in breast cancer mortality in time in nonparticipants

A study by Tabar and colleagues[99] measured the effect of mammography in a population in which service screening was offered to all women 40 years and older. These investigators compared breast cancer death rates in 2 Swedish counties over 3 periods: 1968 to 1977, when virtually no women were screened (prescreening era), 1978 to 1987, when half the population was offered screening in the RCT, and 1988 to 1996, after completion of the trial, when screening was offered to all women, and 85% of the population was being screened. Compared with breast cancer death rates among women aged 40 to 69 years in the prescreening era, breast cancer death rates in 1998 to 1996 were 63% lower for screened women and 50% lower for the entire population (85% screened plus 15% nonscreened) (**Table 4**). During this time, reductions in death rates from breast cancer for screened women were similar to those for women screened during the trial (63% vs 57%, respectively). However, during the RCT trial period (1978–1987), only half of the population was offered screening; for that era, breast cancer death rate reduction in the entire population was only 21%. It seems probable that screening rather than advances in treatment was responsible for nearly all the benefit. The RRs of breast cancer death among nonscreened women aged 40 to 69 years were similar during the 3 consecutive periods (1.0, 1.7, and 1.19, respectively). Moreover, the breast cancer death rate for women aged 20 to 39 years, virtually none of whom was screened, showed no significant difference (1.0, 1.10, and 0.81, respectively) during these 3 consecutive periods. Possibly, women who agree to be screened have selection bias factors, which, apart from the screening process, improved their survival rates. Even assuming the maximum effect of selection bias, screening was shown to reduce breast cancer deaths by at least 50%.

A study by Duffy and colleagues[100] assessed the effect of service screening in 7 Swedish counties. Among women aged 40 to 69 years, according to breast cancer mortality trends, it was estimated that only 12% of the mortality reduction was a result of improved therapy and patient management apart from the screening process. A further study of the 20-year experience in 2 Swedish counties[50] found a significant 40% reduction in mortality with screening at ages 40 to 49 years.

A recent meta-analysis of 7 European IBM service screening studies[98] found statistically significant reductions in breast cancer mortality of 25% among women invited to screening and 38% among those screened (**Table 5**). The 7 nonoverlapping populations and ages screened were from 2 different areas of Finland (50–63),[101,102] Denmark (60–69),[103] Italy (50–69),[104,105] Norway (50–69),[106] Spain (45–69),[107] and Sweden (40–74).[108] Those women from Sweden were from counties other than the 7 counties reported by Duffy and colleagues.[100]

Case-Control Studies

These types of studies involve a retrospective comparison of the presence or absence of screening among women who have died of breast cancer (case patients) and living members of the same population (control patients). Control patients have not died of breast cancer, but they may or may not have the disease. The rational for case-control studies is that if screening reduces breast cancer mortality, then women who die from the disease should be less likely to have a history of screening than matched control patients randomly selected from the population. After the screening history of both case patients and control patients is retrospectively ascertained, reduction in breast cancer mortality as a result of screening can then be estimated.[6,109]

A recent meta-analysis of results from 7 European case-control service screening studies found a statistically significant 31% breast cancer

---

Table 4
Reduction in population death rates from breast cancer in women diagnosed between ages 40 and 69 years in 2 Swedish counties[a]

Screening Status	1979–1987 (Randomized Trial) (%)	1988–1996 (Service Screening) (%)
Screened	57	63
Invited to screening	43	48
Screened plus nonscreened	21	50

[a] Time of diagnosis 1978–1987 or 1988–1996 compared with death rates from cancers diagnosed during 1969–1977 before screening began. All results were statistically significant at 95% confidence level.

Data from Tabar L, Vitak B, Chen HH, et al. Beyond randomized controlled trials: organized mammographic screening substantially reduces breast carcinoma mortality. Cancer 2001;91:1724–31.

Table 5
Summary of results from 7 IBM service screening studies

	RR	95% Confidence Interval	Mortality Reduction (%)
Invited vs not invited	0.75	0.69–0.81	25
Screened vs not screened	0.62	0.56–0.69	38

Data from Broeders M, Moss S, Nystrom L, et al, for the EUROSCREEN Working Group. The impact of mammographic screening on breast cancer mortality in Europe: a review of observational studies. J Med Screen 2012; 19(Suppl 1):14–25.

mortality reduction among women invited for screening and 48% (after correction for possible self-selection) among those screened (**Table 6**).[98] The 7 nonoverlapping populations and ages were Iceland (40–69),[110] Italy (50–69),[111] 3 different regions of Holland (50–74),[112–116] England (50–64),[117] and Wales (50–69).[118]

Trend Studies

Compared with IBM studies and case-control studies, both of which measure breast cancer deaths among different categories of contemporaneous individuals, trend studies compare breast cancer death rates in an entire population before and after the introduction of screening. There are many reasons why trend studies are less reliable than IBM and case-control studies to ascertain the benefit from screening. Results from trend studies are influenced by confounding factors such as changes in breast cancer incidence or treatment methods over time. Trend studies are unable to exclude deaths from breast cancers that were diagnosed before the introduction of screening or at an age younger than the screening age range.

Among 17 trend studies evaluated by the EUROSCREEN Working Group, 5 were descriptive and 12 were quantitative. Six of these 12 studies, had long enough follow-up for meaningful results. Among these 6 studies, 3 compared mortality before and after the introduction of screening. These studies screened women between ages 50 and 69 years in Florence, Italy,[119,120] ages 45 and 65 years, in Navarre, Spain,[107] and ages 50 and 64 years in England.[121] Estimated total reductions in breast cancer mortality were 30%, 36%, and 28%, respectively. The other studies included women ages 50 to 69 in Copenhagen, Denmark,[122]

ages 55 to 74 in Holland,[123] and ages 45 to 65 in Navarre, Spain.[107,124] The average mortality reductions per year (difference in annual mortality prescreening vs during screening/number of screening years) in these studies were 1%, 2.3% to 2.8%, and 9%, respectively.[98]

Results from these many service screening studies indicate that the reductions in breast cancer mortality found in the RCTs can be obtained and exceeded in nonresearch, organized service screening settings. These programs effectively refute the claim by Gotzsche and Olsen that the benefits seen in the RCTs of screening were not real because of supposed flaws in randomization and ascertainment of cause of death.[86,87]

Although there has not been any service screening study in the United States, screening mammography is commonly performed. Seventy percent of women age 40 years and older report having had a mammogram in the past 2 years, and 55% in the past year.[125,126] As a consequence, the average woman with invasive breast cancer is 39% less likely to die from her disease than was her counterpart in the early 1980s when screening was less common.[97] Screening has also resulted in a substantial downstaging of breast cancer, enabling more conservative treatment and allowing every current surgical, medical, and radiation treatment to be more effective.

CAN MODERN TREATMENT SUBSTITUTE FOR EARLY DETECTION?

It is disheartening that new artificial controversies are periodically devised to raise unjustified doubts about the value of screening. Kalager and colleagues[106] reported on the short-term follow-up of Norwegian women aged 50 to 69 years who were offered screening every 2 years along with current (1996–2005) treatment of detected cancers. These women had a 28% mortality reduction compared with historical (1986–1995) breast cancer death rates. Women not offered screening but who received identical current treatment showed an 18% breast cancer mortality reduction compared with the same historical death rates. The investigators concluded that screening accounted for only a 10% mortality reduction (28%–18%) or about one-third (10/28) of the assumed benefit from screen-detected cancers treated with older methods. Thus, the investigators surmised that about two-thirds of the benefit seen in studies such as the Swedish Two-County trial, conducted in the 1980s, could be attained in the absence of screening by means of advances in chemotherapy, surgery, and radiotherapy.

Table 6
Summary of results from 7 European case-control service screening studies

	RR	95% Confidence Interval	Mortality Reduction (%)
Invited vs not invited	0.69	0.57–0.83	31
Screened vs not screened (corrected)	0.52	0.42–0.65	52

Data from Broeders M, Moss S, Nystrom L, et al, for the EUROSCREEN Working Group. The impact of mammographic screening on breast cancer mortality in Europe: a review of observational studies. J Med Screen 2012; 19(Suppl 1):14–25.

As expected in our media-driven society, this study by Kalager and colleagues was quickly publicized in newspaper headlines and television news shows, a flagrant example of the power of sound bites based on a superficial analysis that failed to recognize the faulty methodology of the study.

The main flaw in Kalager and colleagues' study is the mean follow-up period of 2.2 years, which is insufficient to support their conclusions. This extremely short follow-up would be more than adequate for evaluating the treatment of an acute disease, such as the effect of antibiotic agents on pneumonia, but it is inadequate for studying the effect of early detection or treatment on a chronic disease such as breast cancer. No screening mammography trial has ever shown any significant separation of mortality curves between study and control groups in a period shorter than 4 to 5 years after the initiation of screening. Because the maximum length of follow-up for the Norwegian women was 8.9 years, Kalager and colleagues could have analyzed results for the subset of the population who had a mean follow-up of 4 to 5 years, but they did not report any such results.

Moreover, the mean follow-up period was shorter than 2.2 years. Screening in each Norwegian county was implemented gradually over a 2-year period. However, the investigators considered the beginning of the follow-up period as the date that countrywide screening began rather than the date that full or even partial screening was implemented. This gradual introduction of screening in a county also allowed late-stage cancers among screening group women not yet offered screening to be included in the study group merely because of their residence in the county. This problem could have been ameliorated by offering all women in the study group more screening rounds so that any pollution of the screening group by cancers detected either before the patient's screening or only shortly before reaching the clinical threshold would be minimal.

The Kalager and colleagues study did not include any follow-up data after 2005, even although it was published in late 2010. By that time, the Norwegian Cancer Registry could have provided follow-up data to 2008. Inexplicably, the investigators did not avail themselves of that opportunity for a larger, more robust follow-up sample.

Another weakness in the Norwegian study is that only 77% of women offered screening accepted the invitation to be screened, although presumably, 100% of patients with cancer accepted some form of advanced treatment. A related limitation of this study is that an unknown number of women in the control group obtained screening on their own, outside the program.

Although the investigators are unsure how often this screening happened, the comparatively low 12% breast cancer mortality in the control group suggests that such control group contamination may have been significant.

The study by Kalager and colleagues,[106] along with the accompanying editorial by Welch, mistakenly argues that substantial mortality reduction found in earlier mammography service screening studies conducted throughout Scandinavia is no longer valid, because mortality reduction was calculated from historical data from the prescreening era, with insufficient adjustment for advances in treatment.[127]

Shortly after publication of their study, the hypothesis of Kalager and colleagues that the gains from screening mammography could largely be duplicated by advances in treatment was disproved by a subsequent study by Hellquist and colleagues,[128] which reported results from service screening in Sweden. Among the Swedish regions that implemented service screening, about half screened all women aged 40 to 59 years, whereas the remaining areas, because of financial constraints, could offer screening only to those aged 50 to 59 years. This practice allowed a natural experiment, because all regions had access to the same modern treatments through the Swedish national health care system, whereas only some regions screened women younger than 50 years. The investigators found that among women aged 40 to 49 years, death rates for breast cancer were reduced 26% for those offered screening and 29% for those screened. Thus, screening was found to confer a substantial benefit independent of treatment. In contrast to the inadequate 2.2-year follow-up period in the study by Kalager and colleagues from Norway, the Swedish study by Hellquist and colleagues had a follow-up period of more than 16 years.

Review of several other recent service screening studies finds other examples of contemporaneous breast cancer mortality for populations with identical access to modern treatment but different availability of screening. For example, in Finland, nationwide population-based breast cancer screening for women aged 50 to 59 years was introduced between 1987 and 1991 on a near-contemporaneous staggered basis. Women born in even years began screening in 1987 or 1988. Women born in odd years, who began screening in 1989 and 1991, served as controls. An effect of screening emerged in 3 to 4 years of follow-up and rapidly diluted as controls were screened. For this narrow window of time, Hakama and colleagues[102] found that mortality from breast carcinoma was 24% lower among women who were offered screening and 33% lower among women who were screened.

In another service screening study, Jonsson and colleagues[129–131] found a 30% decrease in breast cancer mortality among women aged 40 to 74 years in 2 northern Swedish counties screened in the 1990s. Two adjacent counties where screening was not yet offered and that had otherwise identical breast cancer mortality served as controls.

THE OVERDIAGNOSIS CONTROVERSY

Overdiagnosis refers to the possibility that some cancers detected at screening might not result in death if they had been undetected, and hence, untreated. Presumably, such cancers grow slowly or not at all, metastasize infrequently, or are found in women who are very old or have substantial comorbid conditions, making the primary cause of death something other than breast cancer. The clinical significance of overdiagnosis is that such women may be subjected to unnecessary biopsy, lumpectomy, mastectomy, chemotherapy, and radiation therapy, as well as anxiety from awareness that they have cancer, along with excessive medical costs for them, their families, and society at large.

Overdiagnosis is different from a false-positive biopsy for a lesion that seems suspicious at mammography but is benign on pathologic examination. Overdiagnosis is essentially an epidemiologic rather than a pathologic concept, although such cases might disproportionately be in situ or minimally invasive cancers. The concept of overdiagnosis is related to length-biased sampling, the possibility that slower-growing tumors are more common among screen-detected cancers than among cancers that emerge clinically in an unscreened population. Length-biased sampling, lead time bias, and selection bias are the 3 major reasons why measurement of decreased mortality in RCTs rather than increased survival rates were necessary to provide the initial proof that the benefits from screening are real.

Was there Overdiagnosis in RCTs?

Randomized trials that compare breast cancer mortality for women in study groups offered screening and otherwise comparable control groups preclude any influence of these biases on mortality. Nevertheless, even documentation of mortality reduction, such as the statistically significant 35% mortality reduction among women aged 40 to 74 years at entry into the Swedish Two-County trial, does not prove that overdiagnosis did not occur.[9] To assess possible overdiagnosis in that trial, Yen and colleagues[132] found that the cumulative incidence of breast cancer (invasive and in situ combined) in the study group and the control group were virtually identical on 29-year follow-up of 1 arm of the trial. Similarly, the total number of invasive cancers in each group was the same, as was the total number of in situ cancers in each group. The only indication of possible overdiagnosis was a nonsignificant excess of cancers among study group women aged 70 to 74 years, suggesting that if overdiagnosis occurred, it was mainly confined to the elderly. As desired for the goal of screening, there was a persistent excess of nonadvanced cancers (node negative or <20 mm in size) in the study group and a persistent excess of advanced cancers (node positive or >20 mm or both) in the control group at 29-year follow-up. This study suggests that the level of overdiagnosis from screening mammography is small and is largely confined to older women.

How Frequent was Overdiagnosis in Service Screening Studies?

The major challenge to estimating the frequency of overdiagnosis from direct observation of incidence rates on service screening studies is that screening advances the rate of detection from that encountered in the absence of screening. Thus, the cancer prevalence rate at first screen exceeds the incidence rate in a similar nonscreened population. Subsequent incidence rates on second, third, fourth screens, and so forth approach those of a nonscreened population. After the screening program ends, there is a catch-up point at which the cumulative number of cancers in the screened and nonscreened populations is equal. A second challenge is a possible difference in risk factors between screened and nonscreened women in some service screening studies. Failure to adjust calculations for lead time and risk factors, as well as an insufficient number of follow-up years, explain the widely different estimates for overdiagnosis (0%–54%) among 13 European service screening studies.[133] These disparities have been explained by Puliti and colleagues,[133] who reported that estimates for overdiagnosis among 10 studies lacking adjustment were mostly in the 30% to 54% range. Estimates from the 6 studies that made adjustment were lower, only 2.8% in the Netherlands,[134] 4.6% and 1.0% in Italy,[105,135] 7% in Denmark,[136] and 10% and 3.3% in England and Wales.[121,137]

What Length of Follow-Up Is Needed for an Accurate Estimate of Overdiagnosis?

Although the mean sojourn time (duration during which a nonpalpable cancer is potentially detectable by screening) is approximately 2.85 years for women aged 40 to 74 years, the distribution of lead time (time between detection and palpability) is exponential and has a wide range, as shown in the Swedish Two-County trial.[138] From this range of distribution, Duffy and Parmar[139] have calculated that the number of excess cancers in a hypothetical screening population compared with a nonscreened population does not decrease less than 10% until after 25 years of follow-up, including 10 years after the upper age limit of screening. Applying these criteria for the length of follow-up needed to accurately assess the frequency of overdiagnosis explains why virtually all estimates for overdiagnosis have been too high and must be reduced. For example, Kalager and colleagues[140] estimated an overdiagnosis rate of 18% at 10 years of follow-up of the Norwegian services screening program. However, Duffy and Parmar[139] indicated that a 19% excess cancer rate would be expected from lead time alone.

Use of Trend Studies to Estimate Overdiagnosis

Analyses that crudely assess overdiagnosis from an increase in cancer incidence with the introduction of screening tend to estimate implausibly high rates of overdiagnosis, of the order of 30% to 50%. These estimates are flawed, because they do not fully take account of numerous complicating factors in incidence of breast cancer and its interface with screening. Reasons for increased incidence observed with the introduction of screening include:

1. Continuation of preexisting trends of increasing breast cancer incidence in the late twentieth century
2. Acceleration of these trends by lead time: if screening confers an average lead time of 2 years, for example, 2004 incidence is observed in 2002, 2005 incidence in 2003, and so on
3. Lead time similarly accelerates age effects: age 52 years incidence is observed at age 50 years, and so on
4. A major surge of additional cancers, mostly as a result of lead time, is diagnosed with the prevalence screen when the screening program is introduced
5. A similar surge of prevalence screen tumors occurs continuously as new patients enter the screening program
6. Overdiagnosis is a minor reason for the excess incidence observed at screening

Compared with direct observation of cumulative breast cancer detection rates among screened versus nonscreened women, temporal comparison of cancer incidence rates in the population represents the most unreliable method to gauge the frequency of overdiagnosis. For example, Bleyer and Welch[141] estimated that as a result of screening mammography, 31% of all breast cancers in the United States are being overdiagnosed. These investigators found that breast cancer incidence during 2006 to 2008, when 60% of women age 40 years and older were screened at least once every 2 years, was 31% higher than predicted, assuming a 0.25% per year increase in breast cancer incidence from a 1976 to 1978 baseline, when little screening was being performed.[141] A likely flaw in these investigators' method of calculation was that they ignored the fact that over a longer 40-year period (1940–1980), the increase in breast cancer incidence had been 4 times greater, that is, an increase of 1% per year instead of 0.25% per year.[142] As indicated by Kopans,[143] breast cancer incidence during 2006 to 2008 (128 invasive cancers per 100,000 women) was less than expected (132 cases per 100,000 women per year) from a 1% per year increase. The claim that 31% of breast cancers in the United States are being overdiagnosed was uncritically publicized by the national media and medical journals. Reading these reports can dissuade women from being screened and even influence policies of health care organizations. This episode shows why estimation of overdiagnosis using inappropriate methods of assessment can be problematic.

In another widely publicized study, Esserman and colleagues[144] observed the following: (1) after the widespread introduction of screening in the United States, breast cancer incidence has never returned to prescreening levels, and (2) screening has not caused the relative incidence of regional cancer to decrease commensurate with the increased detection of early-stage cancer. Esserman and colleagues acknowledged that breast cancer mortality has decreased during the screening era in our country but expressed uncertainty about the relative contributions of screening versus treatment to this accomplishment. These investigators too are convinced that there is excessive diagnosis of slow-growing or biologically inert cancers. My critique of their viewpoint is as follows: (1) the increased incidence of breast cancer over the past 30 years is largely related to factors other than screening and (2) the proof of mortality reduction through screening has been established in randomized trials and service screening studies, and proof cannot be negated by distracting observations regarding the higher than expected incidence of regional disease, which is influenced by factors such as overall breast cancer incidence, excessively long screening intervals, tumor growth rates, and inadequate screening compliance rates. It is likely that a disproportionate number of late-stage cancers cited by the investigators occurred in women who were not being screened.

IS DUCTAL CARCINOMA IN SITU A REAL CANCER?

The concept of overdiagnosis has just been discussed. However, detection of ductal carcinoma in situ (DCIS) is worth considering in more detail. Coincident with the increasing use of mammography, there has been a marked increase in the detection of DCIS. Before the era of mammographic screening, DCIS represented less than 5% of all malignancies of the breast.[145] However, DCIS now accounts for between 20% and 40% of all nonpalpable cancers detected at screening and about 20% of all newly diagnosed cancers (screen detected and non–screen detected) in the United States.[145] With appropriate treatment, the survival rate for patients with DCIS should be 99.5%. DCIS may be considered a frequent but nonobligate precursor of fatal breast cancer. All cases of invasive ductal carcinoma are believed to develop from DCIS, but not all cases of DCIS progress to invasive ductal carcinoma. Yet, critics of screening have referred to DCIS as a pseudocancer, false-positive, resulting in harm from screening by leading to unnecessary biopsies and excessive surgery.

Justification for the use of DCIS as an index of the benefit of screening depends on how often and how rapidly DCIS evolves into invasive ductal carcinoma. No direct method exists for determining the natural progression of DCIS. If patients with DCIS were never to undergo biopsy and the DCIS were left to develop into invasive carcinoma, there would be no way to establish that the initial lesion was DCIS. If DCIS is completely excised, its natural history has been stopped, but there is no proof that it would have evolved into invasive ductal carcinoma.

Results from autopsy studies of women with no clinical evidence of breast cancer show 6% to 14% prevalence of DCIS.[145] These rates have been used to suggest that most cases of DCIS may never become clinically apparent. However, there are reasons why this conclusion is not justified. First, most (45%–56%) of the autopsy-detected cases of DCIS could not be identified by radiography performed on the surgical

specimens. An even higher percentage would not have been seen at mammography. If autopsy rates vary around 10% but mammography-detected rates are considerably lower than 1%, it is clear that mammographically detectable DCIS in living women is either a different entity from autopsy-detectable DCIS in dead women, or a special subgroup thereof. The DCIS found at autopsy is not representative of the type of DCIS detected by screening mammography, which would be larger, calcified, and, therefore, a faster-growing lesion. Second, detection rates for invasive ductal carcinoma at prevalence screening (a woman's first screening mammography) are 2 to 3 times higher than the expected incidence, consistent with a 2-year to 3-year detection lead time. In the absence of screening, many cases of high-grade DCIS do not surface clinically as DCIS but rather as invasive carcinoma. Thus, it would not be surprising if the prevalence of mammographically visible DCIS at autopsy were even 10 to 20 times higher than the expected incidence of DCIS. Moreover, some cases classified as DCIS in the autopsy studies, which took place in the 1980s, would be reclassified as atypical hyperplasia according to current histology criteria.

Several follow-up studies of DCIS treated with biopsy alone also shed light on the invasive potential of DCIS. The lesions in these studies were categorized as benign at initial histologic review, and so wide excision was not performed. In 1 study, researchers found development of invasive ductal carcinoma at the biopsy site in 53% of cases within 9.7 years.[145] Another study showed development of invasive ductal carcinoma in 28% of cases by 10 years and 36% cases within 24 years.[145] Recurrence rates for DCIS in series such as these have suggested to some observers that DCIS is unlikely to progress to invasive disease.

However, there are 2 reasons why these studies should lead to just the opposite conclusion. First, these studies underestimate the invasive potential of DCIS, because they involved only cases of low-grade DCIS, that is, all histologic subtypes of DCIS except for comedocarcinoma, the most aggressive subtype. Comedocarcinoma typically accounts for 32% to 50% of all cases of DCIS detected at mammographic screening.[146–148] Second, these studies include both cases in which the DCIS lesion was completely removed and cases in which some DCIS remained in the breast, because biopsy margins were not sufficiently wide. Invasive ductal carcinoma is expected only in this latter subgroup.

Based on a statistical model using the numbers of DCIS and invasive cancers detected at

5 different screening programs, Yen and colleagues[149] estimated that among cases of DCIS detected at prevalence (initial) screening, 63% were progressive and 37% were nonprogressive. At incidence (subsequent) screenings, 96% of detected cases of DCIS were progressive and only 9% were nonprogressive.[149]

Among all cases of DCIS detected at the UK National Health Service Screening Programme,[150] 60% were high grade, 20% intermediate grade, and 20% low grade. It was estimated that 84% of high-grade DCIS would, if undetected, progress to invasive disease in 5 years, most intermediate-grade would progress to invasive disease in 10 years, and low-grade could become invasive in 15 years or longer.

Because screening detects cancers years earlier than they would normally appear clinically, the incidence of invasive cancers is lower than expected for several years after women cease participating in a screening program of limited duration. From observed and expected incidence rates for invasive cancer after cessation of screening in the United Kingdom, McCann and colleagues[151] estimated that 75% of this subsequent decreased incidence and lower mortality was caused by screen-detected invasive cancers and 25% was from screen-detected DCIS. These investigators concluded that "Cancer for cancer, there is as much benefit from detection and treatment of DCIS as from detection and treatment of invasive cancer."

HOW FREQUENTLY SHOULD WOMEN BE SCREENED?

No randomized trial has been designed to compare the relative benefit from different screening intervals. Comparison of mortality reduction among randomized trials having different screening intervals has not been meaningful, because of their confounding factors, such as differences in trial design, screened populations, mammographic technique, and interpretation. Moreover, no single randomized trial has had arms that differed only in length of time between screening.

Much of the evidence for selection of screening intervals has been derived from calculation of tumor sojourn time (duration of preclinical disease).[109] Sojourn time begins when the tumor is potentially detectable by mammography and ends at the start of the clinical phase, which begins when the tumor is found clinically in the absence of screening.

Lead time (mean sojourn time) is the average length of time from the point at which the tumor is detected by mammography to the point at which the clinical phase begins.[109] The lead time is always shorter than sojourn time but approaches the length of sojourn time as screening frequency is increased. Tabar and colleagues[8] estimated that the lead time was 1.7 years for women aged 40 to 49 years and 2.6 to 3.8 years for women aged 50 to 74 years. Effective screening requires that the screening interval should be shorter than the lead time.[75–77]

Mathematical Models

Using a computer simulation model based on observed breast cancer growth rates, Michaelson and colleagues[78] estimated that triennial, biennial, annual, and biannual screening would reduce distant metastases by 19%, 27%, 52%, and 81%, respectively. These investigators found good correlation between screening frequency tumor size and survival. These findings suggest that annual screening could reduce breast cancer death rates by 50% and that screening every 6 months might reduce death rates by 82%.[78]

Using a Markov chain model for progression of breast cancer, based on results from the Swedish Two-County trial, Duffy and colleagues[152] and Chen and colleagues[153,154] estimated that for women aged 40 to 49 years, screening every year, every other year, or every third year might result in reductions in mortality of 36%, 18%, and 4%, respectively. For women aged 50 to 59 years, the same screening intervals might result in reductions of 46%, 39%, and 34%, respectively.[152–154] Thus, older women achieve greater mortality reduction than younger women screened at the same interval. However, older women receive less incremental increase in benefit for progressively shorter screening intervals.

Several investigators have estimated the increased benefits from annual screening versus the observed benefits from screening every 24 months in the Swedish Two-County trial and every 18 months in the Gothenburg, Sweden trial. Such calculations were made from the stage and expected death rates of interval cancers surfacing clinically between screens. In the Two-County trial, the observed mortality reduction was 24% for women aged 40 to 49 years and 39% for those aged 50 to 59 years. Using such data, Tabar and colleagues and Feig, in 2 separate reports, estimated mortality reductions of 35% and 46% for annual screening of these 2 respective age groups.[46,79] In Gothenburg, Bjurstam and colleagues[18,19] found a 45% mortality reduction observed from screening women aged 39 to 49 years every 18 months (80% compliance).

Using data from that trial, Feig estimated that annual screening of these women would have resulted in a mortality reduction between 65% (at 80% compliance) and 75% (at 100% compliance).[80]

Clinical Observational Studies

Several clinical follow-up studies have shown that women aged 40 to 49 years who chose to be screened annually were more likely to be diagnosed with early-stage versus late-stage breast cancer. The Breast Cancer Surveillance Consortium (BCSC) is a large group of breast imaging facilities throughout the United States that are linked to regional tumor registries. Using data from the BCSC, White and colleagues[155] and Kerikowske and colleagues[156] found an increase in late-stage disease among women aged 40 to 49 years screened with a 2-year versus those screened with a 1-year interval. The value of annual versus biennial screening in reducing the likelihood of late-stage breast cancer among women younger than 50 years was also shown in a study of women in Wisconsin by Ontilo and colleagues.[157]

Hunt and colleagues[158] found that women aged 40 to 79 years screened annually at the University of California at San Francisco had invasive cancers that were smaller and lower stage than those among women screened biennially. About 60% of the screeners were aged 50 years or older.

At variance with these conclusions are findings from a 12.8-year follow-up of mortality of women aged 40 to 49 years selected for screening either annually (even year-of-birth cohorts) or triennially (odd year-of-birth cohorts) in Turku, Finland.[159] No differences in incidence based mortality according to screening frequency were found. However, because of lack of a control group with no screening, it cannot be determined whether this result was caused by a low efficacy of mammography in their study, or insufficient follow-up, or lack of incremental benefit for annual versus triennial screening.

Clinical studies of screening frequency for women aged 50 years and older have varied in their conclusions. Using the BCSC database, White and colleagues[155] found that screening at 2-year versus 1-year intervals did not increase the likelihood of late-stage disease at diagnosis but did increase the likelihood of being diagnosed with invasive disease versus DCIS. Using the same database, the lack of effect of screening frequency on late-stage presentation among older women was confirmed by Kerlikowske and colleagues.[156]

It has been observed that weaknesses in the design of both studies may nullify their conclusion that screening every 2 years is sufficient for older women. One criticism regards the definition of late-stage breast cancer: as either positive lymph nodes or metastases by White and colleagues,[155] or as stage 2b or higher or 2 cm or larger by Kerlikowske and colleagues.[156] These cut points may be too high to document benefit from annual screening. Cancers detected by screening mammography are usually stage 1b or earlier. Selection of lower cut points may have led to a different conclusion regarding the optimal screening frequency. It seems logical that reduction of stage 2a or stage 2b to stage 1 or stage 1 to stage 0 should reduce mortality.

Another limitation of these studies is that screening intervals were chosen by the patients or suggested by their physicians rather than made at random. Thus, intervals were subject to selection bias. It is unclear why some women were screened less frequently.

The finding that screening frequency does not influence stage at detection in implausible unless one believes that most breast cancers cease to grow after the patient is aged 50 years. As radiologists, we have observed some cancers, including those presenting as spiculated masses or calcifications, that do not grow over periods of 1 to 4 years.[160,161] However, such cases are exceptional and worthy of reports in the radiologic literature.[162]

Other clinical studies of older women found that those screened annually do have earlier disease than those screened less often. Field and colleagues[163] compared 1-year versus 2-year screening intervals among Michigan women aged 65 years and older. Those screened annually had smaller invasive tumors and a downstaging of their invasion disease and 3 times as many cases of DCIS. Ontilo and colleagues[157] found that women aged 50 years and older in Wisconsin screened at 2-year intervals had a 3 times greater likelihood of stage III or IV breast cancer than those screened at annual intervals. Late-stage breast cancers were also high among the group who had been screened at intervals of 3 years or longer.

USPSTF Controversy

In November, 2009, the USPSTF recommended against mammographic screening for women aged 40 to 49 years except for those at high risk; it recommended screening only every other year rather than annual screening for those aged 50 to 74 years; and it recommended no screening for women 75 years and older.[164,165] The recommendation to screen women in their 40s only if they were at high risk was controversial, because 80% of women with newly diagnosed breast cancers have no significant previous risk factors.[166,167] USPSTF guidelines differ substantially from those of the ACS, American College of Radiology (ACR), Society of Breast Imaging, American College of Obstetricians and Gynecologists, and National Comprehensive Cancer Network, all of which recommend annual screening mammography beginning at age 40 years.[73,168,169]

The USPSTF is a government-supported group of health experts who review published research and make recommendations about preventive health care issues such as screening for carcinoma of the breast, cervix, prostate, and colon. Many members are PhDs and of the few MD members, few are primarily involved in clinical care. There were no breast imagers or breast surgeons on the panel.

Public reaction to USPSTF was immediate and pronounced. Some women mistakenly believed that USPSTF supplanted older guidelines from the ACS, American College of Surgeons, and ACR. Most women were either outraged or confused. A USA Today poll found that 47% strongly disagreed and 29% disagreed, whereas only 5% strongly agreed and 17% agreed with the USPSTF advice.[170] The 2009 USPSTF recommendations were potentially more important than their previous ones issued in 2002, because 1 provision in the then proposed Affordable Healthcare Law forbid Medicare and private insurers from paying for any medical care that did not conform to USPSTF policy. After public outrage, Kathleen Sebelius, Secretary of Health and Human Services, was quick to deny that USPSTF recommendations were government policy.[171] However, concern remains that USPSTF recommendations could encourage insurance companies to reduce their screening mammography coverage.

The USPSTF provided several reasons for its recommendations. First, by USPSTF calculations, RCTs found a breast cancer mortality reduction of only 15% for ages 40 to 49 years and 50 to 59 years compared with 32% for ages 60 to 69 years.[164,165] The reason their calculations derived a lower percentage mortality reduction than those found in the RCTs and service screening studies cited earlier was that the USPSTF included results from the NBSSC, which found no benefit from mammography screening of women aged 40 to 60 years. There are several reasons why inclusion of NBSSC data is unjustified. Unlike all of the other RCTs, NBSSC was not population-based but

rather relied on volunteers. Clinical breast examination was performed by NBSSC staff members before patient allocation to either a study group or control group. As a likely consequence, the trial contained an excessive proportion of symptomatic women, many with advanced palpable cancers, who seem to have been preferentially channeled into the study group rather than the control group.[28–36] In addition, many of the mammographic examinations were judged as technically inadequate by external expert reviewers, even by the standards of the 1980s when the NBSSC was performed.[27–29] Technical problems included poor positioning, poor breast compression, faulty processing, and lack of mammographic grids.

Higher screening recall rates and false-positive biopsy rates relative to cancer detection rates among younger women were also used by USPSTF to justify the recommendation against routine screening for women in their 40s.[172] The USPSTF cited current BCSC data from the United States that the numbers of women recalled from screening to undergo additional imaging in order to find 1 cancer at ages 40 to 49 years, 50 to 59 years, and 60 to 69 years were 47, 22, and 14, respectively.[165,172,173] However, such recall rates are not a valid reason to not screen women in their 40s because more than 90% of all recalls do not result in biopsy and entail nothing more than supplementary mammographic views or ultrasonography.[1] Recall rates are always higher on initial screening than on subsequent screening, in which there are previous mammograms for comparison. Delaying the initiation of screening until age 50 years would only transfer the higher recall rates per detected cancer to that age group. The USPSTF also cited BCSC data that the biopsy positive predictive value (DCIS or invasive cancer per 100 biopsies) was 28% for women aged 40 to 49 years versus 44% for ages 50 to 59 years and 56% for ages 60 to 69 years.[172] The USPSTF neglected to note that 99% of women surveyed considered even 500 or more false-positive mammography examinations to be an acceptable risk to save 1 life and that their anxiety from screening recall and biopsy was slight and transient.[174,175] Then too, biopsy positive predictive value rates of 28% are well within the 20% to 40% range recommend by the US Agency for Healthcare Policy and Research, ACR, and other consensus panels.[1]

Absolute and Relative Benefit

Numerous studies have shown that the relative mortality reduction through screening women aged 40 to 49 years is 30% to 50%, similar to that from screening older women.[9,37,50,51] However, absolute benefit (deaths averted per 1000 women screened) rather than relative benefit (percent mortality reduction) must be used to calculate the cost-effectiveness for screening different age groups, because breast cancer incidence varies according to age. For example, the probability of developing breast cancer in the next 10 years for women aged 40, 50, and 60 years is 1.44%, 2.39%, and 3.4%, respectively.[176] The odds of developing breast cancer in these respective decades are 1 in 69, 42, and 29. Thus, compared with older women, younger women obtain a lower absolute benefit from screening. For these reasons, the USPSTF used both absolute benefit and relative benefit to support their screening recommendations.

USPSTF made serious mistakes in their calculations of both relative and absolute benefit. As discussed, their estimated relative mortality reduction of only 15% for screening women aged 40 to 49 years was too low, because they included results from NBSSC. NBSSC was fatally flawed by poor mammographic technique, recruitment of symptomatic women, and the likely channeling of women with breast masses into the mammography arm. As a consequence, NBSSC was the only screening trial to have excess of late-stage breast cancers in the study group versus the control group. NBSSC was the only trial to find no benefit from screening any age group. These investigators' error in estimation of relative benefit led to another error in estimation of absolute benefit.

Using data from NBSSC and other trials, USPSTF calculated that the number of women needed to be invited to screening at ages 39 to 49 years, 50 to 59 years, and 60 to 69 years to prevent 1 death was 1904, 1339, and 377, respectively. However, excluding NBSSC, these results would have been 950, 670, and 377, respectively. These recalculated values would have been sufficient to recommend screening women in their 40s according to USPSTF's own criteria![176]

The second mistake make by USPSTF was selection of the number of women invited to be screened (NNI) rather than the number of women screened (NNS) for their measure of absolute benefit.

The reality is that not all women invited to screening agree to be screened. In some trials, as few as 32% of women have attended all screening rounds.[72] Thus, NNS is always lower, often considerably lower, than NNI. When reporting USPSTF conclusions, the public media and medical journals often confused NNI with NNS.

This reporting error made screening seem less efficient. Using RCT data, Hendrick and Helvie[177] calculated that NNS at ages 40 to 49 years, 50 to 59 years, and 60 to 69 years were 746, 351, and 253, respectively. These numbers are lower than those for NNI used by USPSTF and thus are more favorable for screening. NNS can be specified in terms of either number of women needed to screen detect 1 cancer, save 1 life, or extend a woman's life by 1 year.

Because of the longer life expectancy of young women, NNS per life year gained (LYG) in these age groups was 28, 17, and 16, respectively. Use of LYG provides even more favorable comparisons of younger versus older women than use of number of deaths prevented.[176] Use of NNS to prevent 1 death or gain 1 life year strongly supports screening all women between ages 40 and 69 years.

Benefits and Costs

Increasing interest in reducing national health care expenditures has led to studies such as a recent one on the aggregate cost for screening mammography by O'Donoghue and colleagues.[178,179] This study estimates costs for 3 different screening strategies: annual (ages 40–84 years), biennial (ages 50–69 years), and USPSTF (high risk ages 40–49 years, biennial ages 50–74 years). The annual cost for each of these plans was estimated at $10.1 billion, $2.6 billion, and $3.5 billion, respectively. Studies such as this raise concerns that cost more than science is responsible for the screening controversies.

The deficiencies in the USPSTF recommendations have already been discussed in detail. Thus, I confine my critique to strategy 2, limiting screening to women aged 50 to 69 years every 2 years.

1. The investigators do not appreciate that annual screening of women aged 40 to 49 years can reduce breast cancer mortality by 40% to 50%. Moreover, 40% of years of life lost to breast cancer may result from cancer appearing during this decade.[7]
2. Most women aged 70 years and older need to be screened, because most still have substantial average life expectancies.
3. Numerous studies have concluded that annual screening is more effective than biennial screening (perhaps not double the benefit of biennial screening, but substantially more). Even USPSTF projected that for women ages 40–69 annual screening would increase life years gained by 37% more than biennial screening.[172]

4. They did not acknowledge that the costs of screening is partly offset by reduced costs for more intensive treatment and long-term care.[2]
5. The investigators estimated the cost per LYG for annual versus biennial screening, but did not indicate their assumed level of benefit entered into their calculation. Their final value exceeded the acceptable upper limit. The more conventional measure of cost per LYG through annual screening has been calculated by other investigators and found to be lower than the commonly accepted upper limit of $50,000 to $100,000 per LYG.[2,180]

SUMMARY

Numerous clinical studies have confirmed that screening women aged 40 years and older reduces breast cancer mortality by 30% to 50%. Several factors including faster breast cancer growth rates and lower breast cancer incidence among younger women, as well as shorter life expectancy and more comorbid conditions among older women, should also be considered in screening guidelines. Accordingly, annual screening beginning at age 40 years and continuing with no upper age limit, as long as a woman has a life expectancy of at least 5 years and no significant comorbid conditions, is recommended by the ACS, the ACR, and the Society of Breast Imaging.

Annual screening is more effective than screening every 2 years for women aged 40 to 49 years and probably for those aged 50 years and older as well. However, the benefit from screening every year is less than double that from screening every other year.

Past controversies regarding the effectiveness of screening women in their 40s have largely been resolved. Differences in recommendations for screening women in this age group are now mostly related to the magnitude of benefit, the lower absolute benefit, the lower cost-effectiveness, and the higher false-positive biopsy rates compared with those in older women.

The previous controversy initiated by Gotzsche and Olsen regarding the validity of screening trial results for women of all ages has been essentially resolved as well. Numerous medical organizations in the United States and Europe concur that the data showing mortality reduction are scientifically sound.

The claim of Kalagar and colleagues that modern treatment can largely substitute for early detection has no scientific support, whereas there is strong evidence that mammography remains indispensable for the substantial decline in breast cancer death rates over the past 30 years.

Most cases of screen-detected DCIS are capable of transformation into invasive disease. There is no reliable way for the radiologist to distinguish these cases from the few cases that represent low-grade DCIS. This is a continuing challenge for the pathologist and surgeon to ensure appropriate treatment.

Overdiagnosis refers to the possibility that some screen-detected cancers may not eventuate in death if undetected by mammography, yet receive unnecessary treatment by surgery, chemotherapy, and radiation therapy. One highly publicized study by Bleyer and Welch claimed that 31% of all breast cancers are misdiagnosed. More reliable calculations by Puliti and colleagues found that the frequency of overdiagnosis is extremely low, between 0% and 5% of all screen-detected cancers.

REFERENCES

1. Feig SA. Adverse effects of screening mammography. Radiol Clin North Am 2004;42(5):807–21.
2. Feig SA. Cost-effectiveness of mammography, MRI, and ultrasonography for breast cancer screening. Radiol Clin North Am 2010;48(5):879–91.
3. Seidman H, Gelb SK, Silverberg E, et al. Survival experience in the breast cancer detection demonstration project. CA Cancer J Clin 1987;37:258–90.
4. Smart CR, Bryne C, Smith RA, et al. Twenty year follow-up of the breast cancers diagnosed during the Breast Cancer Detection Demonstration Project. CA Cancer J Clin 1997;47:134–49.
5. Ries L, Eisner MP, Kosary CL, et al. SEER Cancer Statistics Review, 1973-1998. Bethesda (MD): National Cancer Institute; 2001.
6. Feig SA. Methods to identify benefit from mammographic screening. Radiology 1996;201:309–16.
7. Shapiro S, Venet W, Strax P, et al. Periodic screening for breast cancer, the health insurance plan project and its sequelae 1963-1976. Baltimore (MD): Johns Hopkins University Press; 1988.
8. Tabar L, Vitak B, Chem JJ, et al. The Swedish Two-County Trial twenty years later. Radiol Clin North Am 2000;38:625–52.
9. Tabar L, Vitak B, Chen TH, et al. Swedish Two-County trial: impact of mammographic screening on breast cancer mortality during 3 decades. Radiology 2012;260:658–63.
10. Tabar L, Fagerberg CJ, Gad A, et al. Reduction in mortality from breast cancer after mass screening with mammography. Randomized trial from the Breast Cancer Screening Working Group in the

Swedish National Board of Health and Welfare. Lancet 1985;1:829–32.

11. Andersson I, Aspegren K, Janzon L, et al. Mammographic screening and mortality from breast cancer: the Malmo Mammographic Screening Trial. BMJ 1988;297:943–8.

12. Andersson I, Nystrom L. Mammography screening. J Natl Cancer Inst 1995;87:1263–4.

13. Andersson I, Janzon L. Reduced breast cancer mortality in women under 50: updated results from the Malmo Mammographic Screening Program. J Natl Cancer Inst Monographs 1997;22:63–8.

14. Nystrom L, Andersson I, Bjurstam N, et al. Long-term effects of mammography screening: updated overview of the Swedish randomized trials. Lancet 2002;359:909–19.

15. Nystrom L. Screening mammography re-evaluated [letter to the editor]. Lancet 2002;355:748–9.

16. Frisell J, Eklund G, Helistrom L, et al. Randomized study of mammography screening: preliminary report on mortality in the Stockholm trial. Breast Cancer Res Treat 1991;18:49–56.

17. Frisell J, Lidbrink E, Helistrom L, et al. Follow-up after 11 years: update of mortality results in the Stockholm mammographic screening trial. Breast Cancer Res Treat 1997;45:263–70.

18. Bjurstam N, Bjorneld L, Duffy SW, et al. The Gothenburg Breast Screening Trial: first results on mortality, incidence, and mode of detection for women ages 39-49 years at randomization. Cancer 1997;80:2091–9.

19. Bjurstam N, Bjorneld L, Duffy SW, et al. The Gothenburg Breast Screening Trial. Cancer 1998;83:188–90 [authors' reply].

20. Bjurstam J, Bjorneld L, Warwick J, et al. The Gothenburg Breast Screening Trial. Cancer 2003;97:2387–96.

21. Roberts MM, Alexamder FE, Anderson TJ, et al. Edinburgh trial of screening for breast cancer: mortality at seven years. Lancet 1990;335:241–6.

22. Alexander FE, Anderson TJ, Brown HK, et al. 14 years of follow-up from Edinburgh randomized trial of breast cancer screening. Lancet 1999;353:1903–8.

23. Moss SM, Cuckle H, Evans A, et al. Effect of mammographic screening from age 40-49 years on breast cancer mortality at 10 years follow-up: a randomized controlled trial. Lancet 2006;368:2053–80.

24. Miller AB, Baines CJ, To T, et al. Canadian National Breast Screening Study: 2. Breast cancer detection and death rates among women aged 50-59 years. Can Med Assoc J 1992;147:1477–88 [Erratum appears in Can Med Assoc J 1993;148;718].

25. Miller AB, To T, Baines CJ, et al. Canadian National Breast Screening Study-2: 13-year results of a randomized trial in women aged 50-59 years. J Natl Cancer Inst 2000;92:1490–9.

26. Miller AB, To T, Baines CJ, et al. The Canadian National Breast Screening Study-1: breast cancer mortality after 11 to 16 years of follow-up: a randomized screening trial of mammography in women age 40 to 49 years. Ann Intern Med 2002;137:305–12.

27. Baines CJ, Miller AB, Kopans DB, et al. Canadian National Breast Screening Study: assessment of technical quality by external review. AJR Am J Roentgenol 1990;155:743–7.

28. Kopans DB. The Canadian Screening Program: a different perspective. AJR Am J Roentgenol 1990;155:748–9.

29. Kopans DB, Feig SA. The Canadian National Breast Screening Study: a critical review. AJR Am J Roentgenol 1993;161:755–60.

30. Warren-Burhenne LJ, Burhenne HJ. The Canadian National Breast Screening Study: a Canadian critique. AJR Am J Roentgenol 1993;161:761–3.

31. Bailar JC, MacMahon B. Randomization in the Canadian National Breast Screening Study: a review of evidence for subversion. Can Med Assoc J 1997;156:193–9.

32. Boyd NE, Jong RA, Yaffe MJ, et al. A critical appraisal of the Canadian National Breast Screening Study. Radiology 1993;189:661–3.

33. Boyd NF. The review of randomization in the Canadian National Breast Screening Study: is the debate over? Can Med Assoc J 1997;156:207–9.

34. Sun J, Chapman J, Gordon R. Survival from primary breast cancer after routine clinical use of mammography. Breast J 2002;8:199–208.

35. Mettlin CJ, Smart CR. The Canadian National Breast Screening Study: an appraisal and implications for early detection policy. Cancer 1993;72:1461–5.

36. Tarone RE. The excess of patients with advanced breast cancer in young women screened with mammography in the Canadian National Breast Screening Study. Cancer 1995;75:997–1003.

37. Smith RA, Duffy SW, Gabe R, et al. The randomized trials of breast cancer screening: what have we learned? Radiol Clin North Am 2004;42:793–806.

38. Fletcher SW, Black W, Harris R, et al. Report of the International Workshop on Screening for Breast Cancer. J Natl Cancer Inst 1993;85:1644–56.

39. Smith RA. Breast cancer screening among women younger than age 50: a current assessment of the issues. CA Cancer J Clin 2000;50:312–36.

40. Hurley SF, Kaldor JM. The benefits and risks of mammographic screening for breast cancer. Epidemiol Rev 1992;14:101–30.

41. Chu KC, Smart CR, Rarone RE. Analysis of breast cancer mortality and stage distribution by age for the Health Insurance Plan clinical trial. J Natl Cancer Inst 1998;80:1125–32.

42. Elwood JM, Cox B, Richardson AK. The effectiveness of breast cancer screening by mammography in younger women. Online J Curr Clin Trials 1993. February 25, Doc No 32.

43. Glaszion PP, Woodward AJ, Mahon CM. Mammographic screening trials for women under age 50: a quality assessment and meta-analysis. Med J Aust 1995;162:625–9.

44. Kerlikowske K, Grady D, Rubin SM, et al. Efficacy of screening mammography: a meta-analysis. JAMA 1995;273:149–54.

45. Smart CR, Hendrick RE, Rutledge JH, et al. Benefit of mammography screening in women ages 40 to 49 years: current evidence from randomized controlled trials. Cancer 1995;75:1619–26 [Erratum appears in Cancer 75:2788].

46. Falun Meeting Committee and Collaborators. Breast-cancer screening with mammography in women aged 40-49 years. Swedish Cancer Society and the Swedish National Board of Health and Welfare. Int J Cancer 1996;68:693–9.

47. Hendrick RE, Smith RA, Rutledge JH, et al. Benefit of screening mammography in women aged 40-49: a new meta-analysis of randomized controlled trials. Natl Cancer Inst Monogr 1997;33:87–92.

48. Wald NJ, Murphy P, Major P, et al. UKCCCR multicentre randomized controlled trial of one and two view mammography in breast cancer screening. BMJ 1995;311:1189–93.

49. Evans AJ, Kutt E, Record C, et al. Radiologic findings of screen-detected cancers in a multicentre randomized, controlled trial of mammographic screening in women from age 40 to 48 years. Clin Radiol 2006;61:784–8.

50. Tabar L, Yen MF, Vitak B, et al. Mammography service screening and mortality in breast cancer patients: 20-year follow-up before and after introduction of screening. Lancet 2003;361:1405–10.

51. Coldman A, Phillips N, Warren L, et al. Breast cancer mortality after screening mammography in British Columbia women. Int J Cancer 2007;120: 1076–80.

52. US Bureau of the Census. Statistical abstract of the United States. 212th edition. Washington, DC: US Government Printing Office; 2012.

53. Feig SA. Mammographic screening of elderly women. JAMA 1996;276:446.

54. Mandelblatt JS, Wheat ME, Monane M, et al. Breast cancer screening for elderly women with and without comorbid conditions. Ann Intern Med 1992;116:722–30.

55. Yancik R, Reis LG, Yates JW. Breast cancer in women: a population based study of contrasts in stage, survival, and surgery. Cancer 1989;163:976–81.

56. Faulk RM, Sickles EA, Sollitto RA, et al. Clinical efficacy of mammographic screening in the elderly. Radiology 1995;194:193–7.

57. Wilson TE, Helvie MA, August DA. Breast cancer in the elderly patient: early detection with mammography. Radiology 1994;190:203–7.

58. Constanza ME. Issues in breast cancer screening in older women. Cancer 1994;74:2009–15.

59. Walter LC, Covinsky KE. Cancer screening in elderly patients: a frame-work for individual decision making. JAMA 2001;285:2750–6.

60. Conway BJ, Suleiman OH, Reuter FG, et al. National survey of mammographic facilities in 1985, 1988, and 1992. Radiology 1994;191:323–30.

61. Haus AG. Dedicated mammography x-ray equipment, screen-film processing-systems, and viewing conditions for mammography. Semin Breast Dis 1999;2:30–54.

62. Feig SA. Screening mammography: effect of image quality on clinical outcome. AJR Am J Roentgenol 2002;178:803–7.

63. Young K, Wallis MG, Ramsdale ML. Mammographic film density and detection of small breast cancers. Clin Radiol 1994;49:461–5.

64. Glynn CE, Farria DM, Monsees BS, et al. Effect of transition to digital mammography on clinical outcomes. Radiology 2011;200(3):664–70.

65. Pisano ED, Gatsonis C, Hendrick E, et al. Diagnostic performance of digital versus film mammography for breast cancer screening. N Engl J Med 2005;363:1773–83.

66. Andersson I, Hildell J, Muhlow A, et al. Number of projections in mammography: influence on detection of breast disease. AJR Am J Roentgenol 1978;130:349–51.

67. Anttinen I, Pamilo M, Roiha M, et al. Baseline screening mammography with one versus two views. Eur J Radiol 1989;9:241–3.

68. Bassett LW, Bunnell DH, Jahanshahi R, et al. Breast cancer detection: one versus two views. Radiology 1987;165:95–7.

69. Muir BB, Kirkpatrick AE, Roberts MM, et al. Oblique-view mammography adequacy for screening. Radiology 1984;151:39–41.

70. Sickles EA, Weber WN, Galvin HB, et al. Baseline screening mammography: one vs two views per breast. AJR Am J Roentgenol 1986;147:1149–53.

71. Thurfjell G, Taube A, Tabar L. One-versus two-view mammography screening: a prospective population based study. Acta Radiol 1994;35:340–4.

72. Humphrey LL, Helfant M, Chan BK, et al. Breast cancer screening: a summary of the evidence for the US Preventive Services Task Force. Ann Intern Med 2002;137:347–60.

73. Smith RA, Saslow D, Sawyer KA, et al. American Cancer Society Guidelines for Breast Cancer Screening: update 2003. CA Cancer J Clin 2003; 53:141–69.

74. Feig SA. Determination of mammographic screening intervals with surrogate measures for

women aged 40-49 years. Radiology 1994;193: 311–4.

75. Moskowitz M. Breast cancer: age specific growth rates and screening strategies. Radiology 1986; 161:37–41.

76. Pelikan S, Moskowitz M. Effects of lead-time, length bias, and false-negative reassurance on screening for breast cancer. Cancer 1993;71:1998–2005.

77. Tabar L, Fagerberg G, Day NE, et al. What is the optimum interval between screening examination? An analysis based on the latest results of the Swedish Two-County Breast Cancer Screening trial. Br J Cancer 1987;55:47–51.

78. Michaelson JS, Halpern E, Kopans DB. Breast cancer computer simulation method for estimation of optimal intervals for screening. Radiology 1999; 212:551–60.

79. Feig SA. Estimation of currently attainable benefit from mammographic screening of women aged 40-49 years. Cancer 1995;75:2412–9.

80. Feig SA. Increased benefit from shorter screening mammography intervals for women ages 40-49 years. Cancer 1997;80:2035–9.

81. Tabar L, Fagerberg G, Chen HH. Efficacy of breast cancer screening by age: new results from the Swedish Two-County Trial. Cancer 1995;75: 2507–17.

82. Miettinen OS, Henschke CI, Pasmantier MW, et al. Mammographic screening: no reliable supporting evidence? Lancet 2002;359:404–6.

83. Gotzsche PC, Olsen O. Is screening for breast cancer with mammography justifiable? Lancet 2000; 355:129–34.

84. Olsen O, Gotzsche PC. Cochrane review on screening for breast cancer with mammography. Lancet 2001;358:1340–2.

85. de Koning HJ. Assessment of nationwide cancer-screening programmes. Lancet 2000;355:80–1.

86. Duffy SW. Interpretation of the breast screening trials: a commentary on the recent paper by Gotzsche and Olsen. Breast 2001;10:209–12.

87. Feig SA. How reliable is the evidence for screening mammography? Recent Results Cancer Res 2003; 163:129–39.

88. Tabar L, Fagerberg G, Duffy SW, et al. The Swedish Two County trial of mammographic screening for breast cancer: recent results and calculation of benefit. J Epidemiol Community Health 1989;43: 107–14.

89. Nystrom L, Larsson LG, Rutqvist LE, et al. Determination of cause of death among breast cancer cases in the Swedish randomized mammography screening trials. A comparison between official statistics and validation by an endpoint committee. Acta Oncol 1995;34:145–52.

90. Tabar L, Duffy SW, Yen MF, et al. All cause mortality among breast cancer patients in a screening

trial: support for breast cancer mortality as an end point. J Med Screen 2002;9:159–62.

91. Sjonell G, Stahle L. Mammography screening does not reduce breast cancer mortality. Lakartidningen 1999;96:904–13 [in Swedish].

92. Swedish Board of Health and Welfare. Vilka Effekter Har Mammografic screening?. Referat av ett expert-mote anordnat av Socialstyrelsen och ancerfonden I; Stockholm den 15 February 2002.

93. Rosen M, Rehnqvist N. No need to reconsider breast screening programme on basis of results from defective study [letter to the editor]. BMJ 1999;318:809–10.

94. Health Council of the Netherlands. The benefit of population screening for breast cancer with mammography. The Hague (The Netherlands): Health Council of the Netherlands; 2002.

95. Veronisi U, Forrest P, Wood W. Statement from the chair: global Summit on Mammographic Screening. Milan (Italy): European Institute of Oncology; 2002.

96. International Agency for Research on Cancer. Mammography screening can reduce deaths from breast cancer. Lyon (France): IARC Press; 2002.

97. Feig SA. Effect of service screening mammography on population mortality from breast carcinoma. Cancer 2002;95:451–7.

98. Broeders M, Moss S, Nystrom L, et al. The impact of mammographic screening on breast cancer mortality in Europe: a review of observational studies. J Med Screen 2012;19(Suppl 1):14–25.

99. Tabar L, Vitak B, Chen HH, et al. Beyond randomized controlled trials: organized mammographic screening substantially reduces breast carcinoma mortality. Cancer 2001;91:1724–31.

100. Duffy SW, Tabar L, Chen HH, et al. The impact of organized mammography service screening on breast cancer mortality in seven Swedish counties: a collaborative evaluation. Cancer 2002;95: 458–69.

101. Sarkeala T, Heinavaara S, Anttila A. Breast cancer mortality with varying invitational policies in organized mammography. Br J Cancer 2008;98: 641–5.

102. Hakama M, Pukkala E, Heikkila M, et al. Effectiveness of the public health policy for breast cancer screening in Finland: population based cohort study. BMJ 1997;314:864–7.

103. Olsen AH, Njor SH, Vejborg I, et al. Breast cancer mortality in Copenhagen after the introduction of mammography screening: a cohort study. BMJ 2005;330:220.

104. Paci E, Giorgi D, Bianchi S, et al. Assessment of the early impact of the population-based breast cancer screening programme in Florence (Italy) using mortality and surrogate measures. Eur J Cancer 2002;38:568–73.

105. Puliti D, Zappa M, Miccinesi G, et al. An estimate of overdiagnosis 15 years after the start of mammographic screening in Florence. Eur J Cancer 2009;45:3166–71.

106. Kalager M, Zelen M, Langmark F, et al. Effect of screening mammography on breast-cancer mortality in Norway. N Engl J Med 2010;363:1203–10.

107. Ascunce EN, Moreno-Iribas C, Barcos Urtiaga A, et al. Changes in breast cancer mortality in Navarre (Spain) after introduction of a screening programme. J Med Screen 2007;14:14–20.

108. Swedish Organised Service Screening Evaluation Group. Reduction in breast cancer mortality from organized service screening with mammography: 1. Further confirmation with extended data. Cancer Epidemiol Biomarkers Prev 2006;15:45–51.

109. Morrison AS. Screening for chronic disease. 2nd edition. New York: Oxford University Press; 1992.

110. Gabe R, Tryggvadottir L, Sigfusson BF, et al. A case-control study to estimate the impact of the Icelandic population-based mammography screening program on breast cancer death. Acta Radiol 2007;48:948–55.

111. Puliti D, Miccinese G, Collina N, et al. Effectiveness of service screening: a case-control study to assess breast cancer mortality reduction. Br J Cancer 2008;99:423–7.

112. Otto SJ, Fracheboud J, Looman CW, et al. Initiation of population-based mammography screening in Dutch municipalities and effect on breast-cancer mortality: a systematic review. Lancet 2003;361:1411–7.

113. Otto SJ, Fracheboud J, Verbeek AL, et al. Mammography screening and risk of breast cancer death: a population-based case-control study. Cancer Epidemiol Biomarkers Prev 2012;21:66–73.

114. van Schoor G, Moss SM, Otten JD, et al. Increasingly strong reduction in breast cancer mortality due to screening. Br J Cancer 2011;104:910–4.

115. Paap E, Holland R, den Heeten GJ, et al. A remarkable reduction of breast cancer deaths in screened vs unscreened women: a case referent study. Cancer Causes Control 2010;21:1569–73.

116. Broeders MJ, Verbeek AL, Straatman H, et al. Repeated mammographic screening reduces breast cancer mortality along the continuum of age. J Med Screen 2002;9:163–7.

117. Allgood PC, Warwick J, Warren RM, et al. A case-control study of the impact of the East Anglian breast screening programme on breast cancer mortality. Br J Cancer 2008;98:206–9.

118. Fielder HM, Warwick J, Brook D, et al. A case-control study to estimate the impact on breast cancer death of the breast screening programme in Wales. J Med Screen 2004;11:194–8.

119. Gorini G, Zappa M, Miccinesi G, et al. Breast cancer mortality trends in two areas of the province of Florence, Italy, where screening programmes started in the 1970s and 1990s. Br J Cancer 2004;90:1–4.

120. Barchielli A, Paci E. Trends in breast cancer mortality, incidence, and survival, and mammographic screening in Tuscany, Italy. Cancer Causes Control 2001;12:249–55.

121. Duffy SW, Tabar L, Olsen AH, et al. Absolute numbers of lives saved and overdiagnosis in breast cancer screening, from a randomized trial and from the Breast Screening Programme in England. J Med Screen 2010;17:25–30.

122. Jergensen KJ, Zahl PH, Gotzsche PC. Breast cancer mortality in organized mammography screening in Denmark: comparative study. BMJ 2010;340:c1241.

123. Otten JD, Broeders MJ, Fracheboud J, et al. Impressive time-related influence of the Dutch screening programme on breast cancer incidence and mortality, 1975-2006. Int J Cancer 2008;123:1929–34.

124. Ugarte MD, Goicoa T, Etxeberria J, et al. Age-specific spatio-temporal patterns of female breast cancer mortality in Spain (1975-2005). Ann Epidemiol 2010;20:906–16.

125. American Cancer Society. Cancer prevention and early detection facts and figures, 2011-2012. Atlanta (GA): American Cancer Society; 2013.

126. Available at: http://seer.cancercgov/statfacts/html/breast.html. Accessed March 10, 2010.

127. Welch HG. Screening mammography–a long run for a short slide? N Engl J Med 2010;363:1276–8.

128. Hellquist BN, Duffy SW, Abdsaleh S, et al. Effectiveness of populations-based service screening with mammography for women ages 40-49 years: evaluation of the Swedish Mammography Screening in Young Women (SCRY) cohort. Cancer 2011;117:714–22.

129. Jonsson H, Bordas P, Wallin H, et al. Service screening with mammography in Northern Sweden: effects on breast cancer mortality–an update. J Med Screen 2007;14:87–93.

130. Jonsson H, Nystrom L, Tornberg S, et al. Service screening with mammography of women aged 50-69 years in Sweden: effects on mortality from breast cancer. J Med Screen 2001;8:152–60.

131. Jonsson H, Nystrom L, Tornberg S, et al. Service screening with mammography. Long-term effects on breast cancer mortality in the county of Gavleborg, Sweden. Breast 2003;12:183–93.

132. Yen AM, Duffy SW, Chen TH, et al. Long-term incidence of breast cancer by trial arm in one county of the Swedish Two County Trial of Mammography screening. Cancer 2012;118:5728–32.

133. Puliti D, Duffy SW, Miccinesi G, et al. Overdiagnosis in mammographic screening for breast cancer in

Europe: a literature review. J Med Screen 2012; 191:42–56.

134. de Gelder R, Heijnsdijk EA, van Ravesteyn NT, et al. Interpreting overdiagnosis estimates in population-based mammography screening. Epidemiol Rev 2011;33:111–21.

135. Paci E, Miccinesi G, Puliti D, et al. Estimate of overdiagnosis of breast cancer due to mammography after adjustment for lead time. A service screening study in Italy. Breast Cancer Res 2006;8:R68.

136. Olsen AH, Agbaje OF, Myles JP, et al. Overdiagnosis, sojourn time, and sensitivity in the Copenhagen mammography screening program. Breast J 2006; 12:338–42.

137. Waller M, Moss S, Watson J, et al. The effect of mammographic screening and hormone replacement therapy use on breast cancer incidence in England and Wales. Cancer Epidemiol Biomarkers Prev 2007;16:2257–61.

138. Tabar L, Duffy S, Vitak B, et al. The natural history of breast cancer. What have we learned from screening? Cancer 1999;86:449–62.

139. Duffy SW, Parmar D. Overdiagnosis in breast cancer screening: the importance of length of observation period and lead time. Breast Cancer Res 2013; 15:R41.

140. Kalager M, Adami H, Bretthauer M, et al. Overdiagnosis of invasive breast cancer due to mammography screening: results from the Norwegian screening program. Ann Intern Med 2010;156:491–9.

141. Bleyer A, Welch HG. Effect of three decades of screening mammography on breast cancer incidence. N Engl J Med 2012;367(2):1998–2005.

142. Garfinkel L, Boring CC, Heath CW Jr. Changing trends: an overview of breast cancer incidence and mortality. Cancer 1994;79(Suppl):222–7.

143. Kopans DB. The New England Journal of Medicine article suggesting overdiagnosis from mammography screening is scientifically incorrect and should be withdrawn. J Am Coll Radiol 2013; 10(5):317–9.

144. Esserman L, Shieh Y, Thompson I. Rethinking screening for breast cancer and prostate cancer. JAMA 2009;302(15):1685–92.

145. Feig SA. Ductal carcinoma in situ: implications for screening mammography. Radiol Clin North Am 2000;38:653–68.

146. Lagios MD, Margolin FR, Westdahl PR, et al. Mammographically detected ductal carcinoma in situ. Frequency of local recurrence following tylectomy and prognostic effect of nuclear grade on recurrence. Cancer 1989;63:618–24.

147. Schwartz GF, Finkel GC, Garcia JC, et al. Subclinical ductal carcinoma in situ of the breast. Treatment by local excision and surveillance along. Cancer 1992;70:2468–74.

148. Silverstein M, Waisman JR, Gamigami P, et al. Intraductal carcinoma of the breast (208 cases): clinical factors influencing treatment choice. Cancer 1990; 66:102–8.

149. Yen MF, Tabar L, Smith RA, et al. Quantifying the potential problem of overdiagnosis of ductal carcinoma in situ in breast cancer screening. Eur J Cancer 2003;39:1746–54.

150. UK National Health Service. NHS Breast Screening Programme and Association of Breast Surgery at British Association of Surgical Oncology: an audit of screen detected breast cancers for the year of screening April 2007 to March 2008. UK West Midlands Cancer Intelligence Unit;2009.

151. McCann J, Treasure P, Duffy SW. Modeling the impact of detecting and treating ductal carcinoma in situ in a breast screening programme. J Med Screen 2004;11:117–25.

152. Duffy SW, Chen HH, Tabar L, et al. Estimation of mean sojourn time in breast cancer screening using a Markov chain model of both entry to and exit from the preclinical detectable phase. Stat Med 1995;14:1521–43.

153. Chen HH, Duffy SW, Tabar L, et al. Markov chain models for progression of breast cancer. Part I: tumor attributes and the preclinical screen-detectable phase. J Epidemiol Biostat 1997;2:9–25.

154. Chen HH, Duffy SW, Tabar L, et al. Markov chain models for progression of breast cancer. Part II: prediction of outcomes for different screening regimes. J Epidemiol Biostat 1997;2:25–35.

155. White E, Miglioretti DL, Yankaska BC, et al. Biennial versus annual mammography and the risk of late-stage breast cancer. J Natl Cancer Inst 2004; 96(24):1832–9.

156. Kerlikowske K, Zhu W, Hubbard RA, et al. Outcome of screening mammography by frequency, breast density, and postmenopausal hormone therapy. JAMA Intern Med 2013;173(9):807–15.

157. Ontilo AA, Engel JM, Liang H, et al. Mammographic utilization: patient characteristics and breast cancer stage at diagnosis. AJR Am J Roentgenol 2013;201:1057–63.

158. Hunt KA, Rosen EL, Sickles EA. Outcome analysis for women undergoing annual versus biennial screening mammography: a review of 23,211 examinations. AJR Am J Roentgenol 1999;173:285–9.

159. Parvinen I, Chiu S, Pylkkanen L, et al. Effects of annual vs triennial mammography interval on breast cancer incidence and mortality in ages 40-49 in Finland. Br J Cancer 2011;105:1388–91.

160. Meyer JE, Kopans DB. Stability of a mammographic mass: a false sense of security. AJR Am J Roentgenol 1981;137:595–8.

161. Lev-Toaff AS, Feig SA, Saitas VL, et al. Stability of malignant breast microcalcifications. Radiology 1994;192:153–6.

162. Feig SA. Carcinoma without interval change. In: Bassett LW, Feig SA, Hendrick RE, et al, editors. Breast disease (third series, test and syllabus). Reston (VA): American College of Radiology; 1999. p. 167–79.

163. Field LR, Wilson TE, Strawderman M, et al. Mammographic screening in women more than 64 years old: a comparison of 1- and 2-year intervals. AJR Am J Roentgenol 1998;170: 961–5.

164. US Preventive Services Task Force. Screening for breast cancer: US Preventive Services Task Force recommendation statement. Ann Intern Med 2009;151:716–26.

165. Nelson HD, Tyne K, Naik A, et al, US Preventive Services Task Force. Screening for breast cancer: an update for the US Preventive Services Task Force. Ann Intern Med 2009;151:727–37.

166. Seidman H, Stellman SD, Mushinski MH. A different perspective on breast cancer risk factors: some implications of nonattributable risk. Cancer 1982; 32:301–13.

167. Smith RA. Risk-based screening for breast cancer: is there a practical strategy? Semin Breast Dis 1992;2:280–91.

168. Lee CH, Dershaw DD, Kopans D, et al. Breast cancer screening with imaging: recommendation from the Society of Breast Imaging and the ACR on the use of mammography, breast MRI, breast ultrasound, and other technologies for the detection of clinically occult breast cancer. J Am Coll Radiol 2010;7:18–27.

169. American College of Obstetricians and Gynecologists Breast Cancer Screening (ACOG). ACOG practice bulletin no. 122. Breast Cancer Screening. Obstet Gynecol 2011;118:372–82.

170. Szabo L. Women are insistent on mammograms, poll shows. McLean (VA): USA Today; 2009. p. A1.

171. Sack K, Kolata G. Breast cancer screening policy won't change, US officials say. New York: New York Times; 2009. A1, A3.

172. Mandelblatt JS, Cronin KA, Bailey S, et al, Breast Cancer Working Group of the Cancer Intervention and Surveillance Modeling Network. Effects of mammography screening under different screening schedules: model estimates of potential benefits and harms. Ann Intern Med 2009;151:738–47.

173. Kerlikowske K. Evidence-based breast cancer prevention: the importance of individual risk. Ann Intern Med 2009;151:750–2.

174. Schwartz LM, Woloshin S, Fowler FJ Jr, et al. Enthusiasm for cancer screening in the United States. JAMA 2004;291:71–8.

175. Schwartz LM, Woloshin S, Sox HC, et al. US women's attitudes to false-positive mammography results and detection of ductal carcinoma in situ: cross sectional survey. BMJ 2000;320:1635–40.

176. Feig SA. Number needed to screen: appropriate use of this new basis for screening mammography guidelines. AJR Am J Roentgenol 2012;198(5): 1214–7.

177. Hendrick RE, Helvie MA. Mammography screening: a new estimate of number needed to screen to prevent one breast cancer death. AJR Am J Roentgenol 2012;198(3):723–8.

178. O'Donoghue C, Eklund M, Ozanne EM, et al. Aggregate cost of mammography screening in the United States: comparison of current practice and advocated guidelines. Ann Intern Med 2014; 160:145–53.

179. Elmore JG. The cost of breast cancer screening in the United States: a picture is worth…a billion dollars? Ann Intern Med 2014;160:203–4.

180. Rosenquist CJ, Lindfors KK. Screening mammography beginning at age 40 years: a reappraisal of cost-effectiveness. Cancer 1998;82:2235–40.

BI-RADS Update

Cecilia L. Mercado, MD

KEYWORDS

- Breast • Breast imaging • BI-RADS • BI-RADS atlas • Lexicon

KEY POINTS

- The new edition of BI-RADS has been updated to provide further clarification of lesion interpretation and standardization of lesion terminology and reporting.
- The BI-RADS revision provides a uniformity of terminology in the lexicon across all 3 imaging modalities, mammography, ultrasound, and magnetic resonance imaging.
- Introduction of new descriptive terms in the updated BI-RADS is reflective of new available technologies and evidence provided from current publications.

INTRODUCTION

The American College of Radiology (ACR) Breast Imaging Reporting and Data System (BI-RADS) has undergone revision. The main objectives of the new BI-RADS edition remain the same: to diminish confusion in the interpretation of imaging findings, to standardize reporting, and to simplify outcome monitoring.[1] The overall changes made to the ACR BI-RADS have been designed to give more flexibility for situations where the previous edition of BI-RADS in the past had given much confusion.[2]

The new edition of BI-RADS has made changes to its 3 components, the BI-RADS breast imaging lexicon, the standardized reporting language, and the medical audit and outcome monitoring. The mammography, ultrasound, and magnetic resonance imaging (MRI) lexicons have been made more compatible with each other by using the same descriptors for a lesion across whenever possible all 3 imaging modalities. An increase number of mammography images have been added to the new edition replacing many of the feature illustrations in the previous edition. Also added in this new edition is an increase in number of reference citations, which provides evidence-based justification to the lexicon and management recommendations.[3]

BREAST IMAGING LEXICON

Several changes to the mammography, ultrasound, and MRI lexicon terminology have been made in the new edition.[2] Inconsistencies in some descriptive terms have been addressed, and terms have been deleted, added, or revised in an effort to enhance clarification of appropriate usage.

Mammography Lexicon

Various descriptors in the mammography lexicon were changed to improve clarification of terminology. The previous BI-RADS mammography lexicon used the terms "grouped or clustered" for calcifications less than 1 cc in volume, and the term "regional" for calcifications greater than 2 cc. These terms did not address the group of calcifications measuring 1 cc to 2 cc in volume. The new edition has resolved this inconsistency by expanding the definition of "grouped" to a volume extending up to 2 cc. In addition, the terms "group or clustered", which could be used interchangeably with the previous BI-RADS edition, are being phased out and have been changed to the term "grouped" (historically clustered) with the intension of ultimately changing it to "grouped" in a later revision.[2]

Increased simplification has led to some terms in the new edition to be consolidated, such as the descriptors "lucent-centered", "egg-shell," and "rim" used to describe types of benign calcifications. These are now under one single descriptive term, "rim" (**Fig. 1**). Another term that has been eliminated is the descriptor for mass shape "lobular", which has been replaced by the term

Department of Radiology, New York University School of Medicine, NYU Cancer Institute, 160 East 34th Street, 3rd Floor, New York, NY 10016, USA

E-mail address: cecilia.mercado@nyumc.org

Radiol Clin N Am 52 (2014) 481–487
http://dx.doi.org/10.1016/j.rcl.2014.02.008
0033-8389/14/$ – see front matter

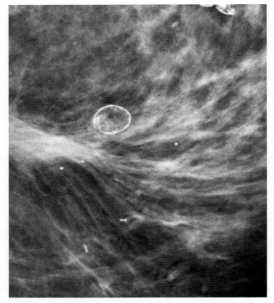

Fig. 1. Updated mammography lexicon terminology. Spot magnification mammography shows rim calcification near lumpectomy site. The descriptors "eggshell" and "lucent-centered" used to describe types of benign calcifications have been consolidated under the term "rim".

"oval" to standardize descriptors across imaging modalities. These changes have been summarized in **Box 1**. Other terms such as "intermediate concern", used for amorphous and coarse heterogeneous calcifications and the term "higher probability of malignancy" used for fine pleomorphic, fine linear, and fine-linear branching calcifications have also been deleted from the mammography lexicon. New published evidence suggests that some of the descriptive terms used to characterize calcifications may not impart the level of suspicion previously believed, and therefore the revised BI-RADS has changed to only using descriptors for lesion characterization.[4]

There are some descriptive terms in the updated BI-RADS that have been expanded, such as the

terms that describe an "asymmetry" often represents summation artifact. In addition, a new term "developing asymmetry", which describes a focal asymmetry that is new, growing, or more conspicuous, has been added to the existing types of asymmetries in the mammography lexicon. Increased clarification has been provided as to the different management recommendations for the 4 types of asymmetries (**Box 2**).

Ultrasound Lexicon

The terminology in the ultrasound lexicon has been expanded in the new BI-RADS edition. Descriptors for tissue composition as characterized on ultrasound have been revised to correlate to the mammographic breast densities. These are "homogeneous-fat", "homogeneous-fibroglandular", and "heterogeneous" tissue composition. As in the previous edition, there are primary descriptors to characterize the shape and margin of masses imaged on ultrasound. Similar to the mammography and MRI lexicon, the ultrasound descriptors were updated to maintain consistency among the 3 modalities. There will be certain terms that will be defined such as that for a complicated cyst, which is defined as a circumscribed, oval, mass parallel orientation containing low-level echoes throughout (**Fig. 2**).

Along with descriptors for the additional section, which include "echo pattern" and "posterior acoustic features", there is a new subsection titled "Associated Features", which will include descriptors for architectural distortion, vascularity, and elastography (tissue stiffness). The descriptive terms for elastography are new and include "soft", "intermediate", and "hard". It is emphasized that the features of elastography do not trump the primary features of morphology, shape, margin, and orientation.[3] These changes have been summarized in **Box 3**.

Magnetic Resonance Imaging Lexicon

Several changes were also introduced into the MRI lexicon. Although previously introduced as a

---

Box 1
Summary of changes to the BI-RADS mammography lexicon

Lexicon Terminology	Updated BI-RADS
Grouped–historically clustered	Replaces "grouped" or "clustered"
Rim	Replaces "lucent-centered", "egg-shell"
Oval	Replaces "lobular"
Developing asymmetry	New

Box 2
Descriptors for types of asymmetry in the mammography lexicon and appropriate assessment category

Types of Asymmetry	Assessment Category
Asymmetry	BI-RADS 1
Global asymmetry	BI-RADS 2
Focal asymmetry	BI-RADS 3
Developing asymmetry	BI-RADS 4

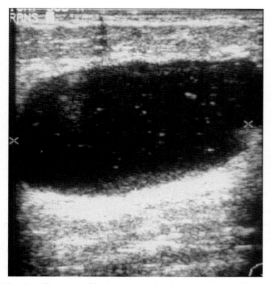

Fig. 2. Ultrasound lexicon terminology updated. Ultrasound images of complicated cysts show a circumscribed, oval mass with parallel orientation containing homogeneous low-level echoes throughout.

concept, background parenchymal enhancement (BPE) has been officially added to the new BI-RADS MRI lexicon and the MRI report. There are 4 terms that describe the amount of BPE: "minimal", "mild", "moderate", and "marked".[5] It is important to recognize that the amount of BPE does not directly correlate with the amount of fibroglandular tissue seen on mammography. However, the amount of BPE depends on the amount of fibroglandular tissue present, and inclusion of terminology that characterizes the amount of fibroglandular tissue as assessed on the noncontrast, nonsubtracted T1 sequence has been added to the BI-RADS revision. These terms are meant to correlate with the amount of fibroglandular parenchyma seen on mammography. The descriptors to describe fibroglandular parenchymal tissue on MRI are "almost entirely fat", "scattered fibroglandular tissue", "heterogeneous fibroglandular tissue", and "extreme fibroglandular tissue".[2,5,6]

Several descriptors have also been changed or deleted from the MRI lexicon to increase

simplification. Terms used to describe mass shape "round", "oval", and "irregular" remain. However, the descriptor "lobular" for mass shape, has been deleted and incorporated in the term "oval" (**Fig. 3**). Mass margin descriptors have also been revised. The term "circumscribed" has replaced "smooth", and the term "irregular" is now a descriptor of mass shape and margin. In addition, terms used to describe the internal enhancement of a mass, "central enhancement", and "enhancing internal septations", have been removed from the lexicon due to lack of usage. Similarly, descriptors used for nonmass enhancement, "reticular" and "dendritic", have also been removed from the lexicon for underutilization. Another descriptor eliminated from the MRI lexicon is "ductal", which has been consolidated under the term "linear" (**Fig. 4**). Other terms "multiple foci" and "stippled", descriptors for nonmass enhancement have been removed from the lexicon as it is now recognized that they represent normal enhancement of fibroglandular tissue and will be described as part of BPE.[5,6] These changes have been summarized in **Box 4**.

A new term to describe nonmass enhancement has been introduced into the MRI Lexicon, "clustered ring enhancement". This finding, although not often seen, has been shown to have a high positive predictive value (PPV) for ductal carcinoma in situ.[7,8] Another new imaging feature introduced into the lexicon describes the characteristics of masses and nonmass enhancement on the T2 noncontrast sequence.[5] This feature assesses the T2 signal intensity of lesions, as increased T2 signal intensity has been mostly associated with benign lesion such as cysts and fibroadenomas,[9,10] and much less with malignant lesions such as mucinous carcinoma. In addition to the changes regarding the morphologic descriptors for mass and nonmass enhancement, the revised edition includes a section on kinetic descriptors, new sections listing nonenhancing findings, and associated findings as well as a new implants section.[5,6]

REPORTING SYSTEM

The new BI-RADS edition has made several changes to the standardized reporting language as well. As in the Breast Imaging Lexicon, some terms have been deleted, added, or clarified. The new edition has eliminated the percent ranges for the breast density categories found in the mammography lexicon. These had been introduced in previous editions in an attempt to provide an equal distribution of breast density assignments throughout all studies performed. However, they were not found to be helpful and were deleted.

Box 3 Summary of changes to BI-RADS ultrasound lexicon	
Lexicon Terminology	**Updated BI-RADS**
Tissue composition descriptors	New
Associative features section	New
Elastography descriptors	New

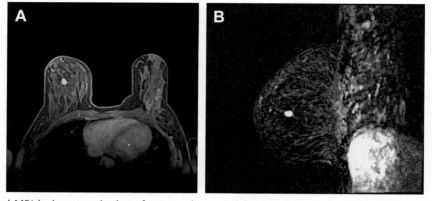

Fig. 3. Revised MRI lexicon terminology for mass shape. Axial post-contrast T1-weighted (*A*) and sagittal post-contrast subtracted T1-weighted (*B*) images show an oval enhancing mass in the central right breast. The descriptor for mass shape "lobular" has been deleted and replaced with the term "oval".

The new BI-RADS also provides clarification of terms used to describe lesion location on mammography. Previously, in cases where a lesion was located in the central breast or at the 12:00 location, a specific quadrant could not be assigned. The new BI-RADS has expanded the terminology for lesion location by adding terms such as "upper/lower/outer/inner central". This terminology has been added to the mammography lexicon and allows for direct correlation of lesion location on ultrasound and MRI. Increased clarification has also been provided to describe the use of subcategories for the BI-RADS assessment Category 4. The new BI-RADS provides specific PPV cut-off points for BI-RADS 4A/4B/4C, which match certain specific imaging findings. The use of these cut-off points remains optional in the new edition but is strongly encouraged.[4]

One of the major changes in the new BI-RADS edition has been the separation of assessment categories and management recommendations that had been "linked" in the previous edition. In most cases, the assessment and management have been paired up appropriately. However, there are some instances where the management recommendations did not go along with the BI-RADS assessment. This is the case in the BI-RADS Category 3/follow-up at 1-year management recommendation given at the third follow-up recommendation for a probably benign finding. The new edition provides flexibility for discordances between the assessment and the management. It also includes situations where a benign finding may require an intervention or surgical management: when a patient presents with a palpable mass without imaging findings still requiring surgical management, or cases of therapeutic cyst aspirations due to patient discomfort. The new BI-RADS edition addresses these discrepancies.

Other specific situations leading to discrepancies that have been addressed include cases of ruptured silicone implants, abscesses, new hematoma, and unexplained edema. In these situations, the imaging findings are benign appearing and lead to a benign recommendation but with

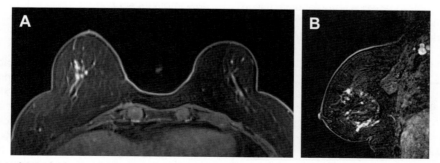

Fig. 4. Updated MRI lexicon terminology for nonmass enhancement. Axial post-contrast T1-weighted (*A*) and sagittal post-contrast subtracted T1-weighted (*B*) images demonstrate linear enhancement in the inferior lateral right breast. The term "ductal" has been eliminated from the lexicon and replaced with the descriptor for nonmass enhancement "linear".

Box 4
Summary of changes to BI-RADS MRI lexicon

Lexicon Terminology	Updated BI-RADS
BPE	New
Amount of fibroglandular tissue	New
Central enhancement	Deleted
Enhancing internal septations	Deleted
Linear, linear branching	Replaces "ductal"
Multiple foci	Deleted
Stippled	Deleted
Reticular	Deleted
Dendritic	Deleted
Clustered ring	New
Nonenhancing lesion section	New
Implant section	New

surgical/clinical management required. By unlinking the assessment from the management, the BI-RADS assessment category then appropriately reflects the imaging finding providing a concordant management recommendation for the assessment. This is then followed by the addition of a separate sentence that explains the discordance and provides the additional management.

AUDITING

The auditing section has also been expanded in the new BI-RADS edition. New and updated performance benchmarks based on more recent published literature have been incorporated in the new edition, as the previous ones were outdated. One of the benchmarks that has been updated is the recall rate. Half of all radiologists do not meet the 10% benchmark for recall rate, and therefore it has been changed to a more realistic number of 12% as more than 75% of radiologists are able to meet it.[11,12]

The definition for "screening interval" has been re-evaluated in the new edition. The revised BI-RADS edition recognizes that the screening interval may differ from country to country and in some countries it may be 1 year or 2- to 3-year intervals. As the definition of "cancer" for purpose of outcome monitoring is cancer diagnosis within the screening interval, the importance of defining the exact length of the screening interval is apparent. A longer screening interval results in a larger number of false negatives as cancers are allowed to grow for a longer period of time before they are discovered.

The new edition also addresses the difference between the 2 types of cyst aspirations: diagnostic versus therapeutic. A diagnostic cyst aspiration is performed to evaluate if a lesion is a cyst and should be accompanied by a suspicious assessment with a recommendation for tissue diagnosis. A therapeutic cyst aspiration is performed on a simple cyst for symptomatic relief and should be accompanied by a benign assessment (Category 2) with an additional phrase added to the recommendation stating why it was performed. Therapeutic cyst aspirations should not be included as biopsies when auditing the practice.[2]

ASSESSMENT CATEGORIES

Changes have been made to the BI-RADS management terminology, which include explanations for each BI-RADS assessment category on its usage. Added explanations provide guidance on how each assessment category should be used and for which specific circumstance. The BI-RADS assessment Category 0 (Incomplete) is used when additional imaging workup is required to make a final assessment, primarily from screening examinations and rarely from a diagnostic study. It can also be used in cases when one is awaiting prior studies for comparison. It states that when used in this situation, re-assessment needs to be performed within 30 days as to avoid delay in reporting. BI-RADS Category 1 (Negative) should be used only when the mammography report describes no specific benign finding, and BI-RADS Category 2 (Benign finding) should only be used when the mammography report describes a benign finding. For both categories, the recommendation remains routine screening.

For BI-RADS Category 3 (Probably benign finding), an explanation is provided on when the assessment category should be used, that is, for lesions that have a less than 2% likelihood of malignancy. A recommendation of short-interval follow-up should be given for lesions assessed as Category 3. The revised BI-RADS edition provides additional guidance as to which particular lexicon descriptor leads to a concordant assessment Category 3 as supported in the literature; these include a group of tiny round/oval calcifications, a noncalcified circumscribed solid mass, and a focal asymmetry.[13,14] A Category 3 assessment should be given only after a full diagnostic imaging evaluation has been performed, almost never if previous examinations are available for comparison, and never from a screening study.

The terminology for recommendations associated with the BI-RADS assessment categories 4, 5, and 6 have changed in the new edition. For Categories 4 and 5, the recommendations have

---

Box 5
Subdivision of category 4 (suspicious abnormality)

Category 4A	Low suspicion for malignancy (>2%–10% likelihood of malignancy)
Category 4B	Moderate suspicion for malignancy (>10%–50% likelihood of malignancy)
Category 4C	High suspicion for malignancy (>50% but <95% likelihood of malignancy)

---

changed to "tissue diagnosis" with a directive that states "Biopsy should be performed in the absence of clinical contraindication". The recommendation "appropriate action should be taken" for Category 6 has also been changed to "Surgical excision when clinically appropriate". The changes to the wording reflect the importance of conveying the appropriate management recommendation when tissue diagnosis is required.

The BI-RADS assessment Category 4 (Suspicious abnormality) is assigned to all findings that are between Category 3 (>2% risk of malignancy) and Category 5 (≥95% risk of malignancy). Most recommendations for tissue diagnosis are Category 4, ranging from aspiration of new complicated cysts to biopsy of very suspicious pleomorphic calcifications.[1] The subdivisions of Category 4 (4A/4B/4C) have been better delineated in the new edition with well-defined cut-off points (**Box 5**). The terminology for Category 4B has changed from "intermediate " to "moderate" and for Category 4C has changed from "moderate" to "high" to reflect new evidence from more recent published literature.[4] The assessment Category 5 (Highly suggestive of malignancy) is assigned to findings that are almost always malignant with more than 95% risk of cancer. It has been recognized that not one single imaging feature can impart such a high risk of malignancy, but rather a combination of findings is required to lead to the assessment Category 5.[2] BI-RADS Category 6 (Known biopsy – proven malignancy) is given when the findings have already been confirmed as malignant by biopsy, and the imaging has been performed before surgical excision. Category 6 lesions should be excluded from the medical audit, as they would inappropriately inflate the cancer detection rate and PPVs.[1]

SUMMARY

The new edition of BI-RADS provides increased clarification of the lexicon terminology by introducing new terms and deleting others when appropriate. It also leads to improved standardization of the reporting language and improved image interpretation. The revision also provides increased guidance in the usage of the BI-RADS management terminology, providing explanations on how the assessment categories should be used and in which specific circumstances. Overall, the changes made in the new BI-RADS give increased uniformity of terminology across the mammography, ultrasound, and MRI lexicons; add compatibility across the lexicons; and promote usage of the same descriptors across all 3 modalities ultimately leading to improved patient diagnosis and patient care.

ADDENDUM

The below is the reference to the new ACR BI-RADS Atlas, 5th Edition which was published later to writing this article. D'Orsi CJ, Sickles EA, Mendelson EB, et al. Breast Imaging Reportng and Data System: ACR BI-RADS Atlas. Reston(VA): American College of Radiology; 2013.

REFERENCES

1. D'Orsi CJ, Mendelson EB, Ikeda DM, et al. Breast imaging reporting and data system: ACR BI-RADS – breast imaging atlas. Reston (VA): American College of Radiology; 2003.
2. Destaunis SV, Sickles EA, Mendelson EB, et al. BI-RADS Update and challenge (an interactive session). Refresher Course the 99th Annual Meeting of the Radiological Society of North America, RSNA. Chicago, December 4, 2013.
3. Hansen B. Inside the New BI-RADS. ACR Bulletin 2011;66(6):22.
4. Torres-Tabanera M, Cárdenas-Rebollo JM, Villar-Castaño P, et al. Analysis of the positive predictive value of the subcategories of BI-RADS(®) 4 lesions: preliminary results in 880 lesions. Radiologia 2012; 54(6):520–31.
5. Edwards SD, Lipson JA, Ikeda DM, et al. Updates and revisions to the BI-RADS magnetic resonance imaging lexicon. Magn Reson Imaging Clin N Am 2013;21:483–93.
6. Available at: http://www.auntminnieeurope.com/index.aspx?sec=sup&sub=wom&pag=dis&ItemID=605318. Accessed December 27, 2012.
7. Uematsu T, Kasami M. High-spatial-resolution 3-T breast MRI of nonmasslike enhancement lesions: an analysis of their features as significant predictors of malignancy. AJR Am J Roentgenol 2012;198(5):1223–30.
8. Tozaki M, Fukuda K. High-spatial-resolution MRI of non-masslike breast lesions: interpretation model based on BI-RADS MRI descriptors. AJR Am J Roentgenol 2006;187(2):330–7.

9. Kuhl CK, Klaschik S, Mielcarek P, et al. Do T2- weighted pulse sequences help with the differential diagnosis of enhancing lesions in dynamic breast MRI? J Magn Reson Imaging 1999;9:187–96.

10. Ballesio L, Savelli S, Angeletti M, et al. Breast MRI: are T2 IR sequences useful in the evaluation of breast lesions? Eur J Radiol 2009;71:96–101.

11. Carney PA, Sickles EA, Monsees BS, et al. Identifying minimally acceptable interpretive performance criteria for screening mammography. Radiology 2010;255(2):354–61.

12. Smith-Bindman R, Chu PW, Miglioretti DL, et al. Comparison of screening mammography in the United States and the United kingdom. JAMA 2003;290(16):2129–37.

13. Leung JW, Sickles EA. The probably benign assessment. Radiol Clin North Am 2007;45(5): 773–89, vi.

14. Gruber R, Jaromi S, Rudas M, et al. Histologic work-up of non-palpable breast lesions classified as probably benign at initial mammography and/or ultrasound (BI-RADS category 3). Eur J Radiol 2013; 82(3):398–403.

Digital Tomosynthesis: Technique

Martin J. Yaffe, PhD*, James G. Mainprize, PhD

KEYWORDS

- Digital tomosynthesis • Digital mammography • Reconstruction • Optimization

KEY POINTS

- Digital breast tomosynthesis (DBT) is an extension of digital mammography (DM) that produces quasi three-dimensional reconstructed images from a set of low-dose x-ray projections acquired over a limited angular range.
- Both filtered back projection and several variants of iterative methods are used for reconstruction, each having distinctive advantages and limitations.
- Although some manufacturers initially defined the examination to include the craniocaudal and mediolateral-oblique tomographic image data sets and conventional projection mammograms for these views, the success in synthesizing two-dimensional images by algorithmic projection through the three-dimensional dataset is likely to obviate the need for the separate conventional exposures, thereby allowing a reduction of dose to the breast.
- An alternative approach to three-dimensional imaging is through dedicated breast CT. DBT and CT each have relative strengths and weaknesses and only clinical evaluation allows the role of each to be more clearly defined.

INTRODUCTION

Digital breast tomosynthesis (DBT) is an extension of digital mammography (DM) and is typically incorporated onto a DM platform. To accomplish tomosynthesis image acquisition, the x-ray tube is moved over a range of angles about a pivot point near the DM detector to obtain a series of low-dose digital projection radiographs. In most designs, the detector remains stationary during image acquisition or (in the isocentric design) it rotates about the pivot point in synchrony with the x-ray source. The x-ray tube may temporarily halt as each projection is acquired (step-and-shoot technique) or may move continuously during acquisition.

From the set of typically between 9 and 25 low-dose projection images, an algorithm reconstructs a quasi three-dimensional representation of the x-ray attenuation properties of the breast tissues. As in computed tomography (CT), the reconstruction algorithm may be based on an iterative approach or it may use Fourier methods or filtered back projection. Constraints can be applied to speed or simplify the reconstruction.

The reconstructed images are often viewed as a "movie-loop" where adjacent x-y planes (parallel to the x-ray detector) are displayed sequentially. Because a complete range of angular data is not obtained, the dataset is highly undersampled, giving rise to artifacts. Typically in DBT the spatial resolution in the x-y plane is quite high, whereas it is coarser in the z (x-ray tube to detector) direction.

The quality of the reconstructed image and the dose to the breast are dependent on the angular range and number of projections, the dose used per projection, and the performance of the x-ray detector and electronics. This article discusses an approach to optimization.

IMAGE ACQUISITION
Geometry

Several configurations of tomosynthesis systems have been developed.[1] These variations are

Sunnybrook Research Insitute, 2075 Bayview Avenue, Toronto, ON M4N 3M5, Canada
* Corresponding author.
E-mail address: martin.yaffe@sri.utoronto.ca

Radiol Clin N Am 52 (2014) 489–497
http://dx.doi.org/10.1016/j.rcl.2014.01.003

distinguished by the path of the x-ray tube and the detector. Arc, linear,[2] and circular[3] x-ray tube paths have been suggested.[1] A "full isocentric geometry"[4] is like that used in true CT systems in which the x-ray tube and the detector rotate in synchrony around a pivot axis. Although some prototype DBT systems used this geometry, most now use a "partial isocentric geometry"[4] in which the x-ray tube rotates in an arc around a pivot centered near the breast support and the detector remains stationary during acquisition (**Fig. 1**). This geometry is relatively easy to use in a modified DM system because no special modifications to the detector housing are required. Several mammography systems already have the mechanics needed to move the x-ray tube head independently of the main gantry. As such, nearly every commercial system and systems that are in preapproval evaluation use this geometry.[5] A notable exception is the DBT system based on the photon-counting MicroDose mammography system (Philips Healthcare, Best, The Netherlands), which uses isocentric geometry but with the isocenter located below the detector.[6]

Step-and-shoot Versus Continuous Gantry Motion

The motion of the x-ray source may be either continuous motion or a step-and-shoot approach in which the x-ray source comes to a complete stop before each x-ray exposure. The continuous motion approach can be accomplished with a simpler mechanical system and, therefore, can move at higher speeds, provided the detector can be read out fast enough. Motion blur in the form of increased focal spot blur in the scanning direction occurs, although this can be ameliorated if short x-ray pulses are used. Pulse duration is limited by the output capability of the x-ray tube

(ie, shorter pulses of x-rays require higher tube current [milliampere] to achieve the same exposure).

In the step-and-shoot approach, the motion of the x-ray source ceases immediately before each x-ray exposure. This eliminates the focal spot motion blur effects associated with continuous motion. However, these systems are necessarily slower, requiring time for the gantry arm to stabilize before each imaging exposure occurs. Vibration may be a problem. With longer imaging times patient motion could occur between projections, resulting in an inconsistent dataset. This could cause loss of detail in the reconstructed image or the introduction of artifacts that could reduce the conspicuity of lesions.

For either approach, a very high degree of geometric accuracy is required, including knowledge of the angular location of the x-ray source for each x-ray exposure. This information is stored in the DICOM header of the acquired projection images to be used by the reconstruction algorithm.

Scan Angle, Angular Sampling, and Number of Projections

The scan angle is the maximum angle traversed by the DBT gantry from first image to last image. The number of projections used in a single scan then determines the angular sampling (the angle between successive projections) for a given scan angle. Various implementations of DBT use scan angles and numbers of projections (angular sampling) that vary quite markedly. Several authors have attempted to optimize these parameters with mixed results.[7–11] Variability in results is largely caused by differences in the metrics used to quantify image quality. These range from simple measures, such as contrast-to-noise ratio and point spread function, to much more complex

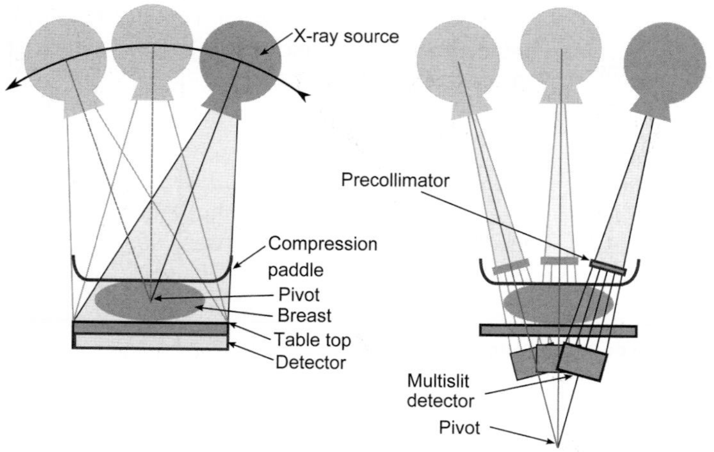

Fig. 1. (*Left*) Schematic of a typical partial isocentric geometry used in DBT. The x-ray source moves in an arc around a pivot axis. The pivot axis is generally placed near the breast support. (*Right*) Geometry used in the MicroDose prototype.

mathematical observer models that attempt to measure real imaging tasks, such as the detection of lesions.[12]

As described by Young,[11] a DBT system can be operated at different dose ranges that limit image quality by one of three conditions. The reconstruction is either (1) quantum noise limited, (2) electronic noise limited at low doses, or (3) anatomic noise limited at higher doses. Anatomic noise refers to the variability of the background fibroglandular tissue structure in breast images that can reduce the conspicuity of lesions. Generally, mammography and DBT systems are operated at sufficient dose levels that images are anatomic noise limited, but attempts to keep the dose below a predefined limit could, in suboptimal situations, result in operation where DBT is either quantum noise or electronic noise limited. Young also noted that the optimization of the acquisition of DBT images depends on breast density.

Increasing the scan angle generally improves the z-resolution[9] but, beyond a certain point, increasing the number of projections does not have a significant effect on resolution. For a breast of average density (25%), Young and colleagues[11] found that increasing the scan angle improved the detectability slightly for 3-mm diameter lesions, but only if the doses were high enough that the images were anatomic noise limited.

The optimal number of projections increases with increasing scan angle and that optimal number is largely independent of radiation dose.[9,11] Using more projections (or equivalently narrower angular sampling) does not significantly improve lesion detectability, although streak artifacts, which could affect lesion characterization, may be reduced.[7,11]

Estimates from optimization studies vary wildly. For example, Chawla and colleagues[7] found that 15 to 17 projections for a 45-degree scan angle were best (although higher scan angles were not investigated), whereas Young[11] found that only seven projections were required for an optimal scan angle of 96 degrees.

Optimal results for microcalcifications and soft tissue masses can be different. Sechopoulos and Ghetti[9] found that the contrast-to-noise ratio for microcalcifications decreased with wider scan angles if doses were held fixed, whereas they improved for masses, where the optimal scan angle was predicted to be 60 degrees. The authors believed that this was because the detection of low-contrast masses greatly benefits from the improved ability to separate tissues in the z-direction by DBT at wide angles, whereas the appearances of microcalcifications would be degraded by increasing image noise because of greater

x-ray attenuation of the increased thickness of the breast at higher angles. However, they noted sensitivity to angle for microcalcifications was relatively small and that the more substantial improvement in mass conspicuity would dictate optimization efforts.

Scatter

Because the angle of incidence of the x-rays on the detectors changes from projection to projection, a conventional grid would cut off the primary x-rays when the x-ray source is located at oblique angles. As a result, a conventional antiscatter grid is not useful. However, scatter plays a role at reducing conspicuity and introducing inconsistent data in the reconstruction.[13] Wu and colleagues[13] demonstrated that cupping artifacts similar to those seen in CT can occur in DBT images because of the recording of scattered radiation.

Technique Selection (Tube Voltage, Tube Current, and Target-Filter Combination)

Because the main goal of DBT is to improve lesion conspicuity by reducing background clutter, the subject contrast of the lesion becomes less important. As a result, DBT can be performed at higher x-ray energies to take advantage of increased penetration and potentially reduced dose. Some systems operate under conditions similar to those of DM (eg, 28 kV Rh/Rh), whereas others use higher kilovolt values and alternative target-filter combinations, such as W/Al or W/Ag.[14,15]

RECONSTRUCTION TECHNIQUES

Several techniques for reconstruction have been implemented successfully for DBT. The simplest technique is a shift-and-add technique that replicates the concept of planar laminography by shifting each projection slightly such that signals from objects at one depth register sharply in each of the projections, whereas those from objects in other planes are spread out and blurred away. The shift-and-add approach, however, requires careful correction if used for partial isocentric geometries.[16]

Many of the reconstruction techniques for DBT rely on the enormous effort expended in the development of CT reconstruction algorithms. However, because of the limited angle–limited view nature of DBT, algorithms must necessarily be modified to accommodate these restrictions.

Filtered Backprojection

Filtered backprojection is the method that arises from Fourier-based or kernel-filtered backprojection techniques used for conventional CT. Specifically, a cone-beam approximate method of filtered back-projection is used.[17] This technique first convolves the projection data with a reconstruction kernel function (equivalent to spatial frequency filtering) and then backprojects the data through a reconstruction volume according to the x-ray geometry with which each projection was originally acquired. This can be accomplished by a ray-driven technique like that of Siddon,[18] which finds the voxels that are intersected by each ray and allocates a weighted fraction of the signal to each voxel.

Filtered backprojection relies on a property of the projection-slice theorem, which states that a projection at angle θ (**Fig. 2**, *left*) contains information regarding the cross-section of the object that is represented by a slice in Fourier domain at angle θ as shown in **Fig. 2** (*right*). In CT, full rotations acquire data such that the Fourier domain is covered by slices that form the spokes of a wheel (see **Fig. 2**, *center*). As can be seen, the density of the spokes at the center of the Fourier domain is much higher than at the edges of the spokes. This imbalance is corrected by weighting or filtering the Fourier data. This filter is known as a reconstruction kernel. This kernel suppresses the low spatial frequency information relative to the high spatial frequency information. The basic kernel for CT reconstruction has a ramp-like shape in Fourier space.[19]

In DBT, however, the maximum angle, θ, is limited and a large portion of the Fourier domain remains unsampled by x-ray projections (see **Fig. 2**, *right*). This means that a large portion of the information corresponding to the z-direction is missing. As the projection angle increases, the x-ray system is better able to interrogate the signals that change along the z-direction. Because of the missing data, especially at high spatial frequencies in the z-direction, resolution is limited. The noise in projections can strongly affect the reconstructed volume. Mertelmeier[20] demonstrated

that tailored angle-specific filtering is used to reduce higher spatial frequency noise for DBT.

Iterative Techniques

Iterative techniques generally involve a cyclic process of (1) estimating the volume, (2) comparing differences between simulated projections to the measured projections, and (3) updating the volume based on those differences. This cycle is repeated until a certain number of iterations is reached or when the differences between the simulated and measured projections are sufficiently small.

The simplest iterative technique is called the algebraic reconstruction method, in which a fraction of the differences between the simulated and measured projection are added back into the volume at every point along the x-ray path through the volume to that detector element.[21,22] Variations on basic algebraic reconstruction method, such as simultaneous algebraic reconstruction method, change the point in the routine at which the simulated projections are updated.[23] Three iterations of a simultaneous algebraic reconstruction method reconstructed slice from a contrast-enhanced (temporal subtraction) tomosynthesis dataset[24] are shown in **Fig. 3** illustrating the improvement in lesion contrast and sharpness with iteration. Iterative algorithms tend to introduce noise artifacts as they attempt to converge the projections through the image updates with the actual measured projection data. Therefore, a key challenge in the development of an iterative algorithm is determining the number of iterations that produces a faithful reconstructed image without undue increase in noise.

More advanced techniques take into account the physics of the process. For example, in a maximum-likelihood routine, the exponential attenuation of signal and the image noise statistics[25,26] are considered. Rather than updating the

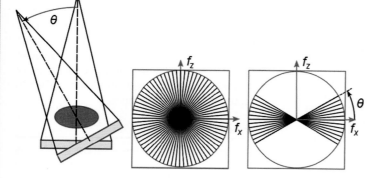

Fig. 2. (*Left*) Definition of projection angle. (*Center*) K-(Fourier) space coverage in CT. (*Right*) corresponding K-space coverage for DBT. Here x is distance along the chest wall in the plane parallel to the detector and z is distance through the breast perpendicular to the detector for $\theta = 0$.

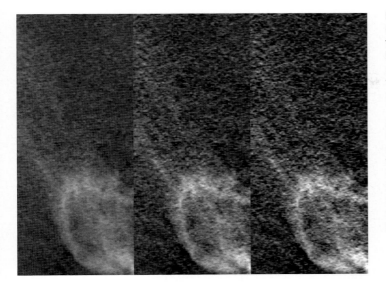

Fig. 3. Examples of tomosynthesis (scan angle 30 degrees, 15 projections) slices of iodine uptake in a rabbit VX2 tumor implanted in the thigh muscle. Reconstruction was performed with a simultaneous algebraic reconstruction method algorithm and 1-mm-thick slices (0.2 × 0.2 mm² pixels) are shown after iteration 1 (*left*), 2 (*center*), and 3 (*right*). Sharpness and contrast of the image features improve with iteration count, but without additional constraints, noise may become enhanced with increasing iterations. (*Courtesy of Melissa Hill, PhD, Sunnybrook Research Institute, Toronto, Canada.*)

volume based on a simple difference, the most probable signal that could create the measured projection is estimated for each iteration. This approach is much more computationally expensive, but accurate models of the imaging chain can produce very high-quality images.

One advantage of iterative techniques is the ability to apply constraints to the update. This may do things such things as impose a smoothness criterion on the volume that reduces the noise in the volume. This is done in such techniques as total variation minimization[27] or penalized maximum-likelihood reconstruction.[28]

Although iterative techniques are computationally demanding, the use of optimized algorithms' modern high-speed computing power makes them practical. Reconstructed image data sets can be available within minutes of acquisition of the projection data.

Artifacts

Because of the limited view nature of DBT, all reconstructions are rife with artifacts. Objects appear to "fade away" as the reader scrolls through slices rather than disappearing. This is especially noticeable for larger objects, which can persist for several slices beyond the known edge of the object (eg, details of the breast can actually be seen several millimeters above the zone of the compression paddle in the reconstruction). Large, high-contrast objects can produce streak artifacts that manifest as overlapping objects that converge as the reader scrolls toward the slice with the true calcification (**Fig. 4**A). A staircase or terracing artifact (see **Fig. 4**B) can occur at

sharp edges that are perpendicular to the scan direction. This is an extension of the general high-contrast artifact for longer object edges. It can also manifest at the edge of the field because of partial volume effects because tissue is covered by only a portion of the projections. Cupping artifacts manifest because of x-ray scatter and beam hardening.[13] This appears as a roll-off in attenuation primarily along the tomosynthesis scan direction from an object edge toward its center (see **Fig. 4**C). This is often apparent on the inferior margin of the breast in a DBT mediolateral oblique view.

Spatial Resolution

In-plane resolution for DBT is largely dictated by the resolution of the detector. To achieve faster readout speeds and reduced detector noise, some systems bin the signal from adjacent detector elements together, resulting in reduction of the resolution by the binning factor (eg, 2 × 2 binning reduces the resolution in each direction by 50%). Systems in which the x-ray source is in constant motion with respect to the breast during image acquisition have an additional resolution loss in the tomosynthesis scan direction equal to the projected distance the focal spot travels during the x-ray pulse. Shorter x-ray pulses can ameliorate this effect.

Because of the incomplete nature of the DBT data, the cross-plane resolution (z-direction) is hard to quantify. In DBT, the z-direction information of small objects is captured better than that of larger objects. This is illustrated by a simple example. Imagine standing in front of a lamppost

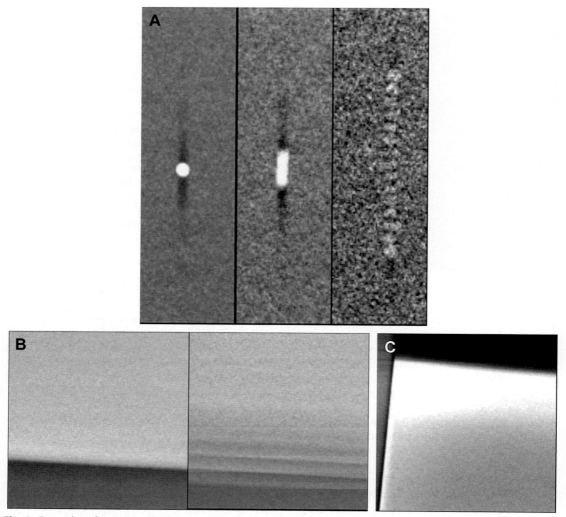

Fig. 4. Examples of image artifacts. (*A*) An in-plane shadow along the tomosynthesis scan direction surrounding a high-contrast object (in this case a 0.8-mm diameter aluminum ball bearing) and a diverging set of shadows above and below the slice. Appearance of the BB is shown in plane (*left*), at 3 mm below the BB (*center*), and 15 mm below the BB (*right*). (*B*) Staircase artifacts can be caused by the edges of sharp objects and by the edges of the reconstruction field. (*Left*) The edge in the reconstructed slice. (*Right*) Artifacts can also be seen in other slices as terracing, shown here at 25 mm below the focus plane. (*C*) Cupping artifacts arise from scatter and beam hardening. This manifests as a strong rolloff in apparent attenuation from the edge of an object to its center. Window and levels on each image have been set to emphasize the artifacts.

and moving left or right by 1 m. Without much difficulty, the thickness of the post can be estimated, even if it has an irregular shape. Now imagine standing in front of a very large tree (large enough to block a significant portion of your visual field). Moving to the side by 1 m likely only provides a very crude guess about the thickness of the tree, and you would have to move a lot further to get a better estimate.

The cross-plane resolution is typically evaluated using an artifact spread function (ASF), which is in many ways similar to the point-spread function, although ASFs are usually measured by imaging relatively large objects (eg, 1-mm ball bearings) rather than pinholes or point objects. As shown in **Fig. 5**, the ASF generally improves with increasing scan angle. Increasing the number of projections generally causes the tail of the ASF to become smoother.

Comparison with Breast CT

There is now one commercial system for breast CT available and at least three clinical prototype

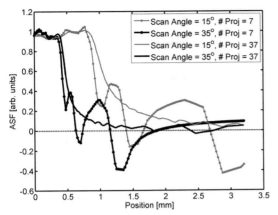

Fig. 5. ASFs for various scan angles and number of projections for a simulated 1-mm diameter ball bearing and a filtered backprojection reconstruction. *Curves* with *dots* and *lines* are for *n* = 7 projections and *line-only* plots are for *n* = 37 projections. *Gray lines* indicate a scan angle of 15 degrees and *black lines* indicate a scan angle of 35 degrees. The width of the ASF is largely determined by the scan angle, whereas the number of projections affects the smoothness of the ASF.

systems under evaluation.[29–31] Breast CT reconstructions are performed with a complete angular set of data and therefore typically use many more angular projections than DBT. Designs are based around a table on which the patient lies prone with the breast pendant into an imaging area containing the x-ray source and an area detector. Therefore, these systems use a cone-beam acquisition approach. Because of the greater number of projections, to avoid a large increase in radiation dose, the reconstructed pixel dimensions tend to be larger than in DBT, although the voxels are typically isotropic with a side on the order of 0.3 to 0.5 mm. As well, higher x-ray energies are used than for DBT; the increased penetration through the breast allowing reduction of what would otherwise be high doses. Breast CT avoids artifacts because of incomplete sampling in k-space, but at the expense of larger pixels and the need for a dedicated table assembly. Designing the system to ensure full imaging access to the axillary aspect of the breast also imposes some challenges.

DOSE AND DOSE OPTIMIZATION

Because DBT has been proposed as a replacement for DM in either a screening or a diagnostic context, a convention of expectation has arisen that the x-ray dose received by the breast for a DBT examination should be approximately equivalent to that for a typical two-view DM screening examination (3–5 mGy). At this point, it is not completely resolved, however, as to what should constitute a complete DBT examination. Should there be one or two DBT views?[32,33] Should there also be one or two standard mammography views with the accompanying increase in dose?[34]

It may be possible to avoid the need for additional two-dimensional mammography views by using a synthesized mammogram. This is created by an algorithm that projects through the three-dimensional DBT reconstructed dataset to form a two-dimensional image.[35] Because of the relatively noisy and artifact-laden nature of the DBT volume, care must be taken to minimize these effects in the synthesized mammogram. One early study has demonstrated that the performance of DBT and a synthesized mammogram compared with a DBT and conventional mammogram was similar (77.2% and 82.6% sensitivity, respectively).[36] The study authors suggested that future improvements in DBT image quality and more advanced synthesized mammogram algorithms could improve their results.

Alternatively, the central projection may be acquired at a much higher dose relative to the other projections (eg, 50% of the dose may be applied to the middle projection).[37] Then, the central projection appears to be very similar to a regular mammogram, although it may appear slightly noisier than a conventional mammogram in a direct comparison.

Researchers have extended this concept of using different dose levels for each projection.[37–40] The hypothesis for the dose-budgeting approach is that the information from each projection is not used equally. For example, it is believed that the central projection contributes the most information and could have its dose budget increased relative to the other projections. Similarly, the highest angle projections only contribute to the vertical separation of large lesions and thus may not require as much dose. Several groups have studied this, and there seems to be some advantage of using unequal amounts of radiation for certain lesion sizes and operating conditions.[40]

SUMMARY

DBT is an extension of DM that produces quasi three-dimensional reconstructed images from a set of low-dose x-ray projections acquired over a limited angular range. The quality of the reconstructed image and the dose to the breast are dependent on the angular range and number of projections, the dose used per projection, and detector resolution and noise characteristics. Most DBT systems use a partial isocentric geometry in which the x-ray tube rotates in an arc around a pivot centered near the breast support and the detector remains stationary during acquisition. The acquisition can be either step-and-shoot or one in which the gantry rotates continuously during imaging. DBT can be performed at a higher x-ray spectral energy to reduce radiation dose. The acquisition motion generally makes it impractical to use a conventional anti-scatter grid and various other approaches to mitigate against the effects of scatter have been considered.

Filtered back projection and several variants of iterative methods are used for reconstruction, each having distinctive advantages and limitations. There are opportunities to use various constraints in the reconstruction to optimize performance. There is also considerable effort being directed at the use of sophisticated filtering techniques to reduce noise and to mitigate against artifacts, the latter mainly associated with the incomplete angular sampling of projection data in DBT.

Although some manufacturers initially defined the examination to include the craniocaudal and mediolateral-oblique tomographic image data sets and conventional projection mammograms for these views, the success in synthesizing two-dimensional images by algorithmic projection through the three-dimensional dataset is likely to obviate the separate conventional exposures, thereby allowing a reduction of dose to the breast.

An alternative approach to three-dimensional imaging is through dedicated breast CT. DBT and CT each have relative strengths and weaknesses and only clinical evaluation allows the role of each to be more clearly defined.

REFERENCES

1. Dobbins JT. Tomosynthesis imaging: at a translational crossroads. Med Phys 2009;36(6):1956.
2. Kuo J, Ringer PA, Fallows SG, et al. Dynamic reconstruction and rendering of 3D tomosynthesis images. Physics (College Park Md) 2011;7961: 796116-1-11.
3. Stevens GM, Birdwell RL, Beaulieu CF, et al. Circular tomosynthesis: potential in imaging of breast and upper cervical spine–preliminary phantom and in vitro study. Radiology 2003;228(2):569–75.
4. Dobbins JT, Godfrey DJ. Digital x-ray tomosynthesis: current state of the art and clinical potential. Phys Med Biol 2003;48(19):R65–106.
5. Sechopoulos I. A review of breast tomosynthesis. Part I. The image acquisition process. Med Phys 2013;40(1):014301.
6. Dahlman N, Fredenberg E, Åslund M, et al. Evaluation of photon-counting spectral breast tomosynthesis. Proc SPIE 2011;7961:796114-1-10.
7. Chawla AS, Lo JY, Baker JA, et al. Optimized image acquisition for breast tomosynthesis in projection and reconstruction space. Med Phys 2009;36(11): 4859.
8. Kempston MP, Mainprize JG, Yaffe MJ. Evaluating the effect of dose on reconstructed image quality in digital tomosynthesis. Lect Notes Comput Sci 2006;4046:490–7.
9. Sechopoulos I, Ghetti C. Optimization of the acquisition geometry in digital tomosynthesis of the breast. Med Phys 2009;36(4):1199–207.
10. Reiser I, Nishikawa RM. Task-based assessment of breast tomosynthesis: effect of acquisition parameters and quantum noise. Med Phys 2010;37(4): 1591–600.
11. Young S, Bakic PR, Myers KJ, et al. A virtual trial framework for quantifying the detectability of masses in breast tomosynthesis projection data. Med Phys 2013;40(5):1–15.
12. Barrett HH. Objective assessment of image quality: effects of quantum noise and object variability. J Opt Soc Am A 1990;7(7):1266–78.
13. Wu G, Mainprize JG, Boone JM, et al. Evaluation of scatter effects on image quality for breast tomosynthesis. Med Phys 2009;36(10):4425.
14. Varjonen M, Strömmer P, Oy P. Optimizing the target-filter combination in digital mammography in the sense of image quality and average glandular dose. Lect Notes Comput Sci 2008;5116:570–6.
15. Dance DR, Young KC, van Engen RE. Further factors for the estimation of mean glandular dose using the United Kingdom, European and IAEA breast dosimetry protocols. Phys Med Biol 2009;54(14): 4361–72.
16. Chen Y, Lo JY, Dobbins JT. Importance of point-by-point back projection correction for isocentric motion in digital breast tomosynthesis: relevance to morphology of structures such as microcalcifications. Med Phys 2007;34(10):3885.
17. Feldkamp L, Davis L, Kress J. Practical cone-beam algorithm. J Opt Soc Am A 1984;1(6):612–9.
18. Siddon RL. Fast calculation of the exact radiological path for a three-dimensional CT array. Med Phys 1985;12:252.
19. Kak AC, Slaney M. Algorithms for reconstruction with nondiffracting sources. Principles of computerized tomographic imaging, Society of Industrial and Applied Mathematics 2001. Available at: http://www.slaney.org/pct.
20. Mertelmeier T. Optimizing filtered backprojection reconstruction for a breast tomosynthesis prototype device. Proc SPIE 2006;6142:61420F-1-12.
21. Kak AC, Slaney M. Algebraic reconstruction algorithms. In: Principles of computerized tomographic

imaging, Society of Industrial and Applied Mathematics. 2001. p. 275–96. Available at: http://www.slaney.org/pct.

22. Wang B, Barner K, Lee D. Algebraic tomosynthesis reconstruction. Proc SPIE 2004;5370:711–8.

23. Zhang Y. Tomosynthesis reconstruction using the simultaneous algebraic reconstruction technique (SART) on breast phantom data. Proc SPIE 2006; 6142:614249-1–9.

24. Hill ML, Liu K, Mainprize JG, et al. Pre-clinical evaluation of tumour angiogenesis with contrast-enhanced breast tomosynthesis. Lect Notes Comput Sci 2012; 7361:1–8.

25. Zhang Y, Chan HP, Sahiner B, et al. A comparative study of limited-angle cone-beam reconstruction methods for breast tomosynthesis. Med Phys 2006;33(10):3781–95.

26. Wu T, Zhang J, Moore R, et al. Digital tomosynthesis mammography using a parallel maximum-likelihood reconstruction method. Proc SPIE 2004;5368:1–11.

27. Sidky EY, Reiser IS, Nishikawa R, et al. Image reconstruction in digital breast tomosynthesis by total variation minimization. Proc SPIE 2007;6510: 651027-1–6.

28. Das M, Gifford HC, O'Connor JM, et al. Penalized maximum likelihood reconstruction for improved microcalcification detection in breast tomosynthesis. IEEE Trans Med Imaging 2011;30(4):904–14.

29. Boone JM, Nelson TR, Lindfors KK, et al. Dedicated breast CT: radiation dose and image quality evaluation. Radiology 2001;221(3):657–67.

30. Madhav P, Crotty DJ, McKinley RL, et al. Evaluation of tilted cone-beam CT orbits in the development of a dedicated hybrid mammotomograph. Phys Med Biol 2009;54(12):3659–76.

31. O'Connell A, Conover DL, Zhang Y, et al. Cone-beam CT for breast imaging: radiation dose, breast coverage, and image quality. Am J Roentgenol 2010;195(2):496–509.

32. Rafferty E, Kopans D, Wu T, et al. Breast tomosynthesis: will a single view do? RSNA 90th Scientific Assembly and Annual Meeting. Chicago, November 28 – December 3, 2004.

33. Wallis MG, Moa E, Zanca F, et al. Two-view and single-view tomosynthesis versus full-field digital mammography: high-resolution X-ray imaging observer study. Radiology 2012;262(3):788–96.

34. Gennaro G, Hendrick RE, Toledano A, et al. Combination of one-view digital breast tomosynthesis with one-view digital mammography versus standard two-view digital mammography: per lesion analysis. Eur Radiol 2013;23(8):2087–94.

35. Bijhold J. Three-dimensional verification of patient placement during radiotherapy using portal images. Med Phys 1993;20(2):347–56.

36. Gur D, Zuley ML, Anello MI, et al. Dose reduction in digital breast tomosynthesis (DBT) screening using synthetically reconstructed projection images an observer performance study. Acad Radiol 2011; 19(2):166–71.

37. Nishikawa RM, Reiser I, Seifi P, et al. A new approach to digital breast tomosynthesis for breast cancer screening. Proc SPIE 2007;6510:65103C-1–8.

38. Hu YH, Zhao W. The effect of angular dose distribution on the detection of microcalcifications in digital breast tomosynthesis. Med Phys 2011; 38(5):2455–66.

39. Das M, Gifford HC, O'Connor JM, et al. Evaluation of a variable dose acquisition technique for microcalcification and mass detection in digital breast tomosynthesis. Med Phys 2009;36(6):1976–84.

40. Young S, Badal A, Myers KJ, et al. A task-specific argument for variable-exposure breast tomosynthesis. LNCS 2012;7361:72–9.

Clinical Implementation of Digital Breast Tomosynthesis

Emily F. Conant, MD

KEYWORDS

- Digital breast tomosynthesis • Digital mammography • Breast cancer • Screening mammography
- Breast imaging

KEY POINTS

- DBT improves specificity and sensitivity in breast cancer screening.
- The conspicuity of masses and areas of distortion is improved with DBT.
- The three-dimensional information from DBT imaging may replace the need for some two-dimensional diagnostic imaging in the evaluation of suspicious lesions.
- Research is ongoing to address the increased x-ray dose of combination DM/DBT and to improve the efficiency of reading the large image sets.

INTRODUCTION

Despite continued controversy over how often and when mammographic screening should occur, the modality remains the mainstay of the early detection of breast cancer. In 2009, the US Preventative Service Task Force on Screening (USPSTFS) published new and controversial guidelines recommending that screening begin at the age of 50 rather than 40 years and that the interval of screening change to every other year rather than yearly. In addition, for the first time, the new guidelines recommended an age at which screening should stop (75 years), when previously no age had been defined.[1]

These controversial guidelines persist in 2013 despite that digital mammography has shown an improved performance over older, analog imaging and that newer, population-based screening trials have shown more than a 30% reduction in breast cancer deaths in patients screened.[2,3] At the heart of the USPSTFS guideline changes are concerns over the risk-benefit ratio of mammography (too many false-positive with few significant cancers detected), the potential for overdiagnosis (finding cancers that probably are not harmful yet are treated aggressively), and that mammography is fraught with false-negatives or misses of clinically significant cancers.

WHY DIGITAL BREAST TOMOSYNTHESIS?

Early data on digital breast tomosynthesis (DBT) has shown that the novel technique may address some of the limitations of conventional mammography by improving the accuracy of screening and diagnostic breast imaging.[4–7] With conventional two-dimensional digital mammographic (DM) imaging, many of the concerning false-positives and -negatives are caused by the same issue: the breast is a three-dimensional structure viewed as a two-dimensional image. In the case of false-positives, normal overlapping tissues of various textures and densities may create a complex appearance that too often mimics suspicious asymmetries or areas of architectural distortion, thus prompting additional imaging and occasionally biopsy (Fig. 1). In the case of false-negatives, overlying normal breast tissue may obscure or mask malignant lesions, preventing detection (Fig. 2).

The technique of DBT allows the breast to be viewed in a three-dimensional format so that in-focus planes, or slices of the breast, can be visualized thus reducing the impact of confounding or

Department of Radiology, Perelman School of Medicine at the University of Pennsylvania, 3400 Spruce Street, Philadelphia, PA 19104, USA
E-mail address: emily.conant@uphs.upenn.edu

Radiol Clin N Am 52 (2014) 499–518
http://dx.doi.org/10.1016/j.rcl.2013.11.013

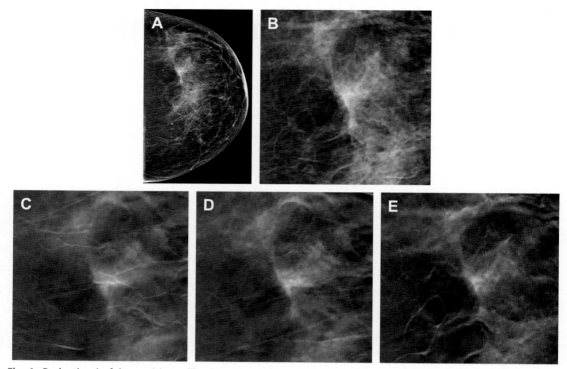

Fig. 1. Reduction in false-positive callbacks with DBT. The DM CC view (*A*) demonstrates focal asymmetry with a suggestion of architectural distortion in the slightly lateral breast. A cropped, enlarged view of the DM focal asymmetry (*B*) better demonstrates the area of possible distortion. Multiple in-plane 1-mm reconstructed slices (*C–E*) from the DBT clearly show that the focal asymmetry seen on the two-dimensional DM study is caused by tissue superimposition rather than a clinically significant finding.

superimposed breast tissue. The multiple, in-plane DBT slices are reconstructed from a series of low-dose exposures acquired as the mammographic x-ray source moves in an arc above the compressed breast.[8–10] The DBT image sets may be acquired from any angle that the x-ray tube moves and may be obtained during the same compression as the two-dimensional mammographic views. This combination of obtaining a two-dimensional image and a tomosynthesis image set together is often called a "combo-mode" acquisition.[11] This combination imaging technique is fast, usually obtained in 3 to 4 seconds (Hologic, Inc. Bedford, MA), and is very well tolerated by patients. In addition, because the two-dimensional and tomosynthesis images are acquired in a single compression, the images are coregistered allowing the reader to toggle back and forth between the image sets to problem solve (see **Fig. 1**). This combination of 2D digital mammography (DM) and DBT imaging was approved by the Food and Drug Administration (FDA) in 2011.[12] **Box 1** summarizes some of the clinical benefits seen with DBT imaging.

Data from reader studies comparing two-dimensional DM with combined DBT and DM show an improvement in sensitivity and specificity[5,13–17] coupled with excellent patient acceptance. Now that DBT has been approved by the FDA and has been implemented in many clinics across the world, prospective clinical data are beginning to emerge. Results from a few of these prospective and observational studies are reviewed here (**Tables 1** and **2**).

SUMMARY OF DBT DATA
DBT in Screening

The early data on the impact of DBT on screening outcomes, although mostly from enriched reader trials, showed up to a 40% reduction in false-positive callbacks[24] with a stable or slightly increased cancer detection rate. Because clinical implementation of DBT began only in the last 2 years, there is little published data from larger, prospective, population-based screening trials to further substantiate these performance outcomes. However, the recently published interval analysis from the prospective Oslo Tomosynthesis Screening Trial provides additional evidence that integration of the combo-mode DBT is associated with improvement in sensitivity and specificity.[6] In

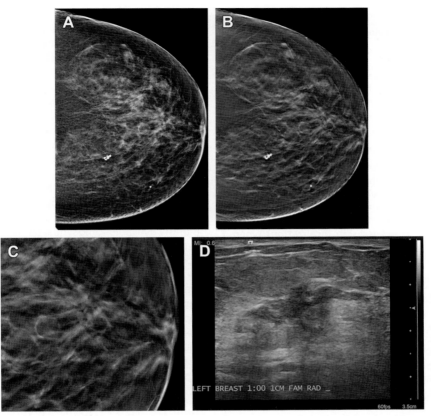

Fig. 2. Malignancy detected on DBT only. (*A*) This patient has scattered fibroglandular densities and no abnormality was detected on the DM imaging. (*B*) The CC DBT view shows an area of architectural distortion in the retroareolar plane. (*C*) An enlarged, cropped view of the DBT in-plane slice of the area of distortion demonstrates the greater conspicuity of the area on tomosynthesis imaging. (*D*) An ultrasound image clearly shows an irregular mass with ductal extension. On biopsy, this was an invasive ductal carcinoma.

this reader- and modality-balanced prospective trial, the participants undergo combined two-view DM plus two-view DBT (Dimensions, Hologic). Thus far, the results from an initial 12,631 women have shown a statistically significant, 27% decrease in false-positive callbacks and an approximately 30% increase in cancer detection. Most importantly, the improvement in the cancer detection rate is caused by a 40% increase in the detection of invasive breast cancer across all breast densities and there was no increase in the detection of ductal carcinoma in situ.[6] Early results from prospective trials in the United States have shown similar reductions in callbacks and improvements in cancer detection.[18–20]

The increase in the detection of invasive cancers and the improvements in specificity gained with the use of DBT begin to address the major concerns regarding screening mammography: the overdiagnosis of clinically insignificant cancers rather than significant, invasive carcinomas, and the high false-positive rates found with routine screening mammography. By shifting the detected cancers with DBT to otherwise occult invasive cancers, there is a greater likelihood that with DBT screening breast cancer mortality and morbidity rates will be improved. By decreasing false-positive callbacks, women are spared unnecessary anxiety, cost, and potentially unnecessary and traumatic biopsies.

Screening DBT: One View Versus Two Views

One might think that because there is three-dimensional information in the reconstructed image stack from a single tomosynthesis projection, a single tomosynthesis acquisition therefore might suffice for screening. However, just as an improvement in cancer detection was seen when the cranial caudal (CC) view was added to two-dimensional screening many years ago,[25] evidence is mounting that the best outcomes in terms of cancer detection and specificity are found when two-view DBT is combined with two-view DM

Box 1
Early evidence on clinical advantages of DBT

Lesion conspicuity

- With DBT, there is subjective improvement in lesion conspicuity for benign lesions (skin lesions, lymph nodes) and for malignant lesions, such as masses and distortion. This ability leads to improved accuracy with DBT.

Three-dimensional localization of lesions

- With the reconstructed slices in a DBT image set, an approximate three-dimensional localization of lesions within the breast is possible. This may allow a decrease in additional diagnostic imaging (ie, ML view for localization or tangential views for skin localization) when DBT is incorporated compared with DM alone.

Slice-by-slice evaluation of the breast

- Ability to work through areas of superimposition by scrolling through the DBT stack contributes to a decrease in false-positive callbacks (because of tissue superimposition) and a potential improvement in cancer detection (because of unmasking of obscured cancers), particularly invasive cancers.

Performance improvement with DBT for all breast densities

- Studies have shown that improvements in sensitivity and specificity are seen across all breast densities, not only in heterogeneous or extremely dense breasts.

(**Boxes 2** and **3**). Both Rafferty and coworkers[26] and Baker and Lo[8] found that approximately 8% to 9% of lesions were visible only on the DBT CC view (**Fig. 3**). Similarly, studies evaluating one-view, mediolateral (MLO) only DBT do not seem to have improved accuracy than standard two-view DM.[13,23,27]

Reader studies using only two-view DBT (without DM) have similar accuracy to standard two-view DM.[4,14,15] Gur and colleagues[14] compared two-view DM alone versus two-view DBT alone versus the combination of the two in an enriched population of 125 cases with 35 cancers. There was a nonsignificant improvement in sensitivity with two-view DBT alone compared with DM alone. As expected, the greatest improvement in specificity was seen with the combination of DM and DBT compared with either DBT alone or DM alone (0.72 vs 0.64 vs 0.60); there was a 30% reduction in false-positive callbacks with the combination DBT mode. However, in this study the combination mode was not associated with an

improvement in sensitivity as has been seen in other, larger, prospective studies. Hologic, in their FDA submission reader study, included an arm of adding one-view DBT (MLO) to two-dimensional DM to keep the dose down compared with the complete combination mode of DBT.[12] Although the modified combination mode had a better performance than two-dimensional alone, the sensitivity and specificity were less that that seen with the full combination set of two-view DBT with two-view DM.

There is definitely a trade-off between increased dose, image quality, and the resultant improvement in screening accuracy when DBT is combined with DM. However, it is important to realize that the available tomosynthesis platforms are still evolving. Just as early DM units used a higher dose than many analog systems and subsequent modifications in digital detectors allowed a substantial dose decrease while maintaining image quality, early DBT imaging is faced with demands for dose reductions if the technology is to become the standard of care for sequential, routine screening. There is extensive, on-going research to address the balance of dose and image quality in DBT (discussed later).

Tomosynthesis Performance Versus Breast Density

Combination DBT shows an improvement in performance over DM alone, irrespective of breast density. Although it is intuitive that the addition of DBT in the evaluation of a heterogeneously dense breast should improve the detection of cancers and the reduction of false-positives, it is not as obvious why DBT improves the screening performance in fatty breasts. However, just as malignant lesions may be obscured by normal, overlapping, tissue in a heterogeneously dense two-dimensional mammography, subtle areas of lower-contrast distortion may be overlooked in fatty or scattered density breast because of confounding areas of low-contrast glandular tissue and Cooper ligaments (**Fig. 4**).

Rafferty and colleagues[5] compared the performance of DM alone with DBT/DM across breast densities, grouped as fatty (BI-RADs density groups 1 and 2) and dense (BIRADs density groups 3 and 4), and found an improvement in the receiver operating characteristic curve for both groups; for fatty breasts the area under the curve (AUC) improved from 0.880 to 0.915; for dense breast, AUC improved from 0.786 to 0.877. An improvement in cancer detection and a significant reduction in false-positive callbacks were seen for both density groups. Although

Table 1
Summary of DBT Screening studies

Author	Study Format	Number of Patients	Callback Rate Reduction	Cancer Detection Rate	Comments
Skaane et al,[6] 2013	Interim analysis of prospective reader, modality balanced	12,631 (expect 18,000)	15% decrease ($P<.001$)	27% increase	40% increase in invasive cancer detection ($P<.001$)
Rose et al,[18] 2013	Prospective clinical practice comparing DBT with years prior of DM	9256 DBT screens compared with the prior 2 y of DM	DBT recall 5.3% compared with DM-only recall 8.7% (-39.5%; $P<.001$)	DBT cancer detection rate 5.83/1000 compared with DM rate of 3.6/1000 ($P = .003$)	Additional cancers mostly invasive
Haas et al,[19] 2013	Prospective clinical practice, indirect comparison of patient from one practice with DBT with another practice without DBT	Practice of 1602 DBT screens vs practice of 4178 DM	DBT recall 7% compared with DM-only recall 10.9% ($P<.01$)	DBT cancer detection rate 5.6/1000 vs DM rate of 3.4/1000 (-35.8%; $P = .24$)	Reduction in recall with DBT largest in patients younger than 50 and/or dense breasts
Conant et al,[20] 2013 RSNA	Clinical practice, prospective comparing DBT with prior year of DM, stable readers	15,633 DBT screens compared with prior year of 10,753 DM	24% reduction in recall ($P<.001$; odds ratio = .80)	Trend of increased cancer detection from 4.4 pre-DBT to 5.48 with DBT ($P = .26$)	There was a statistical significant increase in cancer detected with DBT in women <50 years

DBT showed the greatest performance improvement in the dense breast subset, the AUC was still highest for the fatty breast subset (0.915 for fatty vs 0.877 for dense).[5] This difference in performance is most likely because in extremely dense breasts, there may not be enough fat to create necessary fat-lesion interfaces so that nondistorting lesions may be detected on DBT reconstructed image slices, hence, some cancers are still not detectable. **Fig. 5** shows an example of a woman with extremely dense breast who presented with a palpable mass and neither the two-dimensional nor the in-plane DBT slice shows the lesion. Ultrasound of the area of palpable concern demonstrated an irregular mass that was later proved to be an invasive ductal carcinoma on core biopsy.

Tomosynthesis in Diagnostic Imaging

Incorporating DBT in the diagnostic, or problem-solving imaging of patients has the potential to limit, or possibly replace, much of the additional views performed decreasing the x-ray dose and time of imaging. A few early studies have shown a similar or improved performance for DBT in the analysis of lesion margins compared with conventional DM views, such as spot compression and/or magnification, and 90-degree, medial lateral (ML) views suggesting that tomosynthesis could replace these two-dimensional diagnostic views **(Fig. 6)**.[22,28–31]

Brandt and colleagues[29] compared DBT with conventional diagnostic imaging in the evaluation of 146 women with 158 abnormalities. The

Table 2
DBT Diagnostic studies

Author	Study Format	Patient Mix	Diagnostic Outcomes
Rafferty et al,[5] 2013	Two enriched reader studies.	312	Reduction in callback from 6% to 67% ($P<.03$).
Mitchell et al,[7] 2012	Prospective study, patients recalled from film-screen screening. DM and DBT and callback.	738 patients including 204 breast cancers	Improved accuracy (AUC) when DBT added to film or film with FFDM for masses (not calcifications). Improved cancer detection for fatty and dense breasts.
Skaane et al,[4] 2012	Reader study, mix of symptomatic and patients recalled from screening. Patients had two-view DBT.	129 patients with 27 breast cancer	DBT concordant with no statistical increase in callback; however, two additional cancers detected by DBT alone (8% increase in cancer detection).
Bernardi et al,[17] 2012	Prospective integrating DBT to assess recalled patient from DM screening (7 readers).	158 consecutive patients with 21 cancers	DBT recalled all cancer cases and DBT reduced FP callback by 74%. Similar cancer detection rates.
Nozroozian et al,[16] 2012	Enriched reader study (4 readers) comparing spot compression DM vs DBT in assessment of masses.	67 patients with breast masses (30 cancer, 37 benign)	No statistical difference in accuracy but mass visibility rating slightly better with DBT.
Svahn et al,[13] 2010	Reader study (5 readers) evaluating subtle screen detected or diagnostic lesions.	Comparing two-view DM vs one-view DM/DBT vs one-view DBT only	Highest accuracy with DM plus DBT ($P<.05$).
Poplack et al,[21] 2007	Prospective evaluation of the impact of DBT on consecutive recalls from screening.	98 recalls including 5 breast cancers	40% reduction in FP recall with DBT. No missed cancers. Subjective assessment of lesion conspicuity: DBT equivalent or superior in 89%. However, in calcification-only lesions, DBT inferior.
Tagliaficio et al,[22] 2012	Prospective study, patients recalled from screening (2 readers) compared spot compression vs DBT.	52 consecutive recalls with 9 cancers, accuracy and conspicuity assessed	No statistical difference in DM spot compression vs DBT; however, lesion conspicuity considered significantly better with DBT ($P<.001$).
Gennaro et al,[23] 2010	Reader study (6 readers) evaluating lesions seen on DM to evaluation with one-view, MLO DBT.	200 patients with 63 cancers	Overall performance of one-view DBT was similar to conventional DM.

Box 2
Early evidence: which combinations of DM and/or DBT should be used?

The "combo-mode" (DM plus DBT)

- Two-view DM combined with two-view DBT is associated with an improved accuracy in screening compared with DM alone mostly caused by improvements in specificity (reduction of false-positive callbacks) combined with an equal or slightly improved sensitivity (improved cancer detection rate). The cancers detected by DBT alone are mostly invasive cancers.

What about one-view DBT alone?

- Using only a single DBT projection (usually MLO) alone for screening does not seem to have any improvement in accuracy over conventional two-view DM.

What about two-view DBT alone?

- Using just two-view DBT without any two-dimensional DM has at least an equal accuracy to two-view DM, possibly slightly better.

Box 3
Early evidence: issues to consider with DBT

Dose considerations with combination DM/DBT

- The dose of the combination of two-view DM with two-view DBT is approximately twice that of conventional DM. Research is ongoing to create high-quality, clinically usable, reconstructed or synthetic two-dimensional images from the tomosynthesis acquisition. The FDA has just recently approved one industry's approach to provide reconstructed, "synthetic" 2-D images (see section of dose).

Reading time for DBT

- Reader training necessary and required
- Learning curve should be expected
- Need specific workstations for efficient DBT viewing
- Reading DBT image sets takes approximately twice as long as reading a conventional DM study

Storage of DBT images

- Large data files (up to 1 GB) for DBT images
- May use lossless compression to decrease storage size
- Which image sets should be kept? How long?

Reimbursement

- At present time, no approved CPT code for DBT
- Some sites add unlisted code 76,499 to normal DM codes
- Some sites charge patients out-of-pocket

agreement between the final DBT BI-RADS categories and the final DM BI-RADS categories from conventional imaging was good to excellent for all readers. In addition, for the conventional work-ups, there was an average of three additional diagnostic views per study compared with the DBT evaluation that was considered adequate in 93% to 99% of cases. Waldherr and colleagues[30] found improvement in sensitivity and the negative predictive value of single-view DBT compared with conventional diagnostic imaging in 144 consecutive women referred for diagnostic, problem-solving imaging supporting that DBT will improve the predictive value and diagnostic yield of cancer when incorporated in either screening or diagnostic imaging. Additional studies have shown that DBT is superior to two-dimensional imaging in estimating the extent of malignancies because the margins of the lesions are more conspicuous with tomosynthesis imaging (**Fig. 7**).[7,32,33]

The ability to obtain a three-dimensional location of a lesion in the breast from only one DBT projection is a significant improvement over conventional mammography. In our practice, we have had quite a few cancers that are seen either better or only on one of the two screening DBT projections and not at all on the two-dimensional image set (see **Fig. 3**). When the patient is called back for diagnostic imaging, the next step is then only ultrasound to confirm the location and ease of potential ultrasound-guided core biopsy; no additional mammographic projections are needed to triangulate or confirm the presence of the lesion.

It should also be noted that some of our DBT-only cancers effaced on conventional spot compression views and might have been disregarded if the DBT images were not as concerning. In evaluating these cases, we relied on the concerning appearance of the lesion on DBT and proceeded with an ultrasound irrespective of what spot compression imaging revealed (see **Figs. 3** and **4**). If DBT imaging had not been used, these cancers might have been overlooked.

As demonstrated by Brandt and colleagues,[29] it is conceivable that the total dose from the combo-mode DBT screening could be less than that when a patient who was only imaged with conventional DM is recalled. Because additional diagnostic imaging frequently includes ML, spot compression, and/or magnification views, and sometimes rolled or tangential views, the total dose could add up to

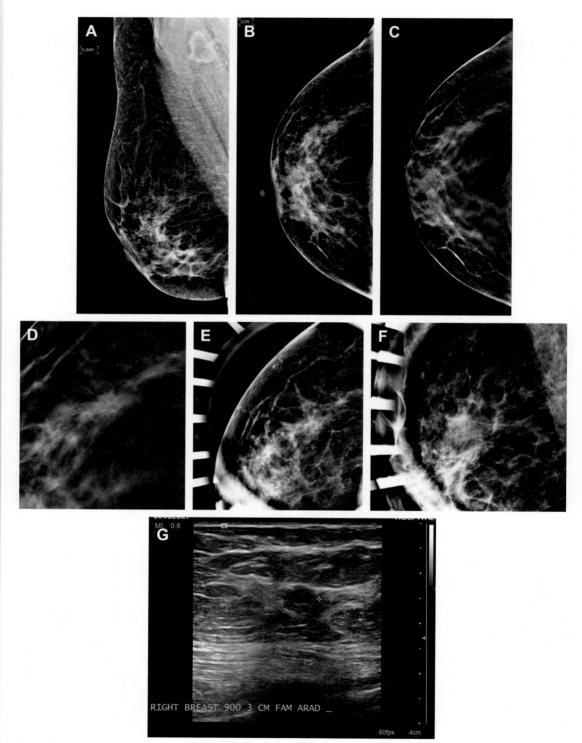

Fig. 3. Cancer seen on only one view of DBT. A 54-year-old woman with normal MLO (*A*) and CC (*B*) two-dimensional mammography has very subtle spiculated mass seen in the lateral breast on the DBT CC view only (*C*). An enlarged, cropped view of the in-plane DBT slice where the subtle speculated mass was detected is shown (*D*). The patient was brought back from screening and additional spot magnification views were performed in the CC (*E*) and MLO views (*F*). There was no definite mass or distortion seen on the diagnostic two-dimensional imaging but on ultrasound (*G*) an irregular mass was visible in the area detected on the CC DBT view. An invasive ductal carcinoma was found on biopsy.

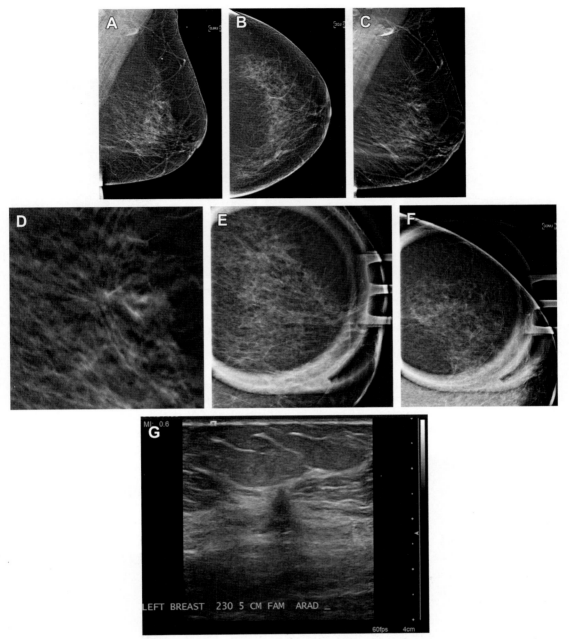

Fig. 4. Cancer seen on MLO DBT view only. A 66-year-old woman presented for screening and has normal two-dimensional DM MLO (*A*) and CC (*B*) views. Note that the breast has very little glandular tissue to obscure lesions. On the DBT MLO view (*C*) a subtle area of distortion is present in the superior breast. An enlarged, cropped view (*D*) of the MLO in-plane DBT slice clearly shows the distortion. Spot magnification two-dimensional views in the MLO (*E*) and CC (*F*) views fail to show a discrete mass or persistent area of distortion. Ultrasound (*G*) was performed based on the three-dimensional localization from the MLO and ML DBT image set. A small, 5-mm intermediate grade invasive ductal carcinoma was found on biopsy.

a similar or greater dose that a combo-DBT. In addition, the DBT imaging might provide more diagnostic information.

However, if tomosynthesis resources are limited and DBT is not performed on all patients at screening, how should one best use DBT in the diagnostic setting? Certainly, if triangulation is needed as part of a diagnostic evaluation of a lesion seen on only one view, a combo-DBT ML gives not only the location in the superior-inferior

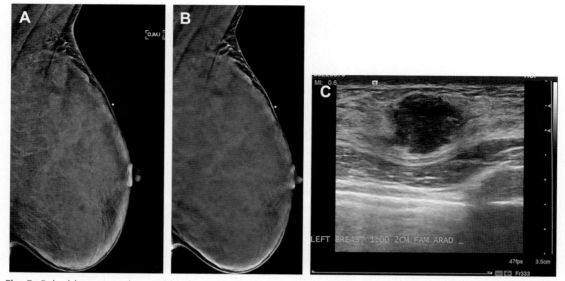

Fig. 5. Palpable cancer obscured by dense tissue even on DBT. A 36 year old presented with a palpable lump in the superior left breast. Before imaging, a metallic BB was placed over the area of palpable concern as seen on the MLO view (*A*). The in-plane slice of the MLO DBT series (*B*) fails to show a distinct mass, presumably because of the very dense breast tissue and lack of fat preventing any clear margin of a suspicious mass to be detected. Targeted left breast ultrasound (*C*) clearly shows a highly suspicious mass in the area of palpable concern. Biopsy revealed a high-grade invasive ductal carcinoma.

dimension but also a good estimate of the location in the medial to lateral dimension from the position of the lesion in the reconstructed DBT stack. In addition, if DBT resources are limited, one might consider performing DBT on all breast cancer survivors, especially those who had a two-dimensional DM occult cancer that presented as a palpable lump. However, it must be noted that

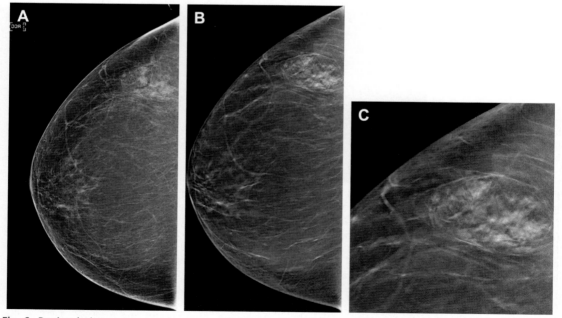

Fig. 6. Benign lesion more conspicuous on DBT. A 53-year-old woman presents for baseline screening and has almost entirely fatty breasts except for focal asymmetry in the lateral right breast on the DM CC view (*A*). On the CC DBT series (*B*) the lesion is clearly a hamartoma; therefore, no further imaging is needed. An enlarged, cropped view (*C*) from the CC DBT series clearly shows the mixed density lesion with a pseudocapsule, typical of a hamartoma. No further imaging was needed and the patient was returned to routine screening.

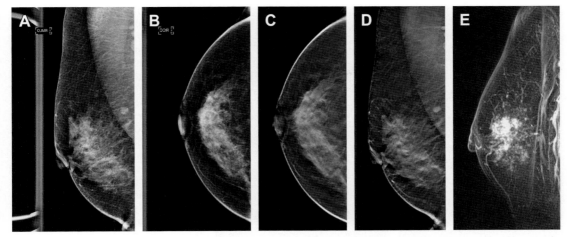

Fig. 7. DBT shows the extent of malignancy better than two-dimensional DM imaging. This patient presented for screening and on the DM MLO view (*A*) no abnormality was seen. On the DM CC view (*B*) there was a subtle approximately 1.5-cm area of distortion seen in the lateral breast. Both the DBT CC and MLO series (*C, D*) show extensive distortion caused by a large mass in the superior subareolar location, much more conspicuous than the subtle, small area seen on the DM CC view. A contrast-enhanced breast MR image (*E*) shows a similar extent of disease as that seen on the DBT study. The patient had a 5-cm invasive ductal carcinoma with an extensive in situ component.

not all cancers will be seen with DBT. Although there are no studies yet published comparing DBT with contrast-enhanced MR imaging in cancer detection, anecdotally we have seen a few cases where fairly large, invasive cancers were not detected on DBT but were seen on MR imaging, presumably because the lesions caused little to no distortion or distinct mass margins.

Calcifications with DBT

There is potentially no greater challenge in DBT imaging than the reconstruction of the tomosynthesis images for the optimal detection and characterization of calcification. If calcifications are small and dispersed, single reconstructed DBT slices may show only a few calcifications of a clinically significant cluster. If calcifications are large, they may cause significant artifacts, appearing on multiple slices as repeating ghost-like, out-of-focus white objects bordered by dark shadows, marching in the direction of the x-ray tube motion (**Fig. 8**).

A few studies have specifically reported on the visibility of calcifications in tomosynthesis imaging with differing results. Poplack and colleagues,[21] in a study comparing DM with DBT image quality in the diagnostic evaluation of lesion subtypes, found that when readers graded a DBT image quality as inferior, 72% of the lesion subtypes on those images were calcifications. However, the study was small and only 14 of 99 lesions evaluated were calcification-only lesions. In addition, the

tomosynthesis unit used in the study had a much longer average scan time (19 seconds vs 4 seconds) than the FDA-approved model now in clinical use. The longer scan times could have led to patient motion and subsequent unsharpness of the calcifications in the reconstructed images.

The characterizing of calcifications continues to be a challenge with DBT imaging and newer studies have found conflicting results regarding the visibility of calcification-only lesions.[34,35] Kopans and colleagues[34] evaluated 119 sequential cases of clinically relevant calcifications and found equal or superior performance of DBT versus DM in 92% of cases studied. However, in contrast to Kopan's results, Spangler and colleagues[35] performed a multireader study comparing DM only with DBT only in the detection and characterization of calcifications using a test set of 20 biopsy-proved malignancies, 40 biopsy-proved benign cases, and 40 negative screening cases. Overall, there was a statistically significant higher detection rate for calcifications on DM than DBT (84% vs 75%); the specificity in evaluating the calcifications was also higher for DM than DBT (71% vs 64%).

For the present time, because two-dimensional DM images are included in the tomosynthesis image set, readers of DBT have the option to scrutinize calcifications in either a two-dimensional format or in the DBT stack of reconstructed images (discussed later). At this point in time, it is very unlikely that DBT imaging can replace dedicated two-dimensional spot magnification views

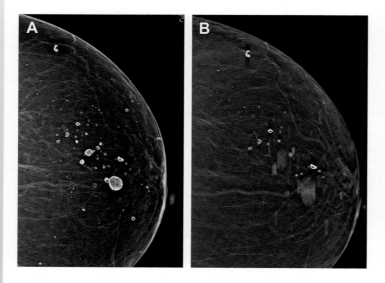

Fig. 8. Artifacts on DBT. The two-dimensional DM CC view (*A*) from a screening mammogram of a woman with an almost entirely fatty breast demonstrates "eggshell" calcifications caused by benign oil cysts. A single reconstructed slice from the CC DBT imaging (*B*) shows a few calcifications in focus but others are out of focus because of their out-of-plane position, above and below the reconstructed plane viewed. One can imagine that such artifacts created by the reconstruction of out-of-plane coarse calcifications or clips from biopsy could obscure the detection of clinically significant findings.

that are often needed for the characterization of calcifications.

BASICS OF DBT INTERPRETATION
What Is in a DBT Image Set?

The DBT/DM image set consists of three images series: (1) the conventional two-dimensional mammogram; (2) the source projection images; and (3) the multiple, reconstructed images presented as the "DBT stack" (see **Fig. 2**). The reconstructed DBT slices, which are typically 1 mm thick, may be displayed either in a cine mode or individually, to be scrolled through manually by the reader. The source, projection images are displayed at the workstation somewhat like a maximum intensity projection image and can be helpful when assessing for gross motion of the patient that might not be evident when viewing the reconstructed DBT stack. In just a click of a button or a toggle between screens, the reader is able to switch back and forth between each image set to compare the coregistered imaging findings quickly and easily.

The DBT slices are generally reconstructed at 1-mm intervals, and therefore the number of reconstructed slices is similar to the thickness of the breast in compression; thick breasts have many more reconstructed slices that thin breasts. At the top or bottom of the DBT stack, the dermis and the cutaneous caves of Kopans,[36] small vertically oriented fat-containing columns, are visible confirming the very superficial location of the first images in the stack. It is in these very early slices that skin lesions, such as moles, skin calcifications, or sebaceous cysts, are clearly visible (**Fig. 9**).

The DBT stack is presented to the reader usually starting with the first reconstructed slice obtained from either side of the breast, medial or lateral for the MLO stack and from the top or the bottom of the breast for the CC view. The choice of which of these starting locations for the first slice of a DBT image stack may be set in the reader preference field of the DBT hanging protocol on the workstation.

Tools for DBT Interpretation

Triangulation
One of the important advantages of tomosynthesis is the ability to localize a finding in the breast in a three-dimensional location. While the reader scrolls through the individual DBT reconstructed images, a numerical and a graphical representation of the slice location is visible (**Fig. 10**). These tools allow the reader to localize from where in the breast each reconstructed slice originates, thus allowing triangulation of breast structures or lesions with only one DBT view. This inference of three-dimensional location is important when a clinically significant lesion is visible in only one two-dimensional DM projection and/or seen only on the tomosynthesis images in one projection. In addition, this ability to localize lesions with DBT imaging may lead to a decrease in diagnostic imaging, such as the 90-degree ML view frequently obtained for diagnostic triangulation or tangential imaging used to localize skin lesions.

Slabbing
Another useful tool for interpreting tomosynthesis images is the ability to sum or "slab" multiple sequential reconstructed slices into one, thicker

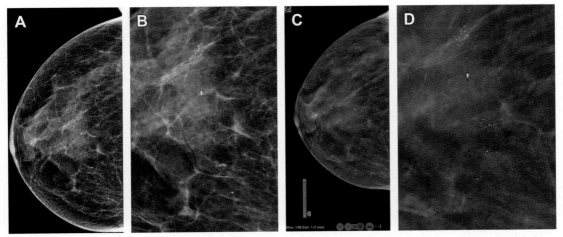

Fig. 9. Three-dimensional localization of skin calcifications with DBT. The two-dimensional DM CC view (*A*) shows multiple clusters of calcifications. An enlarged, cropped two-dimensional CC image (*B*) shows calcifications that are not clearly benign. The CC DBT image (*C*) from the last, inferior or caudal, reconstructed slice (*C*) shows that all the calcifications are localized within the skin. Note the location graphic in the left corner of the image that shows that the slice is the first slice in the series (Slice: 1/46), at the "F" foot or caudal portion of the stack of DBT reconstructed images. Also visible are small round areas of lucency at the edges of the image. These are the caves of Kopans, columns of fat that extend from the dermis to the subcutaneous tissue. These are also seen on the magnified CC DBT view (*D*) again confirming that the calcifications are clearly within the skin and are therefore benign. No additional imaging is needed.

slice. For example, if a small spiculated mass or a cluster of calcifications spans multiple of the 1-mm reconstructed DBT slices, the reader may manually expand the thickness of the reconstruction to include as many slices within the stack as he or she wishes. After a desired thickness is chosen, the slices are summed and can be scrolled through using larger-thickness increments (**Fig. 11**). Although the increased slice thickness increases the number of calcifications seen in the reconstructed slab and may increase the reader's three-dimensional perception of calcifications within a cluster, the spatial resolution of the individual calcifications is decreased with the increased reconstruction thickness. There is great potential for new computer-assisted detection (CAD) algorithms that could help optimize tasks, such as the flagging of concerning calcification clusters on multiple reconstructed slices and the automated volumetric slabbing of zones of calcifications across multiple slices.

How to Incorporate the DBT Images into Hanging Protocols

In our screening practice, the combo-mode hanging protocol is almost identical to the two-dimensional digital screening hanging protocol except that after the two-dimensional mammogram presentation with comparison with prior studies, the CC and MLO DBT views are displayed in full resolution, prompting the reader to scroll through the DBT stack to check for any lesions that might not have been seen on the routine two-dimensional views. These full-screen DBT images are placed in the hanging protocol before the final four-view two-dimensional image set is displayed with any CAD marks. Of course, at any time while the reader is viewing the routine, two-dimensional screening views, he or she may toggle back and forth between the DBT and two-dimensional images of the same projection to problem-solve areas of concern. This ability to rapidly change between the image sets is extremely valuable in assessing areas of calcifications, possible distortions, masses, or focal asymmetries. It is humbling to have reviewed an entire set of two-dimensional screening images that look very normal only to review the DBT image set, which reveals an otherwise occult, spiculated mass.

CONSIDERATIONS IN DBT IMPLEMENTATION
Dose Concerns

Because the only approved use of DBT is in the combo-mode, which in many ways is a double mammogram, one would expect the total dose per breast to be approximately twice that of a conventional DM mammogram. Indeed, Feng and Sechopoulos[37] in a phantom study found that the average dose for a combination DBT/DM study

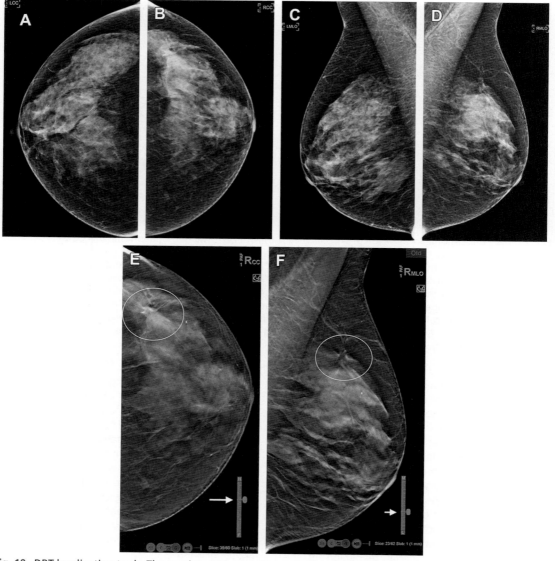

Fig. 10. DBT localization tools. The routine, DM screening mammogram (*A–D*) shows no definite abnormality. On the DBT CC view (*E*) there is an area of architectural distortion in the lateral breast that is localized in the superior portion of the reconstructed stack of slices (Slice: 39/60 and close to the "H" or head, cranial aspect of breast as shown on vertical localizer marker, *arrow*). Now knowing were to search in the MLO DBT reconstructed slices (*F*), a very subtle area of distortion is seen in the superior and lateral aspect of the MLO stack (Slice: 23/62; closer to "L" or lateral side of breast on vertical localizer marker, *arrow*).

of a 5-cm thick breast phantom with 50% glandularity was 2.50 mGy per DBT view, below the 3 mGy per view limit set by the Mammography Quality Standard Act (MQSA). Of course, one must note that the range of dose varies significantly depending on breast size and composition and in the Oslo Screening Trial, using measurements from actual screening patients, the mean glandular dose for the DM and the DBT studies were 1.58 ± 0.61 mGy and 1.95 ± 0.58 mGy, respectively.[6] Therefore, combined together, the average dose for the DM/DBT image set was 3.53 mGy per image set, higher than that calculated by Feng and Sechopoulos[37] and also higher than the MQSA limit.

Much of the desire for the two-dimensional DM when implementing DBT is driven by the need to accurately detect and characterize calcifications but the two-dimensional imaging is also extremely helpful in the transition of implementing DBT clinically when comparing with older DM studies. However, with the combination mode of

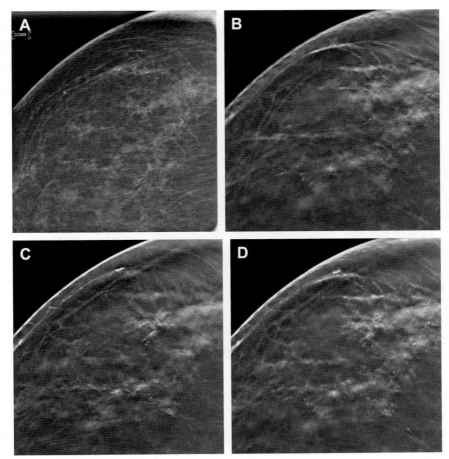

Fig. 11. Slabbing to aid in the analysis of calcifications. A two-dimensional CC DM spot magnification view (*A*) shows suspicious calcifications in the lateral breast. A 1-mm reconstructed DBT slice in the CC projection (*B*) shows some of the lateral, linear calcifications but unsharpness of other calcifications. A different, 1-mm reconstructed DBT slice in the CC projection (*C*) shows additional calcifications that are now in-plane and in focus in an area of subtle architectural distortion. The calcifications seen on the previous slice are not as clearly visible on this 1-mm reconstructed slice. A 10-mm reconstructed "slab" (*D*) better demonstrates the extent of the suspicious calcifications and associated subtle distortion. The slabbing technique may help improve the conspicuity of a larger area of calcifications but also introduces a degree of unsharpness as the reconstruction thickness is increased. On biopsy, this was high-grade ductal carcinoma in situ without invasion.

two-dimensional and DBT, the dose penalty is high and possibly not sustainable for all patients over many years of screening.

To decrease the dose of DBT while still including a two-dimensional formatted image, there is active research in creating synthesized two-dimensional images from the DBT acquisition. Gur and colleagues,[38] in a study of 114 cases with 10 readers, found that there was a loss of sensitivity but an equivalent specificity when synthetic images plus DBT were compared with the full mode of imaging with two-dimensional DM and DBT. It is important to understand that the algorithm used was an early prototype and newer algorithms are under development. Synthesized two-dimensional images are also being evaluated in one arm of the Oslo Tomosynthesis Screening Trial.[39] In mid 2013, the FDA approved the first clinical application of synthetic imaging, or "C-view," for the Hologic tomosynthesis unit (**Fig. 12**).[40] Thus far, full FDA approval has not been granted.

CAD in DBT

Currently, CAD is available for clinical applications only for two-dimensional imaging. Therefore, when DBT is used in the FDA-approved combo-mode, CAD algorithms run on the two-dimensional DM data and CAD marks are displayed at the workstation on the two-dimensional images only.

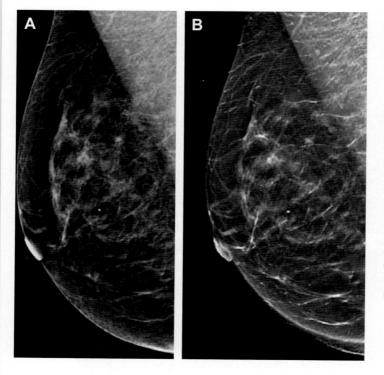

Fig. 12. Synthetic two-dimensional images reconstructed from DBT acquisition. The two-dimensional DM MLO view is shown on the left (A) with the reconstructed synthetic MLO view (B) shown on the right (B). The synthetic image (B) is reconstructed by summing the data obtained from the individual slices that make up the DBT image set. Research and development is ongoing to reconstruct two-dimensional images that provide the necessary two-dimensional information, such as the morphology and distribution of clinically significant calcifications, so that two-dimensional DM imaging and the associated dose could be eliminated in many cases. The synthetic two-dimensional image would be viewed with the DBT image set. (*Courtesy of* Hologic, Inc, Bedford, MA; with permission.)

Although current CAD algorithms for conventional mammography cannot be directly applied to DBT image data, there is active research in this field and data suggest an improvement in three-dimensional CAD performance compared with DM CAD.[11,41–45] This is understandable because on individual DBT slices, the margins of masses and subtle areas of distortion are better depicted, which could lead to more true-positive CAD marks. Additionally, because there are presumably less false-positive focal asymmetries with DBT individual slice data, there may also be less false-positive CAD marks per case. Studies using enriched case sets have reported sensitivities of 85% to 90% for masses with DBT CAD with less than 2.5 false-positive marks per case, per breast volume.[41–44] Reiser and colleagues[45] tested a DBT calcification detection program and found an 86% sensitivity with 1.3 false-positives per breast volume, which was better than DM alone CAD systems.

Because combination DBT/DM image sets do take longer to interpret, DBT CAD could play a significant role in improving workflow efficiency. There is research developing CAD to flag sequential slices of the DBT reconstructed stack containing CAD-detected calcifications so that the reader can quickly target those areas and quickly slab the demarcated thickness to in effect create a volume of slices containing CAD-marked calcifications. This bookmarking of slices containing calcifications detected by the CAD system could help in the efficiency of DBT image interpretation.[11]

Interpretation Time

There is no doubt that the reading time for interpreting a mammogram that includes DBT images is longer than that for a conventional mammogram. The simple math totaling the four images of a routine mammogram plus the approximately 50, 1-mm reconstructed images per stack from each of four DBT projections (two MLO and two CC) of a 5-cm breast, quickly exceeds 200 images for a single case. Several studies have attempted to calculate just how much additional time it will take to interpret combo-mode DBT studies but at the time of writing this review there are very few measures taken from actual clinical experience where readers have fully implemented DBT in their clinical practice. The early published studies have showed a wide range of additional time for the interpretation of DBT studies, which probably reflected the learning curve of the readers and the use of the early, prototype workstations with less than ideal DBT navigational tools.[46] In addition, most of these studies were using test sets that included complicated cancer cases, thus increasing the mean times for interpretation.

Gur and colleagues[38] evaluated DBT reading times in such an enriched test set and found reading times increased from a mean of 1.22 to 2.39 minutes when DBT images were included. More recently Bernardi and coworkers[47] reported that when DBT was incorporated in an enriched screening study, the average reading time increased from 33 seconds to 77 seconds. Early results from the Oslo Tomosynthesis Screening Trial have found similar increases in reading time, with an increase from 45 seconds for DM alone to 91 seconds for the DBT/DM studies.[6]

Assuming that DBT will routinely be incorporated in breast imaging, there is a great need for processing algorithms, robust image display systems, and navigational tools to help optimize image quality and efficiency of display and reading. Similarly, CAD applications that bookmark individual slices and series slices of potential interest in the DBT stack could help with lesion detection and reading efficiency.

Image Storage Issues

The picture archiving system (PACS) storage requirements for DBT studies are significant and before any site begins clinical implementation, preparations must be made to accommodate the large file sizes and the industry-specific file formats. For each DBT examination, the regular DM images and the reconstructed DBT slices must be stored. The number of slices for each DBT view depends on the thickness of breast but an average combination DBT/DM study produces approximately 1 GB of data. If the DBT images are stored with a 4:1 reversible (lossless) compression, the total size of the dataset decreases to approximately 250 MB,[8] which is still substantial compared with a routine DM study and larger than a typical chest-abdomen-pelvis study.[48]

To keep the storage requirements to the minimum, we do not save the raw data or the projection images in our clinical PACS. A valid question that we have not yet addressed is: How long do we save the reconstructed slices for future clinical comparison? Two years? Three years? Certainly, the reconstructed slices need not be saved for eternity if there is a two-dimensional DM study saved.

Learning Curve and DBT Training

As with implementing any new imaging technology, there is a substantial learning curve in interpreting DBT studies. Currently, radiologists, physicists, and technologists are required by MQSA to complete 8 hours of dedicated tomosynthesis training before clinical implementation.[49] Despite this training, our practice had an initial increase in the group's average screening callback rate during the first few months after implementing DBT probably because we began to detect some very subtle, "tomo-only" cancers and began shifting our operating point, calling back screening findings we perceived to be subtle distortion on DBT in hopes of finding additional, "tomo-only" cancers. It is obvious that readers will also need to reset their threshold for passing or calling back what looks extremely benign but seen only on DBT imaging, such as small well-circumscribed masses that are probably cysts or newly unmasked intramammary lymph nodes. We have found that areas of distortion from prior benign biopsies are much more conspicuous with DBT and close correlation with the history of prior procedures and skin scar sites is needed to prevent unnecessary, false-positive callbacks. In addition, we have been surprised with the number of radial scars detected on DBT, high-risk lesions that prompt false-positive biopsies, frequent excision, and occasionally MR imaging.

In our practice, we chose to begin our DBT implementation with large-volume screening so that each reader would develop a template for normal before starting diagnostic imaging. We estimate that it took approximately 1000 DBT screening cases per reader before we had reset our threshold for interpreting DBT at a stable operating point. We have now expanded our DBT practice to include all breast conservation patients and the imaging of the remaining breast in unilateral mastectomy patients.

Reimbursement

DBT is still considered to be investigational and therefore there is no approved CPT code and no standard reimbursement. To receive a level of reimbursement, some centers add the unlisted diagnostic procedure code 76,499 to the appropriate HCPCS Level II "G" codes (G0202, G0204, or G0206) that describes the screening or diagnostic full-field digital mammography performed.[50] The success of obtaining reimbursement with this strategy is unknown. Other sites market the fact that they offer DBT imaging and charge patients up to $50 out of pocket for the addition of DBT to their conventional study.[51,52] Standard reimbursement, at a yet to be determined level, should follow if the results from large, prospective, clinical trials continue to show significant benefits in specificity and improved cancer detection rates.

SUMMARY

Early data, based mostly on small reader studies, suggest that DBT is likely to have a significant impact on breast imaging. The ability to scroll through the tomosynthesis stack to work through areas of tissue superimposition that on two-dimensional imaging appear concerning has led to a decrease in false-positive callbacks. An improvement in lesion conspicuity and the quasi three-dimensional information gained with the tomosynthesis acquisition may also allow more expeditious evaluations of suspicious areas and an increase in cancer detection.

Results emerging from larger, prospective DBT screening trials have supported the findings from the earlier, smaller reader studies by demonstrating significant improvements in specificity and sensitivity. Most significant is the early prospective data that has shown that the increased cancer detection is caused by the increase in detection of invasive cancers, which are more likely clinically significant, rather than an increase in the detection of in situ lesions, which some consider to be adding to overdiagnosis.

There are, however, issues that must be considered when implementing this new technology into daily clinical practice. With the current technology, there are extremely large data files that require PACS storage, there is an approximately double x-ray dose for the combo-mode of DBT/DM, there is an estimated double in the interpretation time needed, and there is no approved reimbursement to cover the additional overhead needed to support this new digital mammography platform.

Despite these issues, it is important to realize that this new technology is only in its clinical infancy and multiple researchers and industries are working to address these issues. There is no doubt that DBT imaging is here to stay and that it will address many of the limitations of conventional 2D mammography. However, additional data from large, multi-site prospective trials is needed so that the true impact of DBT imaging on breast cancer screening outcomes may be realized.

REFERENCES

1. US Preventive Services Task Force. Screening for breast cancer: US Preventive Services Task Force recommendation statement. Ann Intern Med 2009;151(10):716–26.
2. Pisano ED, Gatsonis C, Hendrick E, et al. Diagnostic performance of digital versus film mammography for breast cancer screening. N Engl J Med 2005;353:1773–83.
3. Tabar L, Vitak B, Chen TH, et al. Swedish two-county trial: impact of mammographic screening on breast cancer mortality during 3 decades. Radiology 2011; 260(3):658–63.
4. Skaane P, Gullien R, Bjorndal H, et al. Digital breast tomosynthesis (DBT): initial experience in a clinical setting. Acta Radiol 2012;53:524–9.
5. Rafferty EA, Park JM, Philpotts LE, et al. Assessing radiologist performance using combined digital mammography and breast tomosynthesis compared with digital mammography alone: results of a multicenter, multireader trial. Radiology 2013; 266(1):104–13.
6. Skaane P, Bandos AI, Gullien R, et al. Comparison of digital mammography alone and digital mammography plus tomosynthesis in a population-based screening program. Radiology 2013;267: 47–56.
7. Michell MJ, Iqbal A, Wasan RK, et al. A comparison of the accuracy of film-screen mammography, full-field digital mammography, and digital breast tomosynthesis. Clin Radiol 2012;67:976–81.
8. Baker JA, Lo JY. Breast tomosynthesis: state-of-the-art and review of the literature. Acad Radiol 2011;18(10):1298–310.
9. Helvie MA. Digital mammography imaging: breast tomosynthesis and advanced applications. Radiol Clin North Am 2010;48:917–29.
10. Baldwin P. Digital breast tomosynthesis. Radiol Technol 2009;81:57–74.
11. Available at: http://breasttomo.com/sites/default/files/010-WP-00060-Rev2_June2012-TomoWhite Paper.pdf. Accessed March 30, 2013.
12. Available at: http://www.accessdata.fda.gov/cdrh_docs/pdf8/P080003b.pdf. Accessed March 30, 2013.
13. Svahn T, Anderson I, Chakraborty D, et al. The diagnostic accuracy of dual-view digital mammography, single view breast tomosynthesis and dual-view combination of breast tomosynthesis and digital mammography in a free-response observer performance study. Radiat Prot Dosimetry 2010;139:113–7.
14. Gur D, Adams GS, Chough DM, et al. Localized detection and classification of abnormalities on FFDM and tomosynthesis examinations rated under an FROC paradigm. AJR Am J Roentgenol 2011;196:737–41.
15. Wallis MG, Moa E, Zanca F, et al. Two-view and single-view tomosynthesis versus full-field digital mammography: high resolution X-ray imaging observer study. Radiology 2012;262:788–96.
16. Noroozian M, Hadjiiski L, Rahnama-Moghadam S, et al. Digital breast tomosynthesis is comparable to mammographic spot views for mass characterization. Radiology 2012;262:61–8.
17. Bernardi D, Ciatto S, Pellegrini M, et al. Prospective study of breast tomosynthesis as a triage to assessment in screening. Breast Cancer Res Treat 2012;133:267–71.
18. Rose SL, Tidwell AL, Bujnoch LJ, et al. Implementation of breast tomosynthesis in a routine

screening practice: an observational study. American journal of roentgenology 2013;200(6):1401–8.

19. Haas BM, Kalra V, Geisel J, et al. Comparison of tomosynthesis plus digital mammography and digital mammography alone for breast cancer screening. Radiology 2013;269(3):694–700.

20. Conant EF, McCarthy AM, Kontos D, et al. Digital Breast Tomosynthesis in Combination with Digital Mammography Compared to Digital Mammography Alone: A "Natural Experiment" in General-Population Screening Outcomes in preparation (personal communications) 2014.

21. Poplack SP, Tosteson TD, Kogel CA, et al. Digital breast tomosynthesis: initial experience in 98 women with abnormal digital screening mammography. American Journal of Roentgenology 2007; 189(3):616–23.

22. Tagliafico A, Astengo D, Cavagnetto F, et al. One-to-one comparison between digital spot compression view and digital breast tomosynthesis. Eur Radiol 2012;22:539–44.

23. Gennaro G, Toledano A, di Maggio C, et al. Digital breast tomosynthesis versus digital mammography: a clinical performance study. Eur Radiol 2010;20:1545–53.

24. Rafferty E, Niklason L, Halpern E, et al. Assessing radiologist performance using combined full-field digital mammography and breast tomosynthesis versus full-field digital mammography alone: results of a multi-center multi-reader trial. Presented at the Radiological Society of North America annual meeting. Chicago (IL), 2007.

25. Wald NJ, Murphy P, Major P, et al. UKCCCR multi-centre randomized controlled trial of one and two view mammography in breast cancer screening. BMJ 1995;311:1189–93.

26. Rafferty E, Niklason L, Jameson-Meehan L. Breast tomosynthesis: one view or two? Presented at the Radiological Society of North America annual meeting. Chicago (IL), 2006.

27. Gur D, Abrams GS, Chough DM, et al. Digital breast tomosynthesis: observer performance study. AJR Am J Roentgenol 2009;193:586–91.

28. Zuley ML, Bandoss AI, Ganott MA, et al. Digital breast tomosynthesis versus supplemental diagnostic mammographic views for evaluation of noncalcified breast lesions. Radiology 2013;266: 89–95.

29. Brandt KR, Craig DA, Hoskins TL, et al. Can digital breast tomosynthesis replace conventional diagnostic mammography views for screening recalls without calcifications? A comparison study in a simulated clinical setting. AJR Am J Roentgenol 2013;200(2):291–8.

30. Waldherr C, Cerny P, Altermatt HJ, et al. Value of one-view breast tomosynthesis versus two-view mammography in diagnostic workup of women with clinical signs and symptoms and in women recalled from screening. AJR Am J Roentgenol 2013;200(1): 226–31.

31. Hakim CM, Chough DM, Ganott MA, et al. Digital breast tomosynthesis in the diagnostic environment: a subjective side-by-side review. AJR Am J Roentgenol 2010;195(2):172–6.

32. Fornvik D, Zackrisson S, Ljungberg O, et al. Breast tomosynthesis: accuracy of tumor measurement compared with digital mammography and ultrasonography. Acta Radiol 2010;3:240–7.

33. Meacock LM, Mombelloni S, Iqbal A, et al. The accuracy of breast cancer size measurement: digital breast tomosynthesis (DBT0 vs. 2D digital mammography (DM)). Presented at the European College of Radiology annual meeting. Vienna (Austria), 2010.

34. Kopans D, Gavenonis S, Halpern E, et al. Calcifications in the breast and digital breast tomosynthesis. Breast J 2011;17(6):638–44.

35. Spangler ML, Zuley M, Sumkin J. Detection and classification of calcifications on digital breast tomosynthesis and 2D digital mammography: a comparison. AJR Am J Roentgenol 2011;196:320–4.

36. Kopans DB, Rusby JE. Cutaneous caves and subcutaneous adipose columns in the breast: radiologic-pathologic correlation. Radiology 2008; 249(3):779–84.

37. Feng SS, Sechopoulos I. Clinical digital breast tomosynthesis system: dosimetric characterization. Radiology 2012;263:35–42.

38. Gur D, Zuley ML, Anello MI, et al. Dose reduction in digital breast tomosynthesis (DBT) screening using synthetically reconstructed projection images: an observer performance study. Acad Radiol 2012; 19:166–71.

39. Houssami N, Skaane P. Overview of the evidence on digital breast tomosynthesis in breast cancer detection. Breast 2013;22(2):101–8. http://dx.doi.org/10.1016/j.breast.2013.01.017.

40. Available at: http://www.fda.gov/downloads/AdvisoryCommittees/CommitteesMeetingMaterials/MedicalDevices/MedicalDevicesAdvisoryCommittee/RadiologicalDevicesPanel/UCM328613.pdf. Accessed March 21, 2013.

41. Chan HP, Wei J, Zhang Y, et al. Computer-aided detection of masses in digital tomosynthesis mammography: comparison of three approaches. Med Phys 2008;35:4087–95.

42. Chan HP, Wei J, Sahiner B, et al. Computer-aided detection system for breast masses on digital tomosynthesis mammograms: preliminary experience. Radiology 2005;237:1075–80.

43. Singh S, Tourassi GD, Baker JA, et al. Automated breast mass detection in 3D reconstructed tomosynthesis volumes: a featureless approach. Med Phys 2008;35:3626–36.

44. Reiser I, Nishikawa RM, Giger ML, et al. Computerized mass detection for digital breast tomosynthesis directly from the projection images. Med Phys 2006;33:482–91.

45. Reiser I, Nishikawa RM, Edwards AV, et al. Automated detection of microcalcification clusters for digital breast tomosynthesis using projection data only: a preliminary study. Med Phys 2008;35:1486–93.

46. Good WF, Abrams GS, Catullo VJ, et al. Digital breast tomosynthesis: a pilot observer study. AJR Am J Roentgenol 2008;190:865–9.

47. Bernardi D, Ciatto S, Pellegrini M, et al. Application of breast tomosynthesis in screening: incremental effect on mammography acquisition and reading time. Br J Radiol 2012;85:1174–8.

48. Available at: http://www.auntminnie.com/index.aspx?sec=sup&sub=wom&pag=dis&ItemID=102872&wf=5368. Accessed March 21, 2013.

49. Mammography Quality Standard Act requirements. Available at: http://www.fda.gov/radiation-emittingproducts/mammographyqualitystandardsactandprogram/facilitycertificationandinspection/ucm243765.htm. Accessed March 21, 2013.

50. Available at: http://gm.acr.org/Hidden/Economics/FeaturedCategories/Pubs/coding_source/archives/MayJun2011/QA.aspx. Accessed March 21, 2013.

51. Available at: http://www.okbreastcare.com/tomo.html. Accessed March 21, 2013.

52. Available at: http://www.breastimaginghouston.com/news.html. Accessed March 21, 2013.

High-quality Breast Ultrasonography

Janice S. Sung, MD

KEYWORDS

• Breast • Ultrasonography • Imaging • Image quality

KEY POINTS

- Ultrasonography is an important modality that is frequently used in all aspects of breast imaging, including breast cancer screening, the evaluation of palpable abnormalities, further characterization of lesions seen mammographically, and for determining the method of percutaneous biopsy.
- Understanding the basic technical aspects of ultrasonography equipment is critical to ensure high breast ultrasonography image quality.

INTRODUCTION

Ultrasonography is an important imaging modality for the detection and characterization of lesions in the breast. Appropriate indications for breast ultrasonography as recommended by the American College of Radiology Practice Guidelines include the following:

- Evaluation and characterization of palpable masses and other breast-related signs and/or symptoms
- Evaluation of abnormalities detected on mammography or breast magnetic resonance (MR) imaging
- Determining the method of guidance for percutaneous biopsy
- Supplemental screening to mammography in certain populations

Advantages of breast ultrasonography include that it is a rapid, widely available, and inexpensive modality that does not involve breast compression or ionizing radiation. As with all imaging modalities, ultrasonography's value in the detection and characterization of breast lesions largely depends on the quality of the images. Ultrasonography is highly operator dependent, and erroneous conclusions may be caused by technique or the application or misapplication of image processing algorithms. Although there have been advances in ultrasonography, including the development of three-dimensional transducers and automated whole-breast systems, breast ultrasonography still requires real-time imaging in many situations for accurate interpretation.

In recent years, multiple states have passed legislation mandating that women with dense breasts be notified of their breast density and that they may benefit from supplemental screening. This development has led to the proliferation of whole-breast screening ultrasonography as a supplemental screening modality to mammography in women with dense breasts. Particularly when ultrasonography is used in the screening setting, it is imperative to understand the various technical factors affecting image optimization in order to maximize sensitivity while reducing the number of unnecessary biopsies and recommendations for short term follow-up studies. This article reviews the technical factors that should be considered in order to perform high-quality breast ultrasonography.

PATIENT POSITIONING

The optimal position of the patient should minimize the thickness of the portion of the breast being imaged. During breast ultrasonography, the patient should be positioned with the ipsilateral arm over the head. In general, medial lesions should

Department of Radiology, Memorial Sloan-Kettering Cancer Center, New York, NY 10065, USA
E-mail address: sungj@mskcc.org

Radiol Clin N Am 52 (2014) 519–526
http://dx.doi.org/10.1016/j.rcl.2014.02.012
0033-8389/14/$ – see front matter © 2014 Elsevier Inc. All rights reserved.

be scanned with the patient in the supine position, whereas lateral lesions should be scanned with the patient in a supine oblique position in order to reduce the thickness of the breast.

TRANSDUCER SELECTION

High-quality breast ultrasonography begins with selection of an appropriate transducer. The transducers used in breast imaging must have a high frequency (between 10 and 15 MHz) because of the superficial nature of the breast and the need to resolve small structures (**Fig. 1**). However, higher frequency sound waves are more strongly attenuated by tissue than lower frequency waves. Therefore there is a trade-off between higher resolution and reduced penetration. With proper positioning and the patient in the supine or supine oblique position, most breasts are only a few centimeters thick and high-frequency transducers provide optimum image quality for all of the breast tissue. When evaluating deep tissue in patients with particularly large breasts, it may be helpful to have lower frequency transducers available to be used only in this specific situation.

Bandwidth is another consideration in transducer selection. The bandwidth is the spread of frequency around the central frequency of the transducer, and transducers with a broader bandwidth have improved resolution. Transducers used in breast imaging may either be linear or matrix array, which affects image resolution.

IMAGE RESOLUTION

The goal of equipment selection is to maximize image resolution, which is the ability to distinguish structures that are close together as separate lesions. Image resolution is composed of contrast and spatial resolution (**Fig. 2**). Optimal contrast resolution is necessary to differentiate subtle lesions from the surrounding breast tissue, and these lesions may have subtle variations of gray

scale. Transducers with higher frequencies have improved contrast resolution.

Spatial resolution is composed of both axial and lateral resolution. Axial resolution is the ability to resolve structures along the axis of the ultrasound beam or the Z plane (the depth). Axial resolution depends on pulse length, which is determined by the frequency and the bandwidth of the transducer. A transducer with a higher frequency and a broader bandwidth has a shorter wavelength and pulse length relative to a lower frequency transducer, which improves axial resolution.

Lateral resolution is the ability to resolve structures in the X and Y planes that are at the same depth. Lateral resolution is related to the transducer beam width, and lateral resolution is not adequate when lesions positioned side by side are within the same beam width. Because a higher frequency transducer has a narrower beam width relative to a lower frequency transducer, lateral resolution is improved.

FOCAL ZONE

As discussed earlier, lateral resolution is related to the beam width. In addition to selecting a high-frequency transducer to maintain a narrow beam width, the beam width can be further reduced by adjusting the focal zone.

Linear array transducers have multiple piezoelectric crystals or elements arranged side by side. If a single element is used to both transmit and receive the signal, the beam diverges quickly after traveling a few millimeters, resulting in poor lateral resolution because of beam divergence. Linear array transducers pulse adjacent elements simultaneously as a single element group to overcome beam divergence and then in succession to form the image. Delaying the timing of firing of elements within a single element group adjusts the focal zone so that the beam is narrowed along the long-axis plane. The specific time delay

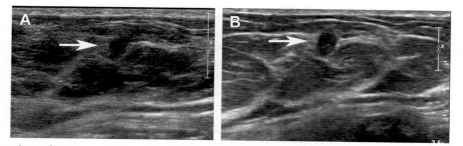

Fig. 1. Transducer frequency. High-quality breast ultrasonography requires the use of high-frequency transducers. The same mass (*arrows*) is imaged using 9-MHz (*A*) and 12-MHz (*B*) transducers. The higher frequency (12 MHz) transducer results in better detail of the mass and the surrounding breast parenchyma.

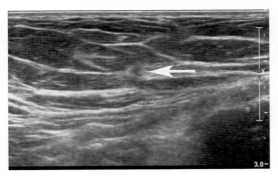

Fig. 2. Image resolution. Static ultrasonography image shows a subtle 2-mm invasive cancer (*arrow*) that would easily have been missed if image quality was not optimized.

determines the depth of focus for the transmitted beam. Matrix array transducers, which have multiple rows of elements, allow focusing in both the short and long axes. The focal zone represents the narrowest part of the beam and is the area where lateral resolution is optimized. Therefore the focal zone should be placed at or slightly below the area of interest (**Fig. 3**). Because of transducer limitations, even the shallowest focal zone setting may not achieve the narrowest beam width possible for lesions near the skin. Therefore a standoff pad may be required to improve resolution (**Fig. 4**).

DEPTH

During an initial survey, the depth on the ultrasonography image should be set so that the breast parenchyma is imaged to the pectoralis muscle, which should be along the far field of view (**Fig. 5**). Once a finding is identified, the depth may be adjusted.

GAIN AND TIME GAIN COMPENSATION

The overall gain control provides uniform amplification of all echo signals returning to the transducer, compensating for increased attenuation of the ultrasound beam as it penetrates deeper into the tissues. Increasing the gain amplifies the intensity of all signals returning to the transducer so that the image is brighter and more visible on the display screen.

The initial gain setting should be adjusted so that the subcutaneous fat is a medium level of gray. Lesions may be mischaracterized if the gain is inappropriately set. For example, a subcentimeter hypoechoic solid mass or a complicated cyst can mimic a simple anechoic cyst if the gain is set too low (**Fig. 6**). In contrast, by inappropriately setting the gain too high, a simple or complicated cyst may appear solid.

Unlike the gain, which adjusts all signals returning to the transducer, the time gain compensation (TGC) function allows selective amplification of weaker signals from areas deeper in the breast. The TGC should be set so that all echoes from similar structures are displayed with the same brightness from the near to far field. For example, the subcutaneous fat should be the same shade of medium gray as the retromammary fat.

SPATIAL COMPOUND IMAGING

With standard imaging, the ultrasound pulses are propagated perpendicular to the long axis of the transducer. Spatial compounding uses electronic beam steering to obtain multiple images at different angles, which are then combined to form a single image in real time.[1] Spatial compounding enhances returning echoes from real structures, thereby improving image resolution, so that image features such as lesion margins may be better characterized. Artifacts, such as posterior acoustic enhancement characteristic of simple cysts and posterior shadowing seen with some solid masses, tend to be averaged out and reduced. However, some small cancers are detected primarily because of their posterior acoustic shadowing. When scanning for a subtle

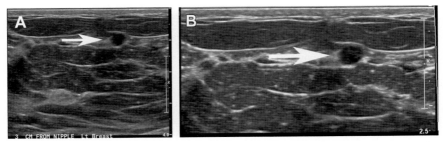

Fig. 3. Focal zone. Images of the same mass with the focal zone set too deep (*A, arrow*) and at the appropriate depth (*B, arrow*). When the focal zone is at the level of the mass, the margins and internal features can be better characterized.

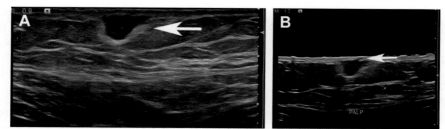

Fig. 4. Focal zone of superficial lesion. Because of transducer limitations, even the shallowest focal zone setting may not achieve the narrowest beam width possible for lesions near the skin. Therefore a standoff pad may be required to improve resolution. (*A*) A superficial hypoechoic mass (*arrow*). With the use of a standoff pad (*B*) allowing optimal resolution at the level of the skin, a skin tract (*arrow*) is now seen, confirming the diagnosis of a benign sebaceous cyst.

lesion, it may be beneficial to use standard ultrasonography imaging, in which the posterior shadowing may help identify the lesion, and then apply spatial compound imaging for analysis once the lesion has been detected.

HARMONIC IMAGING

Harmonic imaging is another signal processing technique to improve contrast and lateral resolution and reduce artifacts.[1] Harmonic imaging applies a filter to remove image harmonics, which are multiples of the transmitted frequency. This technique is advantageous because much of the artifact degrading image resolution is contained within the lower frequency components of the beam (**Fig. 7**).

COLOR DOPPLER AND POWER DOPPLER

Tumor angiogenesis plays a fundamental role in local tumor growth, invasion, and progression to metastases.[2,3] As tumors outgrow their native blood supply, hypoxia ensues, which induces expression of multiple angiogenic factors such as vascular endothelial growth factor. These factors induce the growth of existing capillaries and the formation of abnormal vessels that are often tortuous and disordered, which may be seen on color Doppler.[4] Power Doppler imaging may be used to increased sensitivity compared with color Doppler in detecting small vessels and low flow.

The presence or absence or type of tumor vascularity alone is not sufficient to characterize a lesion as benign or malignant. Features suggesting malignant lesions include hypervascularity, irregular branching central vessels, and more than one vascular pole.[5,6] Demonstrating internal vascularity within a sonographic lesion confirms that it is either solid or at least contains a solid component. Doppler imaging is most useful in distinguishing a high-grade invasive cancer or metastatic lymph node, both of which can appear anechoic, from a simple or complicated cyst (**Fig. 8**). Color Doppler may also be useful in differentiating between debris within a duct and an intraductal mass.

When using Doppler imaging, it is important to apply light transducer pressure to prevent occlusion of slow flow within vessels. The position and size of the color box should also be focused to the lesion of interest to maximize sensitivity to flow.

REAL-TIME IMAGING

Real-time imaging may be essential for accurate interpretation in many situations. In patients with palpable complaints, real-time ultrasonography by

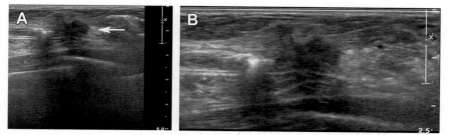

Fig. 5. Depth. The depth should be set so that the image focuses on the area of interest without including the lung, which provides no useful information (*A*). When the depth is set appropriately (*B*), the features of the mass (*arrows*) are better seen.

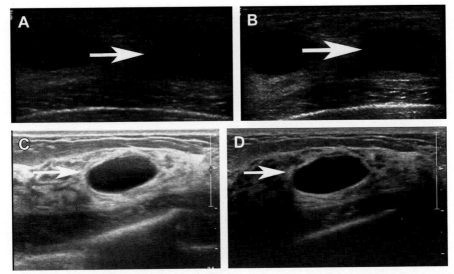

Fig. 6. Gain. Lesions can be mischaracterized if the gain is set too low or too high. (*A*) The gain is set too low and the lesion appears anechoic (*arrow*), suggesting a simple cyst. With the gain set correctly (*B*), low-level internal echoes (*arrow*) are now seen in this complicated cyst. (*C*) The gain is set too high, creating artificial internal echoes (*arrow*) mimicking a solid mass. When the gain is corrected (*D*), the lesion is seen to be a simple cyst (*arrow*).

the interpreting radiologist may be prudent in cases in which initial scanning by the technologist does not identify an abnormality. Another situation in which real-time imaging may be important is when differentiating between mobile debris in a complicated cyst versus a complex cystic mass (**Fig. 9**).

TARGETED ULTRASOUND: LESION CORRELATION

Targeted ultrasonography is often performed in order to identify a sonographic correlate to an abnormality identified on mammography or breast MR imaging before percutaneous biopsy. Ultrasonography-guided biopsy is the method of choice to sample any finding that is sonographically evident. Compared with stereotactic or MR imaging–guided biopsy, ultrasonography-guided biopsy is faster, more comfortable for the patient, and allows greater access to breast tissue, especially for far posterior and medial lesions that may not be amenable to either stereotactic or MR imaging–guided biopsy. In addition, adequate sampling is more consistently obtained because the needle can be seen traversing the target in real time.

When targeted ultrasonography is performed to evaluate a mammographic finding, careful triangulation of lesion location should be performed. Adjustments should be made when using craniocaudal and mediolateral-oblique (MLO) views to determine the clock axis for targeted ultrasonography. The location of the lesion may be higher or lower than expected based on the MLO view for medial and lateral lesions respectively. In addition, careful attention should be paid to both lesion depth

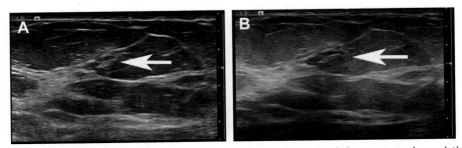

Fig. 7. Harmonic imaging. (*A*) The 12:00 axis of the right breast shows 2 subtle structures (*arrow*) that appear almost isoechoic to the fat. (*B*) Harmonic imaging of the same area allows better delineation of the margins and internal features (*arrow*), which allows the two lesions to be characterized as complicated cysts.

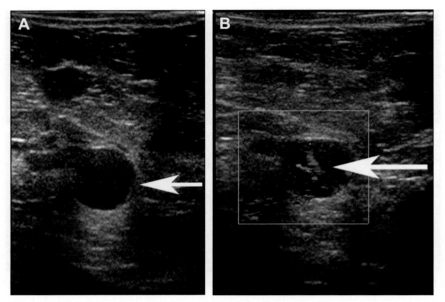

Fig. 8. Color Doppler. (*A*) A hypoechoic mass (*arrow*) in the far field with posterior enhancement, possibly representing a complicated cyst. With color Doppler (*B*), vascularity (*arrow*) is seen within the mass, confirming that it is solid and not a complicated cyst. Biopsy yielded invasive ductal carcinoma.

and the surrounding anatomic landmarks. The patient is positioned differently during breast ultrasonography, MR imaging, and mammogram, which affects lesion location. A superficial mass at the fat-gland interface on mammography or MR imaging should also be at that interface on targeted ultrasonography (**Fig. 10**). Other findings such as an adjacent cyst or dilated duct may also be used as anatomic landmarks.

When sampling a potential sonographic correlate to a mammographic abnormality, a localizing clip should be placed in the biopsied lesion using ultrasonography guidance. A postbiopsy mammogram should be obtained to confirm correlation between the biopsied lesion and the mammographic abnormality.

Targeted ultrasonography is often performed to evaluate for a sonographic correlate to an MR imaging finding in order to facilitate biopsy. A potential correlate is more frequently identified for enhancing masses compared with nonmass

enhancement.[7–11] However, true ultrasonography–MR imaging correlation can only be confirmed if follow-up MR imaging is performed, showing the localizing clip placed at the time of ultrasonography-guided biopsy within the area of enhancement on MR imaging. In one study, the presumed sonographic correlate biopsied yielding a benign, concordant diagnosis did not correspond with the lesion originally detected on MR imaging in 12% of cases.[10] For this reason, 6-month follow-up MR imaging is recommended following benign concordant biopsy of a sonographic correlate to an MR imaging–detected lesion.[12]

AMERICAN COLLEGE OF RADIOLOGY ACCREDITATION

The American College of Radiology offers a Breast Ultrasound Accreditation Program. Accreditation requires the application of many of the concepts discussed in this article to obtain high-quality

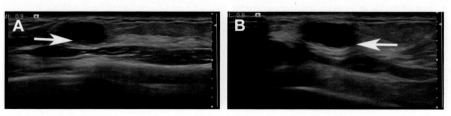

Fig. 9. Real-time imaging. (*A*) In the right breast at the 6:30 axis is a cyst with a possible intracystic mass (*arrow*). (*B*) When the patient is rolled into the left lateral decubitus position, the questionable mass moves into the dependent portion of the cyst (*arrow*), consistent with mobile debris.

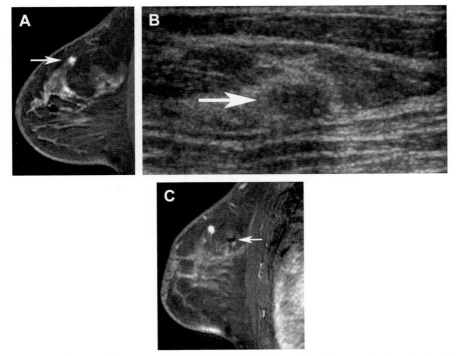

Fig. 10. Lesion miscorrelation. (*A*) A superficial enhancing mass (*arrow*) in the superior breast. Targeted ultrasonography identified a mass (*arrow*) that was thought to represent a correlate (*B*). Although the sonographic mass was of a similar size and clock axis to the MR finding, it was deep within the breast, whereas the MR mass was at the fat-gland interface. Ultrasonography-guided biopsy yielded fibroadenoma. On 6-month follow-up MR imaging, the clip (*arrow*) from ultrasonography-guided biopsy is seen deep to the MR mass (*C*). Subsequent biopsy yielded invasive ductal carcinoma.

images. The center frequency of the transducer must be at least 10 MHz. Unlike breast MR imaging accreditation, in which images from each individual magnet must be submitted, a facility must only provide a single example of a cyst and solid mass in the breast for ultrasonography accreditation regardless of the number of ultrasonography units at that facility. Two orthogonal mammographic views must be submitted with the lesion circled and visible on both views. Sonographic clinical images include the cyst and solid mass on 2 orthogonal views without calibers, and 1 image with appropriate measurements. Images should be taken along the longest axis of a lesion and then an orthogonal image. The longest axis of the lesion is not necessarily in the radial or anti-radial plane, but may be in an oblique position. Criteria for a simple cyst include anechoic, circumscribed margin, and posterior enhancement. For submitted images of cysts, spatial compound imaging should be avoided if the resulting image fails to show posterior enhancement.

SUMMARY

Ultrasonography is an important modality that is frequently used in all aspects of breast imaging, including breast cancer screening, the evaluation of palpable abnormalities, further characterization of lesions seen mammographically, and for determining the method of percutaneous biopsy. Understanding the basic technical aspects of ultrasonography equipment is critical to ensure high breast ultrasonography image quality.

REFERENCES

1. Harvey CJ, Pilcher JM, Eckersley RJ, et al. Advances in ultrasound. Clin Radiol 2002;57(3): 157–77.
2. Schneider BP, Miller KD. Angiogenesis of breast cancer. J Clin Oncol 2005;23(8):1782–90.
3. Weidner N, Semple JP, Welch WR, et al. Tumor angiogenesis and metastasis–correlation in invasive breast carcinoma. N Engl J Med 1991; 324(1):1–8.
4. Less JR, Skalak TC, Sevick EM, et al. Microvascular architecture in a mammary carcinoma: branching patterns and vessel dimensions. Cancer Res 1991; 51(1):265–73.
5. Yang W, Dempsey PJ. Diagnostic breast ultrasound: current status and future directions. Radiol Clin North Am 2007;45(5):845–61, vii.

6. Mehta TS, Raza S, Baum JK. Use of Doppler ultrasound in the evaluation of breast carcinoma. Semin Ultrasound CT MR 2000;21(4):297–307.

7. LaTrenta LR, Menell JH, Morris EA, et al. Breast lesions detected with MR imaging: utility and histopathologic importance of identification with US. Radiology 2003;227(3):856–61.

8. Abe H, Schmidt RA, Shah RN, et al. MR-directed ("Second-Look") ultrasound examination for breast lesions detected initially on MRI: MR and sonographic findings. AJR Am J Roentgenol 2010; 194(2):370–7.

9. Demartini WB, Eby PR, Peacock S, et al. Utility of targeted sonography for breast lesions that were suspicious on MRI. AJR Am J Roentgenol 2009; 192(4):1128–34.

10. Meissnitzer M, Dershaw DD, Lee CH, et al. Targeted ultrasound of the breast in women with abnormal MRI findings for whom biopsy has been recommended. AJR Am J Roentgenol 2009;193(4):1025–9.

11. Beran L, Liang W, Nims T, et al. Correlation of targeted ultrasound with magnetic resonance imaging abnormalities of the breast. Am J Surg 2005;190(4): 592–4.

12. Sung JS, Lee CH, Morris EA, et al. Patient follow-up after concordant histologically benign imaging-guided biopsy of MRI-detected lesions. AJR Am J Roentgenol 2012;198(6):1464–9.

Update on Screening Breast Ultrasonography

Ginger M. Merry, MD, MPH[a,b,*], Ellen B. Mendelson, MD[b]

KEYWORDS

- Screening breast ultrasonography • Breast cancer screening • Dense breast tissue
- Cancer detection rate • Positive predictive value

KEY POINTS

- Handheld screening breast ultrasonography has been shown across multiple studies of patients with dense fibroglandular tissue and/or increased risk of breast cancer to have an average breast cancer detection rate of 3.7 additional cancers detected per 1000 women screened.
- The additional cancers detected by screening breast ultrasonography are at the cost of a low positive predictive value of biopsy (averaging 9.5% across multiple studies) leading to many unnecessary biopsies and at the cost of detection of many Breast Imaging Reporting and Data System 3 probably benign findings that require additional short-interval follow-up.
- As part of widespread implementation of screening breast ultrasonography, appropriate training courses, accreditation criteria, and guidelines should be developed to ensure safe and efficacious use of breast ultrasonography as a screening tool.

Screening mammography is the only modality that has been proved to reduce mortality from breast cancer; however, mammography has limitations and therefore other modalities are being investigated as possible screening tools for breast cancer. Breast ultrasonography and magnetic resonance (MR) imaging are the primary modalities that have been investigated and this article focuses on breast ultrasonography as a screening tool. This article discusses the current recommendations for screening breast ultrasonography, presents a review of the literature, and discusses problems associated with the implementation of screening breast ultrasonography and the political and economic factors influencing the use of screening breast ultrasonography.

CURRENT RECOMMENDATIONS FOR SCREENING BREAST ULTRASONOGRAPHY

The American College of Radiology (ACR) and Society of Breast Imaging currently recommend that screening breast ultrasonography be used, in addition to mammography, in women with a high risk of developing breast cancer who cannot have MR imaging. Breast ultrasonography is considered a possible screening supplement option for women with dense breast tissue who are at an intermediate risk of developing breast cancer.[1,2] High risk is defined as one or more of the following: breast cancer susceptibility genes 1 or 2 (BRCA1 or BRCA2) mutation carrier or untested first-degree relative of a BRCA mutation carrier; history of chest wall radiation between the ages of 10 and 30 years; women with a genetic syndrome that increases the risk of breast cancer; and lifetime risk of breast cancer of 20% or more. Intermediate risk of breast cancer is defined as having a 15% to 20% lifetime risk of breast cancer; this includes risk associated with a personal history of breast or ovarian cancer, and prior breast biopsy diagnosis of lobular neoplasia or atypical ductal hyperplasia.[1,2]

[a] Colorado Permanente Medical Group, 10350 East Dakota Avenue, Denver, CO 80231, USA; [b] Department of Radiology, Lynn Sage Comprehensive Breast Center, Northwestern Memorial Hospital–Prentice 4, Feinberg School of Medicine, Northwestern University, 250 East Superior Street, Chicago, IL 60611, USA
* Corresponding author.
E-mail address: gingermerry@gmail.com

Radiol Clin N Am 52 (2014) 527–537
http://dx.doi.org/10.1016/j.rcl.2013.12.003
0033-8389/14/$ – see front matter © 2014 Elsevier Inc. All rights reserved.

Dense breast tissue is considered a possible indication for screening breast ultrasonography because mammography is less sensitive in detecting breast cancer in dense breast tissue, breast cancer is more likely to develop in areas of denser breast tissue, and having dense breast tissue is a risk factor for breast cancer.[3–6] Breast tissue density is categorized by the Breast Imaging Reporting and Data System (BI-RADS) into 1 of 4 categories based on the composition of glandular tissue seen mammographically: (1) almost entirely fat (<25% glandular), (2) scattered fibroglandular densities (approximately 25%–50% glandular), (3) heterogeneously dense (approximately 51%–75% glandular), and (4) extremely dense (>75% glandular).[7] Although the forthcoming fifth edition of BI-RADS[8] will eliminate the percentage-based subcategorization of breast densities, most published work on ultrasonography screening in women with dense breast tissue defines dense breast tissue as breast tissue with more than 50% glandular tissue (categories 3 and 4) and, unless otherwise stated, this definition applies throughout this article as well.

REVIEW OF THE LITERATURE ON SCREENING WHOLE-BREAST ULTRASONOGRAPHY
Handheld Screening Whole-Breast Ultrasonography

A summary of studies evaluating whole-breast ultrasonography as a screening tool is presented in **Table 1**. Initial small-scale, single-institution, observational studies of supplemental handheld screening breast ultrasonography showed promising results for screening breast ultrasonography using a handheld device as a supplement to screening mammography.[9–14] Berg[15] summarized these results, which included 42,838 examinations from 6 different studies performed between 1995 and 2004. Supplemental screening breast ultrasonography performed in these studies had a mean cancer detection rate of an additional 3.5 cancers per 1000 women screened that were not detected by screening mammography; however, the range was wide (from 2.7 to 9.0 cancers per 1000 women screened).[15,16] Of the cancers seen only by ultrasonography, 94% were invasive and 70% of the invasive cancers were 1 cm or smaller in size.[15] Three of the studies detailed staging and, in total, 36 (90%) of 40 cancers identified only by ultrasonography were stage 0 or I.[15] Also, as predicted, ultrasonography was superior to mammography at detecting cancers in mammographically denser breasts. Women with fatty breast density were excluded from all of these studies, but a disproportionate

number (90%) of the cancers detected only by ultrasonography were in women with dense breasts.[15] These studies also suggested that supplemental ultrasonography was most appropriate in women at increased risk of developing breast cancer. Women at higher risk for breast cancer were 2 to 3 times more likely to have a cancer identified by ultrasonography that was not seen mammographically.[15] The biopsy rate for ultrasonography-only findings in these studies averaged 3.1% and the positive predictive value (PPV) for biopsies (core biopsy or fine-needle aspiration) performed for suspicious findings seen only by ultrasonography was 11.4% with a range of 6.6% to 18%.[15,16] The low PPV for biopsies has caused concern, and many consider this as an unacceptably high percentage of false-positives, with many unnecessary biopsies having been performed as a result.

Although these initial studies showed promise for screening breast ultrasonography as a possible breast cancer screening tool, they were all single-institution studies with varying study designs and several important limitations. One limitation is that the studies were nonblinded; the ultrasonography interpretation was not done independently from the mammography interpretation, with potential bias and leading to screening recalls (targeted ultrasonography evaluations). In addition, these studies only reported prevalence and not rate of incidence; therefore it was not known whether annual screening ultrasonography would provide any additional benefit compared with the initial screening ultrasonography. Follow-up data were incomplete, incremental cancer rates were not reported, and standardized BI-RADS reporting was not uniformly applied. The ability to generalize these studies to current radiology practice is limited because of the single-institution observational nature, variability in interpretive and reporting criteria, and the use of film-screen mammography during these study periods.

The results from these single-institution studies, showing that screening breast ultrasonography is able to detect small, invasive but early stage, mammographically occult breast cancers, was encouraging and in response several larger, prospective, multi-institution studies have been developed. At this point, some questions remained; primarily whether earlier detection of these small invasive cancers can be measured in mortality reduction and whether the results of the studies can be generalized not only across institutions but also among the individuals performing the handheld ultrasonography examinations. A randomized controlled trial (RCT) would have been ideal before implementing ultrasonography

Table 1
Summary of studies of screening breast ultrasonography, biopsies prompted by ultrasonography, positive predictive value of biopsy, and prevalence of cancers seen only on ultrasonography

Investigator, Year	No. Examinations	# Women Biopsied[a] (%)	# Malignant[b] (%)	Prevalence (%)
Single-center Studies				
Gordon & Goldenberg,[11] 1995	12,706	NS	44/279 (16)	44/12,706 (0.35)
Buchberger et al,[9] 2000	8103 867	NS	32/362 (8.8) 8/43 (19)	32/8103 (0.39) 8/867 (0.9)
Kaplan,[12] 2001	1862	97 (5.2)	6/99 (6.1)	6/1862 (0.3)
Kolb et al,[13] 2002	13,547	NS	37/358 (10)	37/13,547 (0.27)
Crystal et al,[10] 2003	1517	38 (2.5)	7/38 (18)	7/1517 (0.46)
Leconte et al,[14] 2003	4236	NS	NS	16/4236 (0.38)
Hooley et al,[30] 2012	935	53 (5.7)	3/63 (4.8)	3/935 (0.32)
Multicenter Studies				
Corsetti et al,[17] 2008	9157	449 (4.9)	37/647 (5.7)	37/9157 (0.40)
Kelly et al,[24] 2010	6425	75 (1.2)	23/75 (30.7)	23/6425 (0.36)
Berg et al,[21] 2012	7473	449 (6.0)	32/449 (7.1)	32/7473 (0.43)
Overall total	66,828	1161/27,369 (4.2)	229/2413 (9.5)	248/66,828 (0.37)

Abbreviation: NS, not stated.
  [a] Biopsies and aspirations prompted by screening ultrasonography.
  [b] Refers to cancers seen only on breast ultrasonography, expressed as percentage of lesions biopsied or aspirated.
  Courtesy of Wendie A. Berg, MD, PhD, Magee-Womens Hospital of UPMC, University of Pittsburgh School of Medicine, Pittsburgh, PA; *Modified from* Berg WA. Supplemental screening sonography in dense breasts. Radiol Clin North Am 2004;42(5):845–51, vi; and Berg WA. Screening ultrasound. In: Berg WA, Yang WT, editors. Diagnostic Imaging - Breast, 2nd edition. Salt Lake City: Amirsys; 2014;9:40.

as a new screening test, but an RCT was thought to be economically unfeasible and clinically impractical. Supported by the positive single-site data, several robust, prospective studies have been undertaken to further document the efficacy of handheld breast ultrasonography for supplemental screening.

Corsetti and colleagues[17] conducted a prospective study with 6 physicians performing ultrasonography examinations in which 9157 women with dense breast tissue and negative mammograms were screened with bilateral whole-breast ultrasonography using a handheld transducer. The study did not indicate that the physician performing the ultrasonography was blinded to the mammogram at the time of the ultrasonography study, but a blinded rereview of all negative mammograms that were associated with an ultrasonography-detected cancer was conducted by 5 radiologists. The incidence of mammographically occult breast cancer detected by ultrasonography was 4 cancers per 1000 women screened, which is similar to all other published work.[17] The results showed that screening ultrasonography may be more beneficial in young women, who tend to have denser breasts. Ultrasonography detected 41.3% of the

cancers in asymptomatic women younger than 50 years and only 13.5% of the cancers in asymptomatic women 50 years of age or older.[17] However, these results have not been consistently reproduced in other studies. PPVs were not reported in this study. Similar to all previously published work, this study showed that ultrasonography detects smaller and earlier stage cancers compared with those cancers detected by mammography alone. This study also showed that breast cancers detected only by ultrasonography were less likely to have axillary lymph node metastases (14% with positive lymph nodes) compared with cancers detected only by mammography (31% with positive lymph nodes). A review of the literature conducted by Nothacker and colleagues[18] identified 3 studies in addition to that of Corsetti and colleagues[17] that reported lymph node status and found that 90% (range, 86%–100%) of breast cancers detected by ultrasonography only did not have axillary metastases at the time of diagnosis.

The American College of Radiology Imaging Network (ACRIN) also recognized the need for a multicenter prospective analysis of screening breast ultrasonography, and the ACRIN 6666 trial started data collection in 2004. The primary aim of the study was to determine whether screening breast ultrasonography performed with a handheld transducer can identify mammographically occult breast cancer and whether the results could be generalized across institutions.[19] The study design was a multicenter prospective study of asymptomatic women at increased risk of breast cancer and with dense breast tissue. These women received 3 rounds of annual screening mammography and screening whole-breast ultrasonography. The interpreting radiologist for each examination was blinded to the results of the other examination, the examinations were performed in a randomized order, and a standardized scanning and interpretation protocol was used. The initial results from the prevalence screening from 2637 women were reported in 2008.[20] Supplemental screening breast ultrasonography showed a prevalence of 4.2 additional cancers detected per 1000 women screened, with a confidence interval of 1.1 to 7.2 cancers per 1000 women screened.[20] Mammography alone detected 78% of cancers, whereas mammography plus ultrasonography detected 91% of cancers.[20] Of the additional cancers detected only by ultrasonography, 92% (11 of 12) were invasive and 89% (8 of 9) were node negative.[20] The PPV1 (the percentage of cancers determined after a positive screening test) was 6.5% for findings seen only on ultrasonography. This result was similar to the PPV1 for findings seen only on mammography, which was 7.6%. The PPV2 (the percentage of cancers after a full diagnostic work-up and a biopsy is recommended) was 8.9% for suspicious findings seen only on ultrasonography, compared with a PPV2 for mammography findings of 22.6%.[20]

More recently, incidence rates of breast cancer from ACRIN 6666's 3 rounds of annual screening ultrasonography were published.[21] The incidence of cancers detected, beyond that of mammography, by annual screening ultrasonography was 3.7 cancers per 1000 women screened. The prevalence in the first screening year was 5.3 cancers per 1000 women screened.[20,21] These results suggest that annual ultrasonography screening can provide additional detection benefit beyond the initial screening year. There was also a low interval cancer rate across the 3 years of the trial, suggesting that the combination of screening mammography and ultrasonography is an effective screening strategy.[21]

The issue of many false-positive results from ultrasonography leading to additional biopsies was also examined in more detail between initial screening and annual screening years. In the first screen year, the PPV3 (the percentage of cancers

among women with a positive screening test who had a biopsy) for mammography alone was 29.2%, for mammography plus ultrasonography it was 11.4%, and for ultrasonography alone it was 9.0%. With the additional screen years, the PPV3 for mammography plus ultrasonography increased to 16.2% and the PPV3 for ultrasonography increased to 11.7%; however, this was still lower than the PPV3 for mammography alone, which increased to 38.1%.[21] This finding indicates that the addition of annual ultrasonography screening continues to result in many false-positives leading to biopsy, although the percentage of false-positive findings from ultrasonography did decrease in the annual incidence screens.

To validate a screening test, an RCT is considered necessary, but surrogate end points for mortality may be acceptable because of the time, number of participants, and high cost associated with an RCT that uses mortality as an end point. The only known RCT in progress is the Japan Strategic Anti-cancer Randomized Trial (J-START), which is a multi-institution prospective RCT being conducted in Japan.[22] Women aged 40 to 49 years are randomized to receive screening mammography alone or a screening mammogram plus screening ultrasonography. Primary end points are sensitivity and specificity, and the secondary end point is the detection rate of advanced breast cancers. Concern over the ability to generalize this study to the general population exists because the study population is restricted to women aged 40 to 49 years, the Japanese population is not representative of Western countries, and the time interval between screening examinations is 2 years.[22]

Ultrasonography Screening Methods: Handheld Versus Automated Whole-breast Ultrasonography

A comparison between handheld and automated breast ultrasonography is presented in **Table 2**. One of the major differences and limitations of screening breast ultrasonography performed with a handheld ultrasound probe is the time required by a highly trained specialist to perform the examination. In most studies published thus far a physician has been the operator. The ACRIN 6666 trial reported a median time for a physician to perform a screening ultrasonography examination to be 17 minutes during the first year which decreased to 13 minutes in the 3rd year.[20] Kolb and colleagues[13] reported an average of 4 minutes 39 seconds performed by a physician, and Kaplan[12] reported an average of 10 minutes

Table 2
Differences between handheld ultrasonography and automated ultrasonography for whole-breast screening

Handheld Ultrasonography	Automated Ultrasonography
Two-dimensional images	Volumetric images (three-dimensional) including whole-breast coronal
PACS workstation or other recording method	Requires dedicated separate workstation
Same equipment as for diagnostic ultrasonography	Requires new equipment only used for screening
Performer of ultrasonography interprets the ultrasonography	Separate performance and interpretation of ultrasonography
Real-time interpretation and decision making	Delayed review and rereview of images possible before decision making

Abbreviation: PACS, picture archiving and communication system.

performed by a technologist. Neither the Kolb and colleagues[13] nor the Kaplan[12] study methodology used a standardized data collection or documentation and reporting system, as recommended in BI-RADS, and therefore these studies may underestimate the time required. The ACRIN 6666 study used a standardized protocol for image documentation, but additional protocol requirements may have extended the time beyond what would be expected in standard practice.[20,23] Overall, 13 to 17 minutes is most likely the closest estimate of the time necessary to perform a handheld screening bilateral whole-breast ultrasonography.

Automated breast ultrasonography screening is one option that has been proposed to overcome the time-consuming and costly nature of handheld, physician-performed screening whole-breast ultrasonography, but there has been limited research on the applicability of this technology. Given the differences in technique, data acquisition, and interpretation, it cannot be assumed that the results from handheld screening breast ultrasonography can be applied to automated breast ultrasonography.

There has been 1 multicenter prospective study, conducted by Kelly and colleagues,[24] comparing screening mammography with the combination of screening mammography plus semiautomated breast ultrasonography in 4419 women with dense breast tissue and/or at increased risk of breast cancer. This ultrasonography system used a standard 12-MHz to 7-MHz linear transducer used for breast ultrasonography attached to a computer-guided mechanical arm. Overlapping strips from superior breast to inferior were obtained, with a sonographer ensuring the appropriate positioning of the transducer and its contact with the skin. The interpreting radiologist for each examination was blinded to the results of the other examination. The results were promising, with an additional 3.6 cancers detected per 1000 women screened, which is similar to the ACRIN 6666 results.[24] The sensitivity for the breast ultrasonography alone was 67% and for mammography alone was 40% but, when the results of the two modalities were combined, the sensitivity increased to 81%.[24] The reported PPVs were higher for this semiautomated breast ultrasonography system compared with previously published work for handheld breast ultrasonography. Kelly and colleagues[24] reported a PPV for biopsy recommendation of 38.4% for all suspicious findings seen using this ultrasonography system and 30.7% for suspicious findings seen when the mammogram was negative. However, a major concern in this study was the high number of interval cancers (19.3%) detected clinically within a year of negative screening mammography and the semiautomated ultrasonography. In total there were 57 cancers detected at the time of initial screening: 15 were seen by both ultrasonography and mammography, 8 were seen only by mammography, and 23 were seen only by ultrasonography. There were 11 cancers that were not seen at initial screening, but on later re-review of the images 9 of these 11 cancers were seen on the ultrasonography images.[24]

Kelly and colleagues[25] also evaluated radiologist reader performance for breast cancer detection in women with dense breasts using this method of automated breast ultrasonography. With minimal (4 hours) training in their technology for semi-automated breast ultrasonography, radiologists were able to improve cancer detection, with an increase of 63% in callbacks of cancer cases and only a 4% decrease in correct identification of true-negative cases. The interpretation time per study was 7 minutes, 58 seconds per study, with a range of 5 minutes 54 seconds to 12 minutes 51 seconds, which is shorter than the physician time reported in the ACRIN 6666 trial, but physician time for ACRIN 6666 included performance of the examination, image documentation, and image interpretation, occurring during the real-time examination.[20,25] These studies highlight several potential advantages of using an automated system as a screening tool compared with handheld breast ultrasonography: reduction of variability in examination performance, less operator dependence, and reduced physician time.

Several studies are underway to evaluate screening whole-breast ultrasonography using a technique that uses a larger transducer head to acquire overlapping images in the transverse plane that are then reconstructed into the sagittal and coronal planes to allow three-dimensional workstation interpretation. An example of a coronal image from this type of technology is given in **Fig. 1**, which shows a small biopsy-proven cancer. Lander and Tabár[26] describe a multicenter prospective study currently being conducted that is designed to assess the sensitivity and specificity of this type of automated whole-breast ultrasonography combined with digital mammography compared with digital mammography alone for cancer detection in asymptomatic women with dense breast tissue. The study has a matched-pair design in which each participant receives a separate interpretation of the mammogram only and a combined interpretation of the mammogram and automated breast ultrasonography.[26] Another prospective, multicenter study with a matched-pair design has been reported using automated breast ultrasonography system with enrollment of at least 20,000 asymptomatic women with dense breast tissue at 10 different sites in the United States.[27] Given the differences in technique, data acquisition, and interpretation between handheld and automated screening breast ultrasonography, these studies are necessary to validate automated whole-breast ultrasonography's equivalence in lesion detection to that of handheld ultrasonography. A summary of published studies for both handheld and automated breast ultrasonography is presented in **Table 1**.

Supplemental Screening Ultrasonography Versus Supplemental Screening MR Imaging

Although this article focuses on ultrasonography as a supplement to screening mammography, the topic of supplemental screening MR imaging cannot be excluded. MR imaging is becoming more available and more efficient while maintaining its status as the most sensitive imaging modality for detection of breast cancer. Its cost remains higher than that of ultrasonography, and, at the current time, MR imaging requires intravenous administration of contrast material. Thus it is necessary to consider the effectiveness, risks, and costs of supplemental ultrasonography versus supplemental MR imaging before a recommendation is made for individual patients.

Numerous studies have shown that for women at high risk for breast cancer the combination of screening mammography and MR imaging has greater sensitivity than the combination of screening mammography and ultrasonography. A review of these studies showed that the combination of screening mammography and ultrasonography identified 52% of cancers, whereas the combination of mammography and MR imaging identified 92% of cancers.[28] These results support the recommendation that supplemental screening MR imaging should be offered to women at high risk for developing breast cancer. Thus, the discussion of supplemental screening breast ultrasonography versus screening MR imaging has been centered on the use of this supplemental screening in women at an intermediate risk of breast cancer. Screening MR imaging detects more breast cancers, but it is unclear whether this additional detection benefit outweighs the costs and risks associated with screening MR imaging. MR imaging is a costly imaging modality that also comes with the disadvantage of a high false-positive rate, leading to the additional economic and emotional cost of performing expensive MR imaging–guided biopsies that are considered to be much

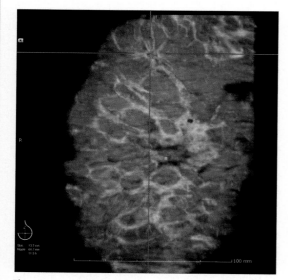

Fig. 1. Breast cancer seen on coronal image from automated breast ultrasonography. A small biopsy-proven invasive ductal carcinoma is seen in the upper left breast, marked by the intersecting lines, on this coronal image from an automated breast ultrasonography examination. The nipple is marked with a yellow square.

less tolerable than an ultrasonography-guided biopsy.

FACTORS INFLUENCING THE IMPLEMENTATION OF SCREENING BREAST ULTRASONOGRAPHY
High Rate of False-positives

Before the implementation of widespread screening breast ultrasonography, there are many factors that need to be addressed (**Box 1**). As discussed earlier, one of the major limitations of implementing a screening breast ultrasonography program is the high rate of false-positive biopsies. **Table 1** provides a summary of studies with an average PPV for biopsies performed of only 9.5%; more than 90% of biopsies performed were benign. Many clinicians consider this an unacceptably low PPV leading to unnecessary harm, discomfort, and emotional distress for the patient. Others argue that ultrasonography-guided biopsies are easy to perform and the benefit of additional cancer detection is worth the small risks. In coming years, recognition and acceptance of sonographic criteria for benign and probably benign lesions may reduce the increased biopsy rate. At present, breast ultrasonography is an option that referring physicians recommend and patients choose, and both the patient and referring physician should be fully informed of the risks and possible benefits before proceeding. In addition, if screening breast ultrasonography becomes more widespread and a standard component of breast screening, as is likely to happen, breast imagers should deepen their knowledge of ultrasonography as they have for other modalities in 8-hour Continuing Medical Education (CME) courses, such as for tomosynthesis or in compliance with accreditation requirements such as those for breast MR imaging.

Probably Benign Findings Requiring Short-interval Follow-up

Another issue that has been addressed in many of the studies is the need for short-interval follow-up of lesions seen sonographically that are considered probably benign (BI-RADS 3), which by definition indicates at least a 98% likelihood of being a benign lesion. Of the initial 6 single-center studies there were 4 studies that reported on short-interval follow-up recommendations with an average of 6.6% and a range of 3% to 10% of women being recommended for a short-interval follow-up examination based on the screening ultrasonography results.[9,11–13,29] The ACRIN 6666 study had similar results, with 8.6% of participating women being recommended for short-interval follow-up of probably benign findings seen on the screening ultrasonography.[20] The experience at Yale University, where studies were performed by sonographers and interpreted by physicians, after the enactment of the Connecticut Public Act 09–41, had a higher percentage of BI-RADS 3 categorizations. A BI-RADS 3 probably benign classification requiring follow-up ultrasonography was given to 20% of the patients, but the investigators stated that, if nonsimple cysts in the setting of multiple cysts as well as solitary, oval, circumscribed complicated cysts less than 5 mm had been classified as benign, then the use of BI-RADS 3 would have been closer to 10%, similar to other published results, without a change in sensitivity.[30]

Malignancy rates of multiple bilateral, circumscribed, similar-appearing masses; clustered microcysts; and solitary circumscribed masses have been shown to be very low. The ACRIN 6666 trial had no malignancies among 127 women with multiple bilateral, similar-appearing circumscribed masses with at least 2 years of follow-up.[31] However, close examination of each mass is essential because these women can develop breast cancer.[31] The ACRIN 6666 malignancy rate for solitary circumscribed masses (complicated cysts; clustered microcysts; circumscribed oval, round, gently lobulated masses) was very low at 0.4% (3 of 836).[31] The results from this trial have led to the suggestion that follow-up diagnostic ultrasonography should be performed at 1 year, instead of at 6 months, for multiple bilateral, circumscribed, benign-appearing masses identified at screening ultrasonography.[31] If 1-year stability is documented, then the patient should

---

Box 1
Factors influencing the implementation of screening breast ultrasonography

- High rate of false-positive biopsies
- Probably benign findings requiring short-interval follow-up
- Increased callbacks from screening if real-time interpretation is not provided
- Increased workforce demands on radiologists and sonographers
- New infrastructure to accommodate demand
- New training and accreditation requirements for radiologists and sonographers
- Reimbursement and insurance coding
- Influence of advocacy groups

return to screening.[31] Additional studies may help reconfirm the validity and safe follow-up intervals recommended in this study. Adoption in practice of the criteria described earlier and follow-up recommendations for probably benign findings may be necessary to have efficient ultrasonography screening programs whose workloads are not overwhelmed by unnecessary short-interval follow-up examinations.

Certification and Accreditation for Screening Breast Ultrasonography

In order to perform screening breast ultrasonography, an imaging center should meet basic eligibility criteria. It has been recommended by the Society of Breast Imaging that any center performing screening breast ultrasonography meet the eligibility criteria set forth by the ACRIN 6666 trial.[32] These eligibility criteria include experience of the person performing and interpreting the ultrasonography examination of 500 breast ultrasonography examinations per year.[33] At a minimum, a radiologist must abide by the ACR requirements, which are initially to have been supervised and/or performed, interpreted, and reported at least 300 breast ultrasonography examinations over a 36-month period. After this initial experience requirement, it is recommended that the radiologist perform and interpret at least 100 examinations per year in order to maintain skills.[23] However, these ACR requirements were specified for training in diagnostic breast ultrasonography before the acceptance of screening among the indications for breast ultrasonography as listed in the ACR's Practice Guideline for the Performance of the Breast Ultrasound Examination.[23] The goal of screening is detection, which requires additional training and experience beyond that for using ultrasonography in lesion confirmation and characterization.

In the absence of practice guidelines, accreditations, and regulatory policies, breast imagers and breast sonographers should amplify their knowledge of ultrasonography through CME. For those who participate in an intensive, skills-based CME course and show proficiency, a certificate of proficiency should be awarded. Radiology residency programs should take action by including breast ultrasonography screening skills within the recommended curriculum.

The ACRIN 6666 trial was designed for physician performance of the ultrasonography screening examination, as has been the practice in Europe and Asia for many decades with variable or no requirements for documentation and with different liability pressures. Screening breast ultrasonography can be time consuming and current inadequate reimbursement may make performance by physicians in the United States the exception rather than the rule. Most studies examining screening breast ultrasonography have used radiologists to perform the ultrasonography examinations, and although it is anticipated, it is not clearly established whether these physician-attained results, which are interpreted as they are scanned, can be applied to sonographers certified in the technique but not in performing interpretation. Although diagnostic breast ultrasonography remains physician performed in some practices, in the United States changing practice patterns are seen, particularly in high-volume settings. Sonographers often perform the initial diagnostic breast ultrasonography with the physician checking the real-time images and asking for additional images or rescanning after the sonographer. It is expected that sonographers will also be asked to perform screening breast ultrasonography and therefore they will need to receive additional training, with possible development of certification in screening by either the American Registry of Radiologic Technologists (ARRT) or the American Registry for Diagnostic Medical Sonography (ARDMS), both of which currently offer certification in breast ultrasonography.

In addition to training requirements, if supplemental screening with ultrasonography becomes widespread concomitant with breast density awareness, practice guidelines for the performance of screening breast ultrasonography need to be developed. Practice standards have been in place for diagnostic breast ultrasonography by the ACR for many years, most recently updated in 2011. These practice guidelines for diagnostic breast ultrasonography include standards for the individual examinations (labeling, lesion characterization, and technical factors), documentation, and equipment specification.[23] Similar guidelines should be developed for screening breast ultrasonography addressing automated ultrasonography as well as the prevailing handheld examination.

Political and Economic Factors

In recent years there has been increased public awareness of breast density and of the research showing that increased breast density decreases the sensitivity of screening mammography. In 2009, Connecticut was the first state to approve a bill that requires reporting of breast density to all patients who receive a mammogram. In the state of Connecticut, if a woman has dense breast tissue (>50% glandular tissue), then the following statement must be included in the mammogram report sent to the patient: "If your mammogram demonstrates that you have dense breast tissue, which could hide small abnormalities, you might benefit from supplementary screening tests, which can include a breast ultrasonography screening or a breast MRI examination, or both, depending on your individual risk factors. A report of your mammography results, which contains information about your breast density, has been sent to your physician's office and you should contact your physician if you have any questions or concerns about this report."[34] Connecticut also requires that insurance companies cover screening breast ultrasonography for women with dense breasts if recommended by a physician. Since this bill was passed in 2009 there has been similar legislation in New York, Texas, Virginia, California, Tennessee, Hawaii, Maryland, Alabama, Oregon, and Nevada.

Since the enactment of the Connecticut bill several retrospective reviews have been published from institutions in Connecticut, all showing similar results.[30,35,36] Hooley and colleagues[30] reviewed the results of women with dense breasts who received supplemental sonographer-performed handheld screening breast ultrasonography at Yale University during the first year after the bill was enacted. The results are an indication of real-world experience in that the interpreting radiologists were not blinded to other imaging results, and they had the option to rescan in real time after a sonographer completed the examination. In this group of women with dense breast tissue, but not selected for any other risk factors, there was a cancer detection rate of 3.2 cancers per 1000 women screened. The PPV for all biopsies or aspirations performed on BI-RADS 4 lesions was 5.6% and the PPV of all biopsies or aspirations performed (including BI-RADS 3 and 4 lesions) was 4.8%.[30] The cancer detection rate was similar to that in other published work, but the PPV was the lowest reported (see **Table 1**). Also, as discussed earlier, there was a high rate of probably benign findings (20%) requiring short-interval follow-up ultrasonography. It will be important to determine whether these numbers will change with additional experience as the demand for screening breast ultrasonography continues to grow.

SUMMARY

Handheld screening breast ultrasonography has been shown by numerous studies to have a potential role in screening for breast cancer in women at increased risk and/or with dense breast tissue. The average cancer detection rate across these studies was 3.7 per 1000 women screened (see

Table 1) and screening breast ultrasonography has been shown to detect mostly small, node-negative, invasive cancers. One of the major drawbacks is the low PPV, with an average of only 9.5% of biopsies being positive for cancer across these studies (see **Table 1**). Automated breast ultrasonography is promising, but data are limited and it is not yet known whether automated ultrasonography will have the same cancer detection yield as handheld ultrasonography. There are many costs associated with implementing a screening breast ultrasonography program, which include establishment of new infrastructure, training of personnel, workflow issues, recall rates, increased number of biopsies, and increased need for follow-up of probably benign findings. As part of widespread implementation of screening breast ultrasonography, accreditation and certification requirements need at least to be defined for those performing and interpreting the examinations. Increasing public awareness of breast density by organizations such as Are You Dense (www.areyoudense.org) will most likely continue to push the medical community to provide screening breast ultrasonography. Although the impact of screening breast ultrasonography continues to be studied and clinicians' experience is increasing, guidelines need to be developed that will ensure safe and efficacious inclusion among breast imaging services.

REFERENCES

1. Lee CH, Dershaw DD, Kopans D, et al. Breast cancer screening with imaging: recommendations from the Society of Breast Imaging and the ACR on the use of mammography, breast MRI, breast ultrasound, and other technologies for the detection of clinically occult breast cancer. J Am Coll Radiol 2010;7(1):18–27.

2. Mainiero MB, Lourenco A, Mahoney MC, et al. ACR appropriateness criteria breast cancer screening. J Am Coll Radiol 2013;10(1):11–4.

3. Mandelson MT, Oestreicher N, Porter PL, et al. Breast density as a predictor of mammographic detection: comparison of interval- and screen-detected cancers. J Natl Cancer Inst 2000;92(13):1081–7.

4. Harvey JA, Bovbjerg VE. Quantitative assessment of mammographic breast density: relationship with breast cancer risk. Radiology 2004;230(1):29–41.

5. McCormack VA, dos Santos Silva I. Breast density and parenchymal patterns as markers of breast cancer risk: a meta-analysis. Cancer Epidemiol Biomarkers Prev 2006;15(6):1159–69.

6. Boyd NF, Guo H, Martin LJ, et al. Mammographic density and the risk and detection of breast cancer. N Engl J Med 2007;356(3):227–36.

7. D'Orsi CJ, Bassett LW, Berg WA, et al. BI-RADS: mammography, 4th edition. In: D'Orsi CJ, Mendelson EB, Ikeda DM, et al, editors. Breast imaging reporting and data system: ACR BI-RADS – breast imaging atlas. Reston (VA): American College of Radiology; 2003.

8. Sickles EA, Bassett LW, D'Orsi CJ, et al. Breast imaging reporting and data system, BI-RADS: mammography. 5th edition. Reston (VA): American College of Radiology; in press.

9. Buchberger W, Niehoff A, Obrist P, et al. Clinically and mammographically occult breast lesions: detection and classification with high-resolution sonography. Semin Ultrasound CT MR 2000;21(4): 325–36.

10. Crystal P, Strano SD, Shcharynski S, et al. Using sonography to screen women with mammographically dense breasts. AJR Am J Roentgenol 2003;181(1): 177–82.

11. Gordon PB, Goldenberg SL. Malignant breast masses detected only by ultrasound. A retrospective review. Cancer 1995;76(4):626–30.

12. Kaplan SS. Clinical utility of bilateral whole-breast US in the evaluation of women with dense breast tissue. Radiology 2001;221(3):641–9.

13. Kolb TM, Lichy J, Newhouse JH. Comparison of the performance of screening mammography, physical examination, and breast US and evaluation of factors that influence them: an analysis of 27,825 patient evaluations. Radiology 2002;225(1):165–75.

14. Leconte I, Feger C, Galant C, et al. Mammography and subsequent whole-breast sonography of non-palpable breast cancers: the importance of radiologic breast density. AJR Am J Roentgenol 2003; 180(6):1675–9.

15. Berg WA. Supplemental screening sonography in dense breasts. Radiol Clin North Am 2004;42(5): 845–51, vi.

16. Feig S. Cost-effectiveness of mammography, MRI, and ultrasonography for breast cancer screening. Radiol Clin North Am 2010;48(5):879–91.

17. Corsetti V, Houssami N, Ferrari A, et al. Breast screening with ultrasound in women with mammography-negative dense breasts: evidence on incremental cancer detection and false positives, and associated cost. Eur J Cancer 2008;44(4):539–44.

18. Nothacker M, Duda V, Hahn M, et al. Early detection of breast cancer: benefits and risks of supplemental breast ultrasound in asymptomatic women with mammographically dense breast tissue. A systematic review. BMC Cancer 2009;9:335.

19. Berg WA. Rationale for a trial of screening breast ultrasound: American College of Radiology Imaging Network (ACRIN) 6666. AJR Am J Roentgenol 2003;180(5):1225–8.

20. Berg WA, Blume JD, Cormack JB, et al. Combined screening with ultrasound and mammography vs mammography alone in women at elevated risk of breast cancer. JAMA 2008;299(18):2151–63.

21. Berg WA, Zhang Z, Lehrer D, et al. Detection of breast cancer with addition of annual screening ultrasound or a single screening MRI to mammography in women with elevated breast cancer risk. JAMA 2012;307(13):1394–404.

22. Ohuchi N, Takanori I, Masaaki K, et al. Randomized controlled trial on effectiveness of ultrasonography screening for breast cancer in women aged 40-49 (J-START): research design. Jpn J Clin Oncol 2011; 41(2):275–7.

23. ACR practice guideline for the performance of a breast ultrasound examination. American College of Radiology. Revised 2011 (Resolution 11). Available at: http://www.acr.org/~/media/52D58307E93E45898B09D4C4D407DD76.pdf. Accessed April 25, 2013.

24. Kelly KM, Dean J, Comulada WS, et al. Breast cancer detection using automated whole breast ultrasound and mammography in radiographically dense breasts. Eur Radiol 2010;20(3):734–42.

25. Kelly KM, Dean J, Lee SJ, et al. Breast cancer detection: radiologists' performance using mammography with and without automated whole-breast ultrasound. Eur Radiol 2010;20(11):2557–64.

26. Lander MR, Tabár L. Automated 3-D breast ultrasound as a promising adjunctive screening tool for examining dense breast tissue. Semin Roentgenol 2011;46(4):302–8.

27. The SOMO-INSIGHT study. 2013. Available at: http://www.somoinsightstudy.org. Accessed June 25, 2013.

28. Sickles EA. The use of breast imaging to screen women at high risk for cancer. Radiol Clin North Am 2010;48(5):859–78.

29. Berg WA. Beyond standard mammographic screening: mammography at age extremes, ultrasound, and MR imaging. Radiol Clin North Am 2007;45(5):895–906, vii.

30. Hooley RJ, Greenberg KL, Stackhouse RM, et al. Screening US in patients with mammographically dense breasts: initial experience with Connecticut Public Act 09-41. Radiology 2012;265(1):59–69.

31. Berg WA, Zhang Z, Cormack JB, et al. Multiple bilateral circumscribed masses at screening breast US: consider annual follow-up. Radiology 2013;268(3): 673–83.

32. Screening breast sonography in dense breasts. SBI statements. Available at: http://www.sbi-online.org/displaycommon.cfm?an=1&subarticlenbr=7. Accessed April 20, 2013.

33. Berg WA, Mendelson EB, Merritt CR, et al. ACRIN 6666: screening breast ultrasound in high-risk women. Published November 9, 2007. Updated November 30, 2007. Available at: http://www.acrin.org/Portals/0/Protocols/6666/Protocol-ACRIN%206666%20Admin%20Update%2011.30.07.pdf. Accessed April 25, 2013.

34. State of Connecticut Substitute Senate Bill No. 458; Public Act No. 09–41: an act requiring communication of mammographic breast density information to patients 2009.

35. Weigert J, Steenbergen S. The Connecticut experiment: the role of ultrasound in the screening of women with dense breasts. Breast J 2012;18(6): 517–22.

36. Parris T, Wakefield D, Frimmer H. Real world performance of screening breast ultrasound following enactment of Connecticut Bill 458. Breast J 2013; 19(1):64–70.

Automated Whole Breast Ultrasound

Stuart S. Kaplan, MD, FACR[a,b,*]

KEYWORDS

- Breast ultrasound screening • Dense breast tissue • Occult breast cancer
- Automated breast ultrasound • Coronal view

KEY POINTS

- Automated breast ultrasound is a developing technology that has recently been approved by the US Food and Drug Administration for use in screening for breast cancer as an adjunct to mammography.
- Given the current national trend toward adopting legislation requiring the reporting of breast density to women having mammography, and the requirement in some of this legislation requiring physicians to provide adjunctive screening such as ultrasound, the need for an efficient, reproducible method to provide such screening is developing.
- Automated breast ultrasound has become a viable option for providing widespread ultrasound screening to fulfill this newly developing demand for adjunctive breast cancer screening.

HISTORY

The use of bilateral whole breast ultrasound for women with dense breast tissue as an adjunct to screening mammography has been a topic of discussion and debate for many years. Several single-institution studies that validated ultrasound's use as an effective screening tool in the subset of women with dense tissue were published in the mid 1990s and early 2000s.[1–4] With these studies as a catalyst, a large multi-institutional trial was published in *The Journal of the American Medical Association* in 2008,[5] confirming the results of the earlier smaller studies. These published studies all showed a 0.3% to 0.5% cancer detection rate. However, in addition to the ability to detect occult breast cancer at an early stage in women with dense breast tissue, these studies shared several issues that have limited ultrasound's widespread implementation as a screening test. The 2 most important of these limitations are the number of false positives generated by ultrasound screening and the difficulty associated with offering and performing the examination because of a lack of adequate personnel, equipment, and time needed to perform and interpret the examination.

Most studies evaluating breast ultrasound for screening that have been published to date were designed using traditional hand-held scanning, with a radiologist having performed the actual scanning.[1,3–5] To date, only 2 studies have been published in which ultrasound scanning was performed by an ultrasound technologist.[2,6] These 2 technologist-performed studies demonstrated equivalent cancer detection results when compared with studies using physician-performed scanning. Despite these results, performance of the examination has remained one of the obstacles for implementing an ultrasound screening program outside of a study protocol. On average, a hand-held bilateral screening ultrasound examination takes 15 minutes to complete,[2]

[a] Breast Imaging, Mount Sinai Medical Center, Comprehensive Cancer Center, 4306 Alton Road, Miami Beach, FL 33140, USA; [b] Department of Radiology, Mount Sinai Medical Center, 4300 Alton Road, Miami Beach, FL 33140, USA
* Breast Imaging, Mount Sinai Medical Center, Comprehensive Cancer Center, 4306 Alton Road, Miami Beach, FL 33140.
E-mail address: skaplan659@aol.com

Radiol Clin N Am 52 (2014) 539–546
http://dx.doi.org/10.1016/j.rcl.2014.01.002
0033-8389/14/$ – see front matter © 2014 Elsevier Inc. All rights reserved.

though 1 study demonstrated the examination could be completed in 5 minutes.[1] In most patient populations, at least 40% of patients will have dense breast tissue, and therefore would be candidates for screening ultrasound. Radiologists working in medium- to high-volume centers do not have the time necessary to spend scanning the number of patients recommended for the examination. Although training ultrasound technologists to perform the examination is a viable option, most radiologists have been reluctant to introduce this concept into their normal daily practice.

The necessity for radiologists to offer screening breast ultrasound has become more of an issue in recent years. The diligence of advocacy groups has increased public awareness with regard to the concept that dense breast tissue limits mammography's ability to detect breast cancer. The nonprofit organization Are You Dense is the most active of these groups. This organization has been instrumental in helping to pass legislation in several states that requires a patient to be informed of her breast density as part of the mammography report sent to both the physician and the patient. In addition, breast density has been established as an independent risk factor for breast cancer. As the number of states adopting these laws continues to increase, the demand for supplemental ultrasound screening will grow. In addition, attempts are being made to pass a federal law requiring breast density reporting to all patients throughout the United States. If this legislation is passed, widespread offering of supplemental screening ultrasound will become necessary.

A recent technological advance may provide the impetus (or the solution if mandated by law) for the widespread implementation of ultrasound as an adjunct to mammography for breast cancer screening. Automated breast ultrasound (ABUS) is a technology in which ultrasound scanning is performed mechanically, eliminating the effect of operator dependence on image quality and reproducibility.

EQUIPMENT/SYSTEMS

Currently, there are several types of automated breast ultrasound systems available. Thus far, only 1 system has been granted US Food and Drug Administration (FDA) approval specifically for use in breast cancer screening in the United States.

One system uses a standard ultrasound transducer mounted onto an articulating arm (**Fig. 1**). Scanning is then accomplished by mechanically moving the articulating arm over the breast, in a way similar to the way in which hand-held ultrasound is performed. Imaging data are acquired continuously throughout the scanning process, and stored on a computer hard drive for review and interpretation on a workstation by a radiologist at his or her convenience. This technique does not allow for 3-dimensional manipulation or reconstruction of the raw data. The imaging is reviewed in real time, in the same fashion as any standard ultrasound examination would be reviewed, either at the time the examination is performed, or later if the examination were recorded and stored. Several studies have been published in which this type of automated system was utilized, with results similar to those studies using hand-held ultrasound for screening.[7,8]

Another type of automated scanner currently available has been FDA approved for screening and operates in a different fashion from handheld ultrasound. These units acquire raw data via a larger transducer similar in size and shape to a standard mammography compression paddle (**Fig. 2**). The transducer paddle is placed over the breast, with a small amount of compression

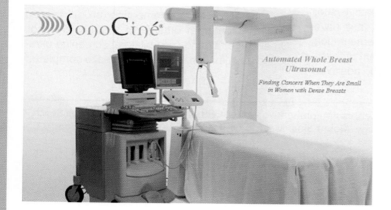

Fig. 1. FDA-approved ABUS using an articulating arm for scanning. This system works in conjunction with a standard ultrasound transducer and unit. (*Courtesy of* SonCiné, Reno, NV; with permission.)

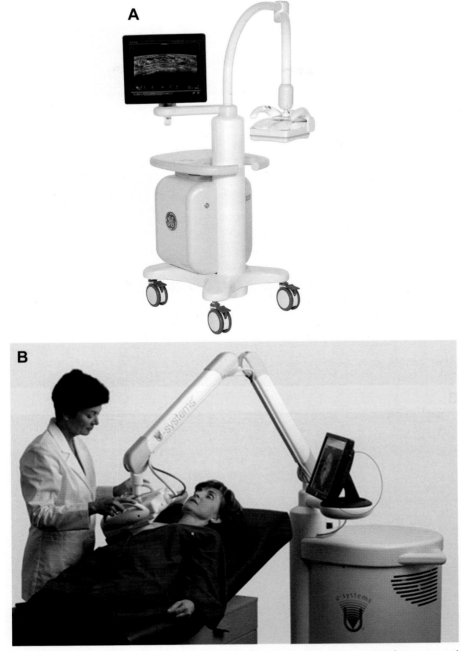

Fig. 2. (*A, B*) FDA-approved ABUS using a transducer similar in size to a mammography compression paddle. This ABUS is a stand-alone unit that acquires and processes the ultrasound images. (*Courtesy of* GE Healthcare, Wauwatosa, WI; with permission.)

applied to stabilize the breast. Three image acquisitions of each breast are usually sufficient to image virtually all of the breast tissue, excluding the axilla. In women with larger breasts, 4 or 5 acquisitions of each breast may be needed. The total time to complete the examination is on average 15 minutes. Once the imaging data are obtained, the data are processed using computer algorithms and stored on a hard drive. The images can then be reviewed on a standard workstation. During interpretation, images can be displayed in the transverse, coronal, or sagittal planes using 3-dimensional reconstruction of the data (**Fig. 3**). These systems therefore provide additional clinical information not available with standard hand-held ultrasound.

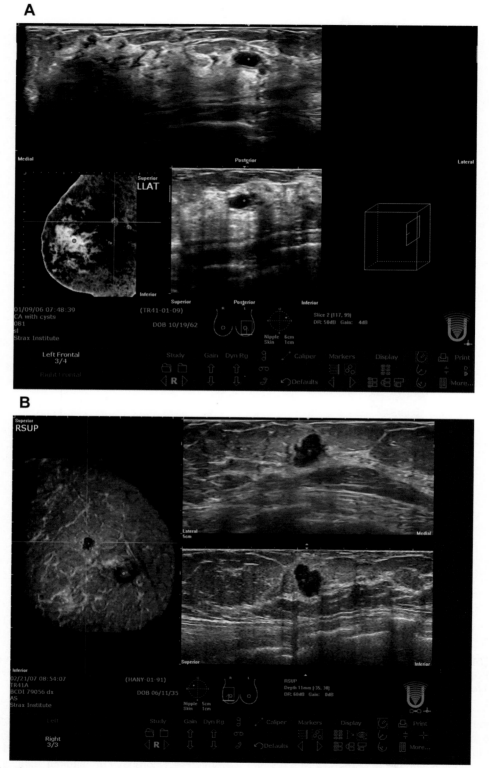

Fig. 3. (A, B) Work station screen display showing ABUS images. The lower left image in (A) and the left image in (B) are coronal views. Localization, measurement, and other image manipulation tools are seen in the lower portion of the screen. (*Courtesy of* GE Healthcare, Wauwatosa, WI; with permission.)

Other automated ultrasound units in development utilize a scanning procedure with the patient lying prone on the table (**Fig. 4**). Scanning is performed in a rotational manner, with the transducer configured to obtain circumferential data acquisition. The raw data are then processed and reconstructed to allow for 3-dimensional rendering.

TECHNOLOGY

The technology involved in generating images for automated breast ultrasound is virtually the same as in traditional hand-held ultrasound. Images are displayed in typical gray scale. Currently, neither Doppler applications nor elastography is available for automated ultrasound. The transducer footprint is large, approximating the size of a standard mammography compression paddle. A proprietary material is used on the portion of the transducer in contact with the breast, which in combination with scanning gel, allows for maximum skin contact and minimal artifact due to air gaps. A curved transducer designed to follow the contour of the breast has been developed, which further maximizes image quality and access to the maximum amount of breast tissue. The transducer used for scanning currently is a 14 MHz linear transducer. The current versions of ABUS systems allow only for automated scanning; however, future developments will likely also provide a hand-held attachment to allow for targeted scanning of areas of interest detected on the automated scan while the patient is still present in the department or clinic, thus reducing the necessity for the patient to be called back. This would also allow for ultrasound-guided interventional procedures to be performed using a single ultrasound unit, eliminating the need for facilities to have an additional ultrasound system for targeted scanning and interventional procedures.

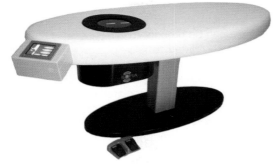

Fig. 4. ABUS in development. This system has a scanning window in the tabletop for prone imaging using standard ultrasound transducers. (*Courtesy of* iVu Imaging Corporation, Grapevine TX; with permission.)

There are some limitations in automated ultrasound technology. Artifacts that occur during data acquisition remain an issue that can cause false-positive results or can obscure actual findings. The area where the most significant artifact usually occurs is in the subareolar region, due to shadowing artifact caused by the nipple. The equipment manufacturers have worked diligently to reduce and potentially eliminate these artifacts, and have made significant improvements in this area. As the technology continues to evolve, the degree of artifact present in the scans should continue to diminish. Another limitation is anatomic in nature, as the scanning paddle cannot adequately include the axilla. Therefore, given the current design, there is incomplete assessment of the entire breast when performing an automated scan. Further strategies and methods to more completely include the axillary breast tissue are needed.

CLINICAL USE/WORKFLOW

Regardless of the type of automated system used, automated ultrasound offers several advantages over traditional hand-held ultrasound scanning. First, there is consistency and reproducibility when using an automated system. Hand-held ultrasound is operator dependent, meaning that the ability to detect and accurately document clinically significant findings is dependent upon experience and expertise of the person performing the scanning. Because this skill is highly variable, the quality of the examination can vary between different technologists, and between technologist- and physician-performed scanning.

Second, operation of the automated system to acquire the scanning data does not require the use of an ultrasound technologist. Although an ultrasound technologist can operate the system, because knowledge of ultrasound physics and artifacts, breast anatomy, and scanning technique are not necessary to obtain the raw data, anyone can be trained to operate the equipment for scanning. Given their familiarity with assisting patients and with positioning compression paddles on the breast for mammography, a mammography technologist can perform the scanning. Because mammography technologists are an integral component of a breast center, the hiring of additional personnel may not be necessary when introducing automated ultrasound into a breast imaging practice. Alternatively, if mammography technologists are not available to perform the automated ultrasound examination, virtually any other breast center personnel can be trained to perform the examination. The elimination of the need to hire high-salaried ultrasound technologists to successfully perform screening ultrasound is an appealing feature of ABUS.

Another advantage involves the time to acquire the raw data, which is more consistent in ABUS. The total acquisition time averages 15 minutes for a patient with average-sized breasts, and slightly longer if more than the standard 3 views of each breast are needed in women with larger breasts. This timing is consistent, since only acquisition of data is being performed while the patient is on the scanning table. This differs from hand-held ultrasound, during which the technologist needs to document, label, and measure all significant findings, extending the time to perform the examination significantly. Knowing that a consistent amount of time is needed to complete the process of scanning a patient is an advantage to breast centers, in that they can allocate the proper time slot for each patient, with confidence that there will not be unexpected delays, thus improving efficiency of patient throughput. Newer systems in development have been demonstrated to reduce the scanning time even further, thus allowing for even faster patient throughput.

A significant difference in automated versus handheld screening ultrasound involves the amount of physician time spent performing and interpreting the examination. In a setting in which the technologist performs hand-held scanning, the physician time involves only interpretation, which is usually minimal. For a negative examination, the physician only needs view the images to confirm there are no overlooked findings, and then complete the report, which should take under 1 minute. Even when there are significant findings, typically there is only one or a few that need to be evaluated. The technologist has already done all measurements, and often presents a written summary or diagram to the radiologist along with the images for interpretation. The radiologist can then easily review the case and issue the report. Although longer than a negative examination, this process still only takes a few minutes in the majority of cases. Using ABUS, it is the radiologist who must review the raw data, scrolling through all images and searching for significant findings. As with all new technologies, there is a learning curve involved in this process. Initially, it may take 10 to 15 minutes for a radiologist to complete the assessment of a single ABUS case, even when negative. When there are significant findings, the radiologist must determine the location of the findings and perform measurements, which add to interpretation time. With experience, the efficiency of this process increases. On average, when a radiologist becomes comfortable reviewing and interpreting ABUS images, the time to read a negative examination should take approximately 3 minutes. The time should increase to approximately 5 minutes when there are 1 or 2 significant findings. Occasionally, a case may still require 10 minutes or longer to fully interpret and report.

There are a few factors that can alter the amount of time needed to interpret an ABUS examination. Some radiologists have advocated the use of the coronal view to triage the case for areas needing more detailed evaluation. The coronal view is unique to ABUS in breast ultrasound evaluation, as it can only be obtained through 3-dimensional reconstruction of the raw data (see **Fig. 3**). Using the coronal view is a way to quickly evaluate the case, and then spend time on areas of interest. The coronal view is especially useful in detecting areas of architectural distortion, which can be difficult to appreciate on standard axial (transverse/longitudinal) images. However, caution must be taken in placing too much confidence using only the coronal view when interpreting a case. After initially viewing the coronal images, the entire data set should also be scrolled through in the traditional axial (transverse/longitudinal) view before providing a final interpretation.

A scenario that would significantly diminish the time required of the radiologist in ABUS interpretation would involve the use of an ultrasound technologist or Radiology physician assistant (P.A.) in the initial viewing of the ABUS images. This would serve a similar function to the technologist's role in current handheld ultrasound screening. The technologist or P.A. would review the entire data set, and perform any necessary measurements and location determination of significant findings. The radiologist could then perform a less detailed review than necessary if interpreting the case without assistance. In this situation, a review of only the coronal view, and evaluation of specific lesions if present as indicated by the technologist or P.A., may suffice. Peer reviewed research of this possible interpretation model are needed before it can be brought to clinical use.

Concerns related to false positives have been the most significant limiting factor preventing widespread adoption and implementation of screening breast ultrasound. An associated concept that has been discussed is the "call back rate" from whole breast ultrasound. The acceptable call back rate from screening mammography has been established as 6–13%.[9] However, this performance level has been achieved via implementation of screening mammography throughout the United States for almost 50 years. The established standard for callback rate from mammography needed to evolve to an acceptable level over time, as Radiologists became more experienced and technology improved. Screening ultrasound has not yet had the benefit of long term experience to allow for reduction of call back rates or false positive rates to more acceptable percentages, which should happen naturally as more Radiologists perform and interpret the exam. Additionally, recall rates have been shown to be significantly higher on baseline exams than in situations where comparison exams are available. Almost all of the data related to call back and false positive rates for screening ultrasound have been established based on the performance of a single, or "baseline" exam. Again, as the technique evolves, having comparisons should lower the necessity for follow-up and biopsy of screening ultrasound findings.

To examine this issue further, the definition of what constitutes a "call back" needs to be established. In most settings where hand-held screening ultrasound is performed, a Radiologist reviews the images from the study while the patient is still present in the Breast Center. Therefore, patients do not need to be "called back" from screening, as significant findings can be evaluated by the Radiologist by personally scanning the patient when necessary. Although this constitutes a "call back" based on current guidelines, in many cases verification results in confirmation that the finding is benign, and requires nothing more than routine follow up. This situation would not add significant anxiety or other emotional responses by the patient, as has been suggested as a negative outcome from breast ultrasound screening. Even in situations where a short-term (6 month follow up) or biopsy are recommended, the patient can be given this information at the time of the exam, limiting anxiety related to delay in communication of results. In a recent article discussing the "breast density conundrum",[10] D'Orsi discusses the concept that any additional images taken beyond what constitutes a routine exam should be considered an abnormal test for auditing purposes. This concept, although accurate if following the established auditing definition of a negative screening exam, introduces unfair assessment of ultrasound screening regarding call back rate or positive screening data. The fact that a technologist documents a benign, simple cyst should not make that test a positive screen, any more so than seeing benign calcifications should result in a screening mammogram being considered a positive screening finding. This auditing issue needs further discussion and evaluation to establish a consistent and fair assessment of ultrasound screening.

Unlike real-time hand-held ultrasound, automated ultrasound may result in patients needing to be recalled for additional evaluation of findings detected on the screening exam. This is because interpretation is performed after the exam has concluded and the raw data and has been processed for interpretation, in a similar fashion to the way screening mammography is interpreted. Once the radiologist reviews the images, the patient may be recalled for targeted ultrasound of specific findings that may not be conclusive based on the screening exam. This would be similar to the situation in which a patient is recalled for further evaluation of findings on a screening mammogram.

To date, there has been little data published regarding call back rates from screening ultrasound. In the ACRIN 6666 multi-institutional trial, the call back rate from ultrasound screening is reported as 5.4%,[5] and is described as patients that were "recommended for additional imaging". As previously discussed, in spite of the screening recall rate from the ACRIN trial, this occurrence should be infrequent with handheld scanning, assuming the radiologist is available to review the images prior to the patient leaving the Breast Center. This issue needs further evaluation regarding automated ultrasound, as there is no current published data demonstrating recall rates from automated scanning. It is possible that with automated ultrasound, the call back rates may be lower than with handheld, given the ability to use 3D reconstruction and view masses and other findings in all imaging planes. With these advantages, it may be easier to make determinations regarding biopsy versus short-term or routine follow up of findings without the need to re-scan the patient. Furthermore, the advent of computer assisted detection/diagnosis for use with both handheld and automated ultrasound may enhance diagnostic abilities further.

Another important issue regarding ABUS and screening breast ultrasound in general is reimbursement for performance and interpretation of the examination. At this time, no insurance code exists specifically reimbursing for ultrasound used for screening. This has been a significant limitation in the implementation of ultrasound for breast cancer screening. Although the FDA has approved the use of the U-Systems technology (GE Healthcare, Wauwatosa, WI, USA) for screening, accompanying CPT and ICD-9 codes were not developed. There is a diagnosis code that does exist that accounts for inconclusive mammography due to dense tissue (ICD-9-cm 793.82), and the CPT code 76645 can be interpreted to include ultrasound for screening,[11] so many practitioners have adopted these codes for use in ultrasound screening in order to get properly paid. However, there is a difference between applying existing codes and definitions to justify payment for screening and having an actual, specific code for the diagnosis and the examination. Some states that have adopted legislation requiring the reporting of breast density also include a requirement to provide ancillary screening, usually with ultrasound. In these states, payment for performance of the examination is also mandated through the legislation. Additionally, even if the existing codes are used and are accepted, many argue that the reimbursement resulting from the use of these codes is not sufficient to justify the expense in technology and personnel required to implement a breast ultrasound screening program. Radiologists, hospital and outpatient facility administrators, and legislators are addressing these issues. Equipment manufacturers are equally participating in the endeavor to develop an insurance code for screening. As the demand for screening ultrasound increases, the issue of reimbursement will need to be settled.

In summary, ABUS is a developing technology that has recently been FDA approved for use in screening for breast cancer as an adjunct to mammography. Given the current national trend toward adopting legislation requiring the reporting of breast density to women having mammography, and the requirement in some of this legislation requiring physicians to provide adjunctive screening such as ultrasound, the need for an efficient, reproducible method to provide such screening is developing. ABUS has become a viable option for providing widespread ultrasound screening to fulfill this newly developing demand for adjunctive breast cancer screening.

REFERENCES

1. Kolb TM, Lichy J, Newhouse JH. Occult cancer in women with dense breasts: detection with screening US—diagnostic yield and tumor characteristics. Radiology 1998;207:191–9.
2. Kaplan SS. Clinical utility of bilateral whole-breast US in the evaluation of women with dense breast tissue. Radiology 2001;221:641–9.
3. Buchberger W, Niehoff A, Obrist P, et al. Clinically and mammographically occult breast lesions: detection and classification with high-resolution sonography. Semin Ultrasound CT MR 2000;21:325–36.
4. Gordon PB, Goldenberg SL. Malignant breast masses detected only by ultrasound: a retrospective review. Cancer 1995;76:626–30.
5. Berg WA, Blume JD, Cormack JB, et al. Combined screening with ultrasound and mammography vs mammography alone in women at elevated risk for breast cancer. JAMA 2008;299(18):2151–63.
6. Hooley RJ, Greenberg KL, Stackhouse RM, et al. Screening US in patients with mammographically dense breasts: initial experience with Connecticut Public Act 09-41. Radiology 2012;265(1):59–69.
7. Kelly KM, Dean J, Comulada WS, et al. Breast cancer detection using automated whole breast ultrasound and mammography in radiographically dense breasts. Eur Radiol 2010;20(3):734–42.
8. Kelly KM, Richwald GA. Automated whole-breast ultrasound: advancing the performance of breast cancer screening. Semin Ultrasound CT MR 2011; 32(4):273–80.
9. Rosenberg RD, Yankaskas BC, Abraham LA, et al. Performance benchmarks for screening mammography. Radiology 2006;241:55–66.
10. D'Orsi CJ. The Breast Density Conundrum. Radiology 2013;269(3):646–7.
11. Kolb GR. Payment puzzle. Imaging Economics 2012;26–7.

High-Quality Breast MRI

R. Edward Hendrick, PhD

KEYWORDS

- Breast cancer detection • Contrast agent • Spatial resolution • Temporal resolution
- Technical quality

KEY POINTS

- High-quality breast magnetic resonance imaging (MRI) requires the competing factors of high spatial resolution, good temporal resolution, high signal-to-noise ratios (SNRs), and complete bilateral breast coverage.
- High-quality breast MRI requires a modern MR scanner with a magnetic field strength of 1.0 T or higher, good magnetic field homogeneity, a bilateral breast coil with prone positioning, strong magnetic gradients with short rise times, and good fat suppression over both breasts.
- The key pulse sequence for high-quality breast MRI is a multiphase 3D gradient-echo sequence performed bilaterally with submillimeter in-plane spatial resolution, thin slices, and temporal resolution of 1 to 3 minutes to correctly capture the morphology and time-enhancement pattern of enhancing breast lesions.

INTRODUCTION

Early breast magnetic resonance imaging (MRI) studies conducted in the early to mid-1980s attempted to distinguish malignant breast lesions from benign lesions and normal breast tissues based on inherent tissue T1 and T2 values.[1,2] Malignant breast lesions were found to have higher T1 and T2 values than normal breast tissues, but shorter T1 and T2 values than most benign breast lesions such as fibroadenomas.[3–5] Significant overlap in both T1 and T2 values between benign and malignant breast lesions, however, discouraged the use of noncontrast breast MRI for cancer detection and diagnosis. It is now an accepted standard that high sensitivity to breast cancer requires contrast-enhanced breast MRI both without and with a gadolinium (Gd)-based paramagnetic contrast agent to identify enhancing lesions.[6–10] Most recent studies of contrast-enhanced breast MRI have reported sensitivities to breast cancer between 90% and 100%, depending on the subject cohort, imaging techniques, including other imaging tests performed along with breast MRI, and criteria for breast cancer.[11–16]

One of the limitations of contrast-enhanced breast MRI has been the lack of standardized imaging protocols, contrast agent administration, image postprocessing, and image review. A major step forward has been standardization of breast MRI reporting terminology through publication of the fourth edition of the American College of Radiology's (ACR's) Breast Imaging Reporting and Data System (BI-RADS), which included reporting terminology for breast MRI and breast ultrasound, as well as mammography.[17] Another recent step forward has been the initiation of the ACR's Breast MRI Accreditation Program, which is described briefly at the end of this article.

This article provides specific recommendations for achieving high-quality breast MRI. Because of different MRI hardware, software, and scanning capabilities, it is not possible to achieve complete uniformity of protocols, but fairly specific guidelines for equipment requirements and scanning protocols are given for performing bilateral contrast-enhanced breast MRI with high spatial resolution, good temporal resolution, and high signal-to-noise ratio (SNR). This article describes the technical parameters needed to achieve

Department of Radiology, School of Medicine, University of Colorado–Denver, Anschutz Medical Campus, 12700 E. 19th Avenue, MS C-278, Aurora, CO 80045, USA
E-mail address: edward.hendrick@gmail.com

Radiol Clin N Am 52 (2014) 547–562
http://dx.doi.org/10.1016/j.rcl.2013.12.002

consistently high-quality contrast-enhanced breast MRI.

EQUIPMENT REQUIREMENTS

MRI systems used for breast cancer detection and diagnosis should include (1) adequate magnetic field strength with good magnetic field homogeneity across both breasts, (2) adequate magnetic field gradients to permit fast gradient-echo imaging, (3) a bilateral breast coil enabling prone positioning, and (4) good fat suppression over both breasts.

These requirements are discussed individually.

Adequate Magnetic Field Strength and Homogeneity

The magnetic field strength of whole-body MRI systems ranges from 0.064 T to 8 T (1 T = 10,000 G; the naturally occurring magnetic field at the earth's surface ranges from 0.25 to 0.65 G). MRI systems approved by the Food and Drug Administration (FDA) for clinical use have magnetic field strengths up to 3.0 T. Above a few tenths of a Tesla, image SNRs per voxel go up approximately linearly with magnetic field strength, if receiver coil design, voxel size, and imaging parameters other than field strength remain constant.[18] Thus, higher magnetic field strength (B_0) should provide higher SNR per voxel for breast imaging for the same pulse sequence, although the linear increase in SNR with field strength is moderated somewhat by the increase in tissue T1 values at higher field strengths. T1 values increase by about 20%, going from 1.5 T to 3.0 T.[19]

Most breast MRI is done on 1.5-T scanners, with a few sites performing breast MRI at 1.0 to 1.2 T and a growing number of sites performing breast MRI at 3.0 T. Although SNR per voxel is nearly doubled for the same pulse sequence at 3.0 T, compared with 1.5 T, 3.0 T systems have some additional technical challenges.[20] It is more difficult to get uniform fat suppression on 3.0-T systems than on 1.5-T systems (**Fig. 1**). In addition, artifacts are often more pronounced at 3.0 T than at 1.5 T. Most importantly, higher-frequency radio waves used for tissue excitation are more highly attenuated. Because 3.0-T systems have double the resonant frequency of 1.5-T systems, the penetration of radiofrequency (RF) waves transmitted to excite breast tissues, the B_1-field, is less uniformly distributed within breast tissues at 3.0 T because of greater absorption by external tissues. This causes nonuniformity of signal excitation and, thus, nonuniform measured signals.

Kuhl and colleagues[21] compared contrast-enhanced breast MRI at 1.5 T and 3.0 T in the same group of 37 patients. Overall image quality scores were slightly higher and differential diagnosis of enhancing lesions was made with greater confidence at 3.0 T, as shown by larger areas under the receiver operating characteristic curve.[21] The investigators pointed out, however, that technical problems exist at 3.0 T beyond those observed at 1.5 T.[22] These included increased nonuniformity of transmitted B_1 RF waves, particularly between left and right breasts with the larger field-of-view (FOV) used for transaxial scanning. This in turn led to reduced enhancement of lesions located in "low B_1 areas."[22] The investigators used a 2-dimensional (2D) gradient-echo pulse sequence, pointing out that the adverse effects of low B_1 areas on lesion enhancement should be reduced with the 3D (volume) sequences more commonly used in the United States because of the shorter repetition times (TRs) used in 3D imaging. Others have pointed out that B_1 nonuniformities can be reduced by using 3D techniques, careful choice of flip angle to match the TR of the imaging sequence, smaller FOV (eg, sagittal rather than transaxial acquisitions), and optimized shimming of the acquisition volume.[23]

Another reason for performing breast MRI at magnetic field strengths of 1.0 T or greater, beyond higher SNR, is to ensure higher static magnetic field homogeneity over the entire imaged volume. High magnetic field homogeneity for breast imaging means that the static magnetic field strength (B_0) should remain nearly constant across both breasts, including the chest wall and axillae. Because hydrogen nuclei in water and fat differ in resonant frequencies by 3.4 parts per million (ppm), the magnetic field homogeneity must be significantly less than 3.4 ppm to achieve good chemically selective fat suppression of hydrogen signals from fat, while preserving hydrogen signals from water.

The standard criterion to ensure that chemically selective fat suppression is effective is that the magnetic field strength should vary by less than 1 ppm over the entire volume of tissue being imaged. At 1.5 T, a nonuniformity of 1 ppm would amount to a magnetic field difference of 1.5 μT (microTesla), or a resonant frequency difference of 63.9 Hz, compared with the water-fat frequency difference of 224 Hz (3.4 ppm). The static magnetic field should be homogeneous to this level across a FOV 30 to 35 cm in diameter encompassing both breasts. This is generally not possible for low-field to midfield scanners (less than 1.0 T), and is a challenge even for high-field scanners, as the location

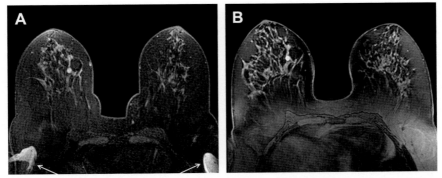

Fig. 1. Same slice of a fat-suppressed T1-weighted transaxial scan of volunteer imaged on a 1.5-T scanner (*A*) and 3.0-T scanner (*B*). All acquisition parameters other than magnetic field strength were matched between the 2 scanners. Note the more uniform fat-suppression in (*A*) and higher SNR in (*B*). Aliasing artifacts (signal wrap) of the volunteer's arms from the opposite sides (*arrows*) are visible in (*A*).

of the breasts in prone-positioned breast MRI typically is not at the isocenter of the magnet. Instead, in most magnets, the breasts are below isocenter to allow prone positioning of the patient, with breasts in the breast coil, and to allow adequate space for the patient's torso in the magnet bore.

A Bilateral Breast Coil with Prone Positioning

Bilateral imaging is recommended for the following reasons: (1) Clinical comparison of both breasts is as important in breast MRI as it is in mammography. Bilateral comparison helps identification of focal enhancement and helps prevent overcalling of physiologic enhancement, which tends to occur bilaterally, especially in premenopausal women and postmenopausal women on hormone replacement therapy.[24,25] (2) Data from recent breast MRI studies indicate that when a breast cancer occurs, there is a 3% to 5% chance that breast MRI will detect a mammographically occult cancer in the contralateral breast.[26–31] (3) Unilateral imaging in the transaxial or coronal plane can incur image wrap (or aliasing) artifacts from the contralateral breast, especially if phase encoding is set left-to-right (as it typically is in transaxial imaging), a bilateral breast coil is used, and the field-of-view is narrowed to include only the breast being imaged.

Bilateral breast imaging is typically performed using the body coil as the RF-transmit coil and a prone-positioned bilateral breast coil as the RF-receiver coil. A few systems, such as the Aurora breast MRI system, have bilateral breast coils serving as RF-transmit-receive coils. Modern breast coils, whether receive-only or transmit-receive coils, have multiple-channel elements. Bilateral breast coils currently have between 2 channels (1 channel for each breast) and 18 channels (9 channels for each breast). In multichannel coils, the received signals are recorded simultaneously using multiple amplifier and analog-to-digital converters. Multiple-channel receiver elements require a scanner capable of simultaneously recording multiple channels of data, so it is important to make sure that scanner hardware and software can accommodate the number of channels in the breast coil.

Multiple receiver channels were developed to boost coverage and signal uniformity, but acquired a single dataset for image reconstruction. A technique developed over the past decade, parallel imaging, modifies data acquisition so that different channels or sets of channels simultaneously acquire different datasets simultaneously.[32,33] In parallel imaging, each coil element (or set of coil elements) acquires different pieces of the image simultaneously, or in parallel; then, more complex image reconstruction techniques are used to recombine the different partial datasets into planar images or volumes. Parallel imaging also requires a short prescan to map out the sensitivity profile of each coil element (or set of coil elements) on each patient. This is done in a separate acquisition on some scanners and within the parallel imaging pulse sequence itself on other scanners. Some parallel imaging techniques acquire multiple channels of data in physical space, whereas others acquire multiple channels of data in spatial frequency (or k-) space.[32,33] Parallel imaging speeds image acquisition by a prespecified factor (eg, 2, 3, or 4), but requires longer for image reconstruction after all data have been acquired. Parallel imaging typically is done with an acceleration factor of 2, which cuts the acquisition time nearly in half. Use of higher-acceleration factors in breast imaging tends to cause image reconstruction artifacts (**Fig. 2**) and has been avoided in most clinical practices.

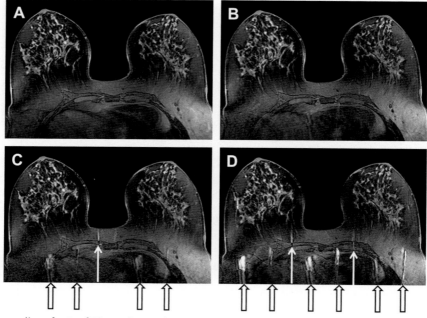

Fig. 2. The same slice of sets of 3D gradient-echo sequences acquired on the same volunteer using a 3.0-T scanner without (*A*) and with (*B–D*) parallel imaging using acceleration factors (AF) of 2 to 4. All were acquired with the same FOV, matrix, and slice thickness. Total acquisition time for each 3D gradient-echo acquisition covering both breasts was 102 seconds without parallel imaging (*A*), 57 seconds with AF = 2 (*B*), 42 seconds with AF = 3 (*C*), and 34 seconds with AF = 4 (*D*). Note the presence of parallel imaging reconstruction artifacts in (*C*) and (*D*) (*arrows*). As a result of more artifacts with higher AF values, most sites performing parallel imaging in breast MRI use an AF of 2.

Adequate Magnetic Field Gradients

Magnetic field gradients are produced by additional coils that generate magnetic fields (each pointing along the static magnetic field, B_0) that intentionally vary the magnetic field strength linearly along each of the 3 perpendicular axes: x, y, and z (**Fig. 3**). Gradient fields are switched on and off rapidly during each repetition of the pulse sequence to spatially resolve the source of signal by briefly altering the precessional frequencies of hydrogen nuclei at different locations as a function of x, y, or z location. The knocking noise heard from MR units as they scan is due to magnetic field gradients being turned on and off.

Two parameters characterize the performance of magnetic field gradients: (1) Maximum gradient strength, expressed in milliTesla per meter (mT/m), plays a role in determining how small voxels can be made. Modern MR scanners have magnetic field gradient strengths of up to 50 mT/m. (2) Gradient rise times describe the time interval needed for a magnetic gradient to go from zero to maximum strength, which in turn determines

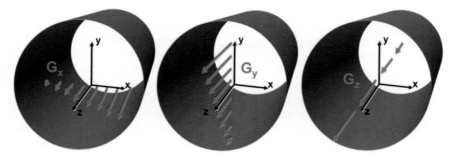

Fig. 3. The x, y, and z gradients shown within the bore of a solenoidal magnet. The main static magnetic field, B_0, points along the z direction, which is also the direction of the magnetic field of each gradient; x, y, or z gradients, when applied, alter the strength of the magnetic field pointing along the z-axis as a function of the x, y, or z direction, respectively.

how quickly pulse sequences can be performed. The shorter the gradient rise time, the shorter TR and echo time (TE) can be made in 2D or 3D gradient-echo imaging. Modern MR scanners have gradient rise times as short as 200 microseconds, yielding TR values as short as 4 ms and TE values as short as 1 ms. Generally, to achieve adequate spatial resolution and short enough imaging times in 3D gradient-echo imaging, TR needs to be shorter than 10 ms and TE needs to be less than 4 ms. In gradient-echo sequences without or with incomplete fat suppression, TE should be carefully chosen to minimize chemical-shift artifacts.[33]

Good Fat Suppression Over Both Breasts

In 2D or 3D MRI, fat suppression is typically achieved by applying a frequency-selective 90° saturation pulse that acts only on the hydrogen nuclei in fat (**Fig. 4**). In 2D imaging, this saturation pulse is applied to each slice at the start of each pulse sequence repetition; in 3D (volume) imaging, this saturation pulse is applied to the entire volume of tissue within the RF-transmit coil. If applied uniformly across both breasts, the fat suppression pulse effectively eliminates fat signal from signal measured during the pulse sequence repetition that follows. **Fig. 5** shows examples of T1-weighted bilateral breast MRI without fat suppression, with good fat suppression, and with incomplete fat suppression. Fat suppression is useful in contrast-enhanced breast MRI because it reduces the signal from fat in both precontrast and postcontrast scans. In postcontrast scans, lack of

fat suppression makes it more difficult to separate enhancing breast lesions from fat, because fat and enhancing breast lesions have similar signal intensities. In subtracted images (postcontrast images minus precontrast images), even a small amount of motion or misregistration between precontrast and postcontrast scans causes structured noise artifacts that complicate interpretation and, in some cases, simulate enhancing lesions. Good fat suppression in both precontrast and postcontrast images minimizes the structured noise of misregistration artifacts in subtracted images, allowing detection of smaller enhancing lesions or nonmasslike lesions with greater reliability.

PULSE SEQUENCE REQUIREMENTS

Beyond good equipment, high-quality breast MRI requires the use of appropriate pulse sequences. Breast MRI pulse sequences should include several noncontrast series, performed before contrast administration, along with a multiphase series of pulse sequences applied just before and several times after contrast agent administration. Recommended pulse sequences include (**Fig. 6**):

1. Scout images obtained in transaxial, sagittal, and coronal planes.
2. A T1-weighted non–fat-saturated series obtained bilaterally, including axillae and chest wall, to distinguish fat from water-based tissues including fibroglandular tissue, cysts, lymph nodes, and other benign lesions, muscle, and cancers.

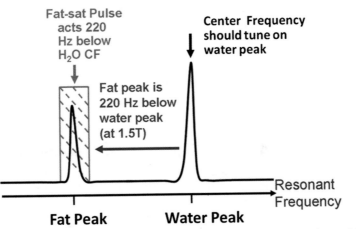

Fig. 4. Schematic of the resonant frequency difference between hydrogen nuclei in fat and hydrogen nuclei in water at 1.5 T. The MR scanner's center frequency is tuned to the resonant frequency of hydrogen nuclei in water. When fat-saturation is selected, a saturation pulse is applied with a narrow frequency range to cancel the signal from hydrogen nuclei in fat molecules, which resonate at about 220 Hz (1 Hz = 1 cycle per second) lower frequency than the hydrogen nuclei in water at 1.5 T. At 3.0 T, the frequency shift between hydrogen fat and water peaks doubles to about 440 Hz.

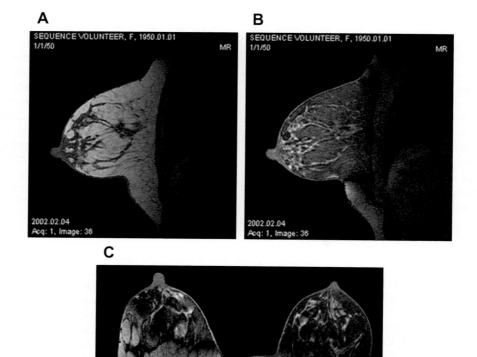

Fig. 5. T1-weighted breast MRI: (*A*) sagittal plane image without fat suppression; (*B*) sagittal plane image with uniform chemically selective fat suppression; (*C*) transaxial image with incomplete fat suppression. Fat saturation was adequate distally, but failed near the chest wall and on the lateral side shown on the left.

3. A T2-weighted fat-saturated series obtained bilaterally to distinguish cysts from solid lesions. A STIR (short inversion time [TI or tau] inversion recovery) series can be used in place of a T2-weighted series (**Fig. 7**) if TI is set correctly to minimize the signal from fat. A TI of about 180 ms at 1.5 T, or about 215 ms at 3.0 T, should do a good job of suppressing fat signal.[33] Good fat-suppression is important in either T2-weighted or STIR images, so that the brightest tissues in the image are fluid-filled cysts or blood vessels.

4. A multiphase 3D Fourier transform (3DFT or volume acquisition) gradient-echo T1-weighted pulse sequence acquired once before and multiple times after contrast agent administration, preferably with chemically selective fat-suppression, is used to identify the vascular bed and any enhancing lesions in the breast. T1-weighting is achieved by setting the pulse sequence TR short relative to the T1-values of tissues being imaged, setting the TE as short

as possible, and using a flip angle that is relatively small and based on the TR value to optimize SNR.[33]

Any modern MR scanner should be able to deliver the first 3 pulse sequences without difficulty. Scout images acquired in all 3 perpendicular planes are routine and should take less than 1 minute to acquire and display. Both T1-weighted non–fat-saturated and T2-weighted fat-saturated series can be obtained using accelerated spin-echo sequences, called fast spin-echo (FSE) or turbo spin-echo (TSE) sequences, in a time of less than 3 to 4 minutes for each series. If parallel imaging with an acceleration factor of 2 can be applied to these noncontrast series, scan times can be decreased by nearly a factor of 2, to about 2 minutes per series.

The key pulse sequence for breast cancer detection and lesion characterization is the multiphase 3D gradient-echo T1-weighted series acquired before and several times after MR contrast-agent

A

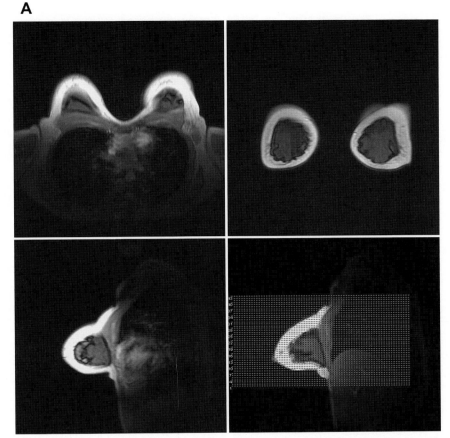

Fig. 6. (*A*) Scout images obtained on a woman with double-lumen implants. Scout images were obtained in the transaxial, coronal, and sagittal planes through both breasts. The second sagittal scout shows slice locations for subsequent transaxial T1-weighted and T2-weighted acquisitions. (*B*) One slice of 42 non–fat-saturated T1-weighted images using a 2D FSE sequence. (*C*) The same single slice of 42 fat-suppressed T2-weighted STIR images. Note on both T1-weighted and T2-weighted series a cyst anterior to the right implant with signal similar to that in the inner (saline) portion of the double-lumen implant. The cyst is dark on T1-weighted images and bright on T2-weighted or STIR images. (*D*) A single slice through the left breast in a bilateral multislice precontrast T1-weighted 3D gradient-echo image set. (*E*) The same slice from the first postcontrast series, acquired using the same bilateral multislice 3D gradient-echo series as in the precontrast set. On core biopsy, the enhancing lesion just anterior to the left implant was found to be a 4-mm Grade 3 invasive ductal carcinoma. (*F*) Subtraction of the precontrast slice shown in (*D*) from the postcontrast slice shown in (*E*), making more apparent the rim effect of contrast uptake in the enhancing lesion. (*G*) MIP reconstructed from the entire set of subtracted images of the left breast. The dataset is projected in a direction rotated nearly 180° from the primary sagittal acquisitions to better display the enhancing invasive ductal carcinoma. Note the absence of signal in the implant area of both subtracted and MIP images, since no contrast uptake occurred in that region. Note also that rim enhancement of the lesion, an important indicator of malignancy, is more clearly seen in postcontrast and subtracted series than in MIP images.

administration. Stronger gradients permitting very short TR and TE values, along with multichannel coils and scanner software permitting parallel imaging, have sped multiphase acquisitions, allowing improved spatial resolution by using a higher matrix (that is, more phase-encoding and frequency-encoding steps), while maintaining adequate SNRs per voxel. This has enabled breast MRI to meet all of the spatial resolution and temporal resolution goals listed below when proper pulse sequence techniques are used.

The important features of a contrast-enhanced multiphase T1-weighted series are as follows:

1. Consistent Gd-chelate contrast agent administration based on patient mass or weight: 0.1 mmol/kg, followed by a 20-mL saline flush.
2. Bilateral acquisition with prone positioning.
3. A multiphase 3D gradient-echo T1-weighted pulse sequence (1 precontrast and multiple postcontrast series extending at least 6 minutes after contrast injection).

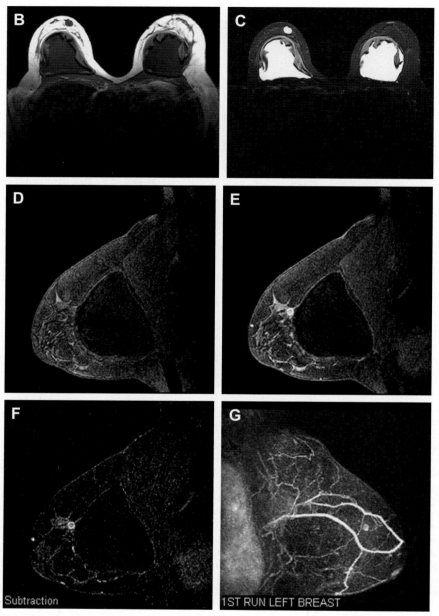

Fig. 6. (*continued*)

4. Adequately thin slices of 3 mm or less.
5. Pixel sizes of less than 1 mm in each in-plane direction.
6. Phase-encoding direction chosen to minimize artifacts across the breasts.
7. Total acquisition time for each series (or "phase" of the multiphase series) of 1 to 3 minutes.
8. Adequate SNR to visualize small enhancing vessels on 3D maximum intensity projection (MIP) images.

Each of these items is described in more detail in the following sections.

Gd-chelate Contrast Agent Administration: 0.1 mmol/kg Followed by 20 mL of Saline

Although MR contrast agents are not labeled specifically for breast cancer detection, use of an appropriate contrast agent is essential for high sensitivity to breast cancer. There are 6 MR contrast agents that are FDA-approved for use in the brain and spine (**Table 1**) and suitable for breast MRI. All are labeled for a recommended dose of 0.1 mmol/kg of patient body mass. All but one (Gadavist, Bayer Healthcare Pharmaceuticals Inc, Wayne, NJ, USA) are packaged in

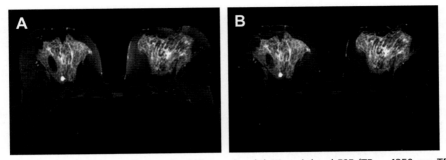

Fig. 7. The same slice of 44 transaxially acquired slices using (A) T2-weighted FSE (TR = 4350 ms, TE = 111 ms, echo-train length [ETL] = 15) and (B) fast STIR images (TR = 6080, TE = 59 ms, TI = 180 ms, ETL = 13). Tissue contrast is similar in both scans. Note the bright cyst near the chest wall of the left breast in both. Fat-suppression typically is more uniform in STIR images than in T2-weighted images, because in STIR images fat-suppression is based on the TI setting. Fat-suppression in T2-weighted images depends on achieving uniform chemically selective fat-suppression over the entire FOV, which in turn depends on the uniformity of the static magnetic field B_0 and the uniformity of transmitted RF excitations.

a concentration of 0.5 mmol/mL; therefore, in terms of packaged contrast agent volume, the recommended dose is 0.2 mL per kg of body mass. For example, a 140-pound woman has a body mass of 64 kg (140 lb/2.2 lb/kg = 64 kg) and her administered dose of MR contrast agent packaged at a concentration of 0.5 mmol/mL should be 13 mL (64 kg * 0.2 mL/kg = 12.8 mL) rounded to the nearest milliliter. A simple rule to follow to administer label-recommended doses of 0.1 mL/kg of body mass for agents packaged at 0.5 mmol/mL is to inject 1 mL (or 1 cubic centimeter, cc) of contrast agent for every 11 pounds of body weight. Using the previous example, a 140-lb woman should receive 140 lb * (1 mL/11 lb) ≈ 13 mL of Gd-chelate contrast agent.

Gadavist is packaged at a higher concentration of 1.0 mmol/mL, so half a much Gadavist should be administered for a given body mass to achieve a dose of 0.1 mmol/kg of body mass. A simple rule with Gadavist is to administer 1 mL (or 1 cc) of agent for every 22 lb of body weight.

Contrast agent should be administered with a controlled flow rate (most sites use a rate of 2 mL per second) followed immediately by a bolus of 20 mL of saline administered at a similar rate. This is best done with an dual-headed MR-compatible power injector that can administer both contrast agent and saline flush sequentially at controlled flow rates.

Bilateral Acquisition with Prone Positioning

Prone positioning in a dedicated bilateral breast coil positions the breasts pendently and reduces breast motion due to respiration and cardiac pulsation.

Table 1
Gd-chelated contrast agents approved for central nervous system indications in the United States (and used for breast cancer detection)

Agent	Common Name	Molecular Weight	Molarity, mol/L	Viscosity, cP, 37°C	Relaxivity α_1, L/(mmol·s)
Magnevist (Gd-DTPA)	Gadopentetate dimeglumine	938	0.5	2.9	4.1–4.9
Prohance (Gd-HP-DO3 A)	Gadoteridol	559	0.5	1.3	4.1–5.4
Omniscan (Gd-DTPA-BMA)	Gadodiamide	574	0.5	1.4	4.3–5.4
Optimark (Gd-DTPA-BMEA)	Gadoversetamide	662	0.5	2.0	4.7
Multihance (Gd-BOPTA)	Gadobenate dimeglumine	1058	0.5	5.3	6.7–9.7
Gadavist	Gadobutrol	605	1.0	5.0	5.2

Viscosities are measured in centipoises (cP) at 37°C (viscosity of water is 1.002 cP); Relaxivity α_1 is the relaxation rate (the inverse of relaxation time, T_1) per unit concentration of agent and is expressed in mmol/L)$^{-1}$s^{-1} or L/(mmol·s). Magnevist (Bayer Healthcare Pharmaceuticals Inc, Wayne, NJ, USA); Prohance (Bracco SpA, Milan, Italy); Omniscan (GE Healthcare, Princeton, NJ, USA); Optimark (Mallinckrodt Inc, St. Louis, MO, USA); Multihance (Bracco SpA, Milan, Italy).
Data from manufacturer's labeling and Rohrer M, Bauer H, Mintorovitch J, et.al. Comparison of magnetic properties of MRI contrast media solutions at different magnetic field strengths. Invest Radiol 2005;40(11):715–24.

Because the patient is supported by the coil at the sternum, lateral chest, and above and below the breasts, most respiratory and cardiac motion affects chest tissues posterior to the breasts. Any motion between precontrast and postcontrast scans or during scanning causes misregistration in subtracted breast images. By positioning the patient comfortably and by properly instructing the patient before the multiphase T1-weighted series (rather than during the series, such as just before administration of contrast agent), the MR technologist can help minimize breast and patient motion. Keeping total scan time reasonably short (20 minutes or less) will also help decrease patient discomfort and motion during scanning.

A 3D Fourier Transform Gradient-Echo T1-Weighted Pulse Sequence

T1-weighted pulse sequences are used in contrast-enhanced breast MRI because Gd-chelates, while shortening both T1 and T2, cause a greater fractional change in T1 than T2 (or T2*).[34] In gradient-echo imaging, T1 weighting is achieved by using a short TR, very short TE, and a relatively low flip angle that is matched to the TR.[33] For 3D Fourier transform (3DFT) imaging, extremely short TR values are used to keep the scan times for each phase of the multiphase series reasonably short, ideally 3 minutes or less. Although 2DFT pulse sequences acquire image data from a single plane at a time, 3DFT pulse sequences acquire image data from an entire volume at a time. Multislice 2DFT imaging typically has small gaps between individual slices, with Gaussian slice profiles. The 3DFT imaging acquires contiguous slices within the 3D volume, with rectangular slice profiles, so that no signal gaps occur between slices.

For 3DFT imaging, total acquisition time is $T_{total} = (TR)(N_{pe})(N_{acq})(N_{slices})$, where TR is the basic pulse sequence repetition time, N_{pe} is the number of in-plane phase-encoding steps to resolve signal in a single in-plane direction, N_{acq} is the number of times each phase encoding step is repeated (usually set to 1 in 3DFT imaging), and N_{slices} is the number of slices, which equals the number of phase-encoding steps used to separate the 3D volume in the third (slice-select) direction (in 2DFT imaging, N_{slices} is automatically set to 1). It is because of this additional factor, N_{slices}, which can be as high as 160 with slices comparable in thickness to the in-plane pixel size (isotropic voxels), that gradient-echo sequences with very short TR values are needed in 3DFT imaging. The 3DFT sequences have a signal-to-noise advantage over 2DFT sequences because signal is acquired from the entire excited volume of tissue, including both breasts, instead of from just a single plane, at each signal measurement. The 3DFT sequences require more phase-encoding steps (by the factor N_{slices}) to resolve not just a plane of tissue, but an entire volume of tissue, into individual voxels.

Adequately Thin Slices of 3 mm or Less

Slice thickness sets the limit on the smallest lesion that can be imaged without slice partial volume effects decreasing lesion contrast. Although slice thickness may not impair visualization of high-contrast lesions that enhance dramatically, it can play an important role in the detection of low-contrast lesions. To image a low-contrast lesion of a given diameter without partial volume effects, which would decrease its contrast relative to surrounding tissues, a slice thickness of half the lesion's diameter or less should be used. For example, to be sensitive to a low-contrast 5-mm enhancing lesion, a slice thickness of 2.5 mm or less should be used (**Fig. 8**). Thin slices are particularly important for minimizing partial volume effects on diffuse, non-masslike enhancing lesions, such as those sometimes associated with ductal carcinoma in-situ (DCIS) (**Fig. 9**).[33]

Pixel Sizes of Less than 1 mm in Each In-Plane Direction

Pixel sizes smaller than 1 mm in each in-plane direction can be achieved by selecting an acquisition matrix (number of phase-encoding and frequency-encoding steps) that exceeds the FOV (in mm) in both the phase-encoding and frequency-encoding direction. For example, in transaxial imaging with a 30 × 30 cm (300 × 300 mm) FOV, an acquisition matrix of 300 × 300 or greater should be used. If a 384 × 384 matrix were used for this FOV, each in-plane pixel would be (300 mm)/384 = 0.78 mm in each direction, which would give excellent spatial resolution. Sub-millimeter in-plane pixels are important for good lesion margin visualization, which helps distinguish benign from malignant enhancing lesions based on their morphology.[35]

Phase-Encoding Direction Chosen to Minimize Artifacts Across the Breasts

A primary cause of image artifacts (structured noise in MR images), is patient motion, including cardiac and respiratory motion. These motion artifacts propagate across the image in the in-plane phase-encoding direction, regardless of the direction of motion in the patient.[33] Therefore, it is essential to orient the in-plane phase-encoding direction to minimize artifacts across the breast. For

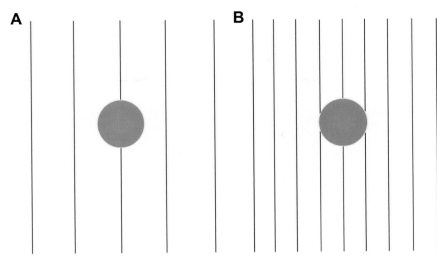

Fig. 8. Relationship between slice thickness and minimum lesion size seen without, or with minimal, partial volume effects. (*A*) Slice thickness equals lesion size. In this case, partial volume effects will significantly decrease lesion conspicuity. (*B*) Slice thickness equals one-half lesion size. Regardless of alignment of lesion and slices, in this case at least one slice will display the lesion without, or with minimal, partial volume effects.

sagittal plane acquisitions, the phase-encoding direction should be head-to-foot (or superior-inferior) (**Fig. 10**). For transaxial plane acquisitions, phase-encoding should be oriented left-to-right to ensure that cardiac and respiratory motion obscure a minimal amount of breast tissue (**Fig. 11**). For coronal plane acquisitions, phase encoding can be either left-right or head-to-foot, as cardiac and respiratory motion will not propagate across the breasts in either in-plane direction.

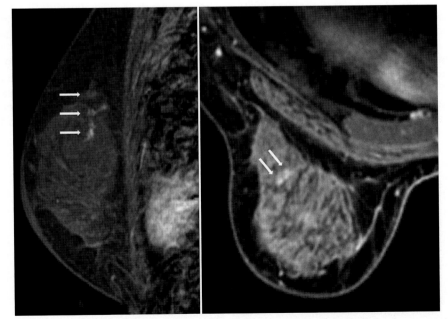

Fig. 9. Surveillance breast MRI in a 48-year-old woman revealed a subtle non-masslike enhancement in a linear/ductal, clumped pattern (*arrows*) in sagittally acquired and axially reconstructed images. Core biopsy demonstrated the enhancing lesion to be intermediate-grade cribriform and solid DCIS. Note that the enhancing lesion appears less sharp in the reconstructed axial image than in the originally acquired sagittal image because the slice thickness of acquired sagittal images exceeded the in-plane pixel size. The thicker slices in sagittally acquired images lowered spatial resolution in the slice-select direction, which is left-to-right in the reformatted axial images. (*Courtesy of* Robyn Birdwell, MD, Breast Imaging, Brigham and Women's Hospital, Boston, MA.)

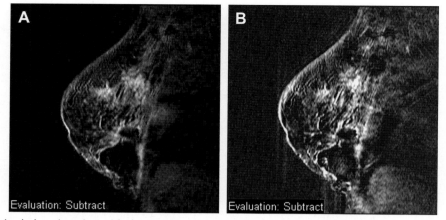

Fig. 10. Sagittal plane imaging with the phase-encoding direction: (*A*), correctly selected in the head-to-foot (or superior-inferior) direction, and (*B*), incorrectly selected in the anterior-posterior direction. Note in (*B*) that motion and wrap artifacts are propagated across breast tissue.

Phase-encoding is usually chosen to be head-to-foot for coronal imaging because it requires less spatial coverage than left-to-right, minimizing the number of phase-encoding steps needed.

Total 3DFT Acquisition Time for Each Series of 1 to 3 Minutes

The temporal resolution required for breast MRI is determined by the time course of contrast agent uptake. Peak contrast enhancement in malignant lesions typically occurs between 60 and 120 seconds after injection.[36] It is important to capture contrast uptake at or near its maximum with one of the postcontrast series. To do that, it is also important to know that 3DFT acquisitions have maximum contrast-weighting at the low spatial frequency acquisitions (ie, when the center of

k-space is being acquired), which occurs at one-third to one-half of the total pulse sequence acquisition time, depending on the manufacturer (eg, 3DFT sequences on Siemens acquire the center of k-space about one-third of the way into the full acquisition, on GE and Philips at half-way through sequence acquisition). The goal is to select imaging parameters that place the maximum contrast-weighting of the first postcontrast series at or near the time of peak contrast agent uptake. Assuming that peak enhancement of breast lesions occurs 90 seconds after contrast injection, you would like the center of k-space of the first postcontrast series to occur 90 seconds after the end of contrast injection. If you were using a Siemens 3DFT series with a 2-minute series scan time, peak contrast-weighting would occur at one-third of 2 minutes, or 40 seconds, into the series,

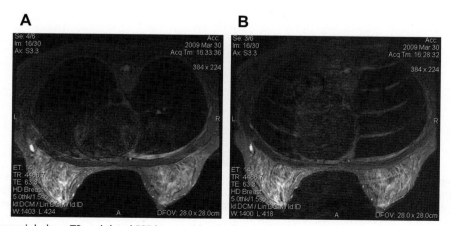

Fig. 11. Transaxial plane T2-weighted FSE images identically acquired, except with the phase-encoding direction: (*A*) correctly selected in the left-to-right direction, and (*B*) incorrectly selected in the anterior-posterior direction. In (*B*), cardiac and respiratory motion artifacts propagate across breast tissue.

so to properly time the center of k-space 90 seconds after injection, you would wait 50 seconds after injection to begin the first postcontrast series. If you were using a GE or Philips scanner with, for example, a 3-minute 3DFT acquisition, peak contrast weighting would occur at the midpoint of the series, so you would begin scanning immediately after injection to place maximum contrast-weighting at 90 seconds.

Typically, a precontrast series and several postcontrast series are acquired with identical acquisition parameters so that subtractions of precontrast from postcontrast images reveal only temporal changes. Thus, all precontrast and postcontrast series should be identical. A single precontrast scan should be acquired, followed immediately by contrast agent injection. A pause of scanning during, and perhaps after, contrast injection might be needed, depending on the calculation outlined previously to place peak contrast at the center of k-space of the first postcontrast series. Then, several postcontrast series should be acquired without pauses or delays between them, extending so that the last measurement samples the center of k-space at least 6 minutes after the end of contrast injection. This is done so that the detailed shape of the time-enhancement curve can be determined for any significantly enhancing lesions. Contrast agent uptake is best characterized by dividing enhancing

lesions into 3 categories: continuous uptake (Type 1), plateau (Type 2), or washout (Type 3) (**Fig. 12**). Kuhl and colleagues[37] demonstrated in a study of 266 enhancing lesions (101 breast cancers) that only 6% of lesions with Type 1 curves were malignant, 65% of lesions with Type 2 curves were malignant, and 87% of lesions with Type 3 curves were malignant. Characterizing lesions by both their morphology, which does not require multiple postcontrast time points, and their time-enhancement curve shape, which does, adds specificity to contrast-enhanced breast MRI. Thus, it is important to collect data with adequate temporal resolution, and adequate duration, to accurately capture the time course of lesion enhancement.

Initially, European breast MRI protocols emphasized the need for high temporal resolution, on the order of 1 minute per series, to gain specificity.[8] A subsequent article by Kuhl and colleagues[35] demonstrated that temporal resolution could be relaxed to approximately 2 minutes without sacrificing specificity, especially if that added time was used to improve spatial resolution to submillimeter in-plane pixels. More recent work by Gutierrez and colleagues[38] indicated that 3-minute temporal resolution was adequate to correctly characterize time-enhancement curve shapes when the center of k-space was properly positioned at approximately 90 seconds after contrast

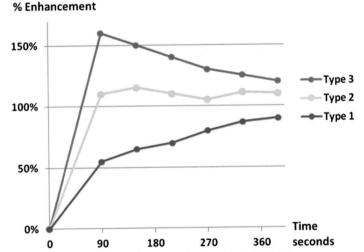

Fig. 12. Three time-enhancement curve types typical of enhancing breast lesions. Lesions with Type 1 curves have continuous uptake and have the lowest probability of malignancy. Lesions with Type 2 curves enhance by at least 80% to 100% from their noncontrast signal values and then demonstrate a plateau behavior, not gaining or losing signal appreciably from their peak value. Lesions with Type 2 curves have a moderate (40%–70%) suspicion of malignancy. Lesions with Type 3 curves have rapid uptake of contrast within 3 minutes of administration, then washout, and have a high (60%–80%) suspicion of malignancy. Images producing these curves were acquired every 60 seconds (1-minute temporal resolution), with the first postcontrast series acquired 90 seconds after contrast administration.

injection. In addition, the longer acquisition time per series of 3-minute acquisitions captured greater peak signal than 90-second acquisitions. Based on their findings, it appears that 3-minute temporal resolution is adequate to add specificity by correctly characterizing time-enhancement curve shapes. Going faster than 1 minute per series fails to add additional information about curve shape and decreases SNR per series.[33,39] Other studies, such as Schnall and colleagues,[39] have shown that, although curve shape and degree of lesion enhancement are important, lesion morphology assessment is an even more important factor in the overall accuracy of breast MRI for cancer detection.

Adequate SNR to Visualize Small Enhancing Vessels on 3D Maximum Intensity Projection Images

The ability to visualize small enhancing vessels (2–3 mm in diameter) on maximum intensity projection (MIP) images is a good surrogate for the ability to visualize small enhancing lesions on subtracted or MIP images. Failure to see relatively small blood vessels on subtracted or MIP images gives the radiologist little confidence that small or subtle enhancing lesions would be detected, if present. **Fig. 13** provides examples of good, SNR-deficient, and SNR-starved MIP images: good, marginal, and poor-quality breast MR images.

THE ACR BREAST MRI ACCREDITATION PROGRAM

The ACR Breast MRI Accreditation Program (BMRAP) began accrediting facilities that perform breast MRI on May 10, 2010. As of May 1, 2013, 1264 facilities have been accredited, with 72 facilities under review. The repeat rate for facilities is 20%. Like other ACR accreditation programs, the BMRAP includes requirements for personnel (radiologists, MRI technologists, and medical physicists), equipment, quality assurance, and

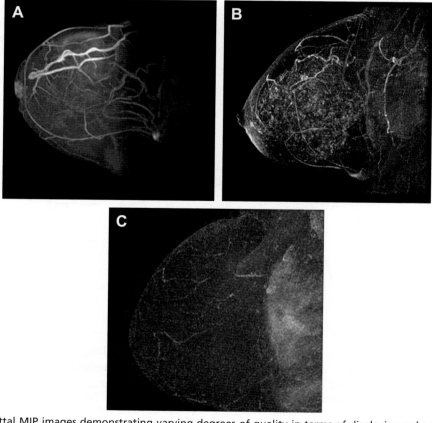

Fig. 13. Sagittal MIP images demonstrating varying degrees of quality in terms of displaying enhancing vessels (and lesions, if they were present): (A) good MIP image, where small vessels are clearly displayed; (B) marginal MIP image, where visibility of small vessels is limited due to low SNR; and (C) poor MIP image, due to extremely low SNR and no display of large or small vessels. The poor image quality in (C) gives low confidence that this scan would demonstrate a small or diffusely enhancing lesion, if present.

accreditation testing based on submission of clinical images to assess breast MRI scanning protocols and clinical image quality. A complete discussion of the BMRAP is beyond the scope of this article, but is available at http://www.acr.org/Quality-Safety/Accreditation/BreastMRI, including a complete list of BMRAP requirements, a Breast MRI Clinical Image Quality Guide, and complete procedures for applying for ACR Breast MRI Accreditation.

SUMMARY

Current MRI systems are capable of meeting the stringent technical requirements of performing multiphase T1-weighted contrast-enhanced scanning with high in-plane spatial resolution ($\leq$1 mm pixel sizes), thin slices ($\leq$3 mm thick), adequate temporal resolution (1–3 minutes), bilateral breast coverage, and adequate SNR to detect small or diffusely enhancing breast lesions. Careful attention to breast MRI equipment selection and breast MRI protocols is required to achieve all of these requirements simultaneously. The ACR's BMRAP provides a peer-review system for validating that breast MRI personnel, equipment, quality-control procedures, scanning protocols, and image quality are adequate to perform high-quality breast MRI.

REFERENCES

1. Ross RJ, Thompson JS, Kim K, et al. Nuclear magnetic resonance imaging and evaluation of human breast tissue: preliminary clinical trials. Radiology 1982;143:195–205.
2. El Yousef SJ, Alfidi RJ, Duchesnau RH, et al. Initial experience with nuclear magnetic resonance (NMR) imaging of the human breast. J Comput Assist Tomogr 1983;7:215–8.
3. McSweeney MB, Small WC, Cerny V, et al. Magnetic resonance imaging in the diagnosis of breast disease: use of transverse relaxation times. Radiology 1984;153:741–4.
4. Wiener JI, Chako AC, Merten CW, et al. Breast and axillary tissue MR imaging: correlations of signal intensities and relaxation times with pathologic findings. Radiology 1986;160:299–305.
5. Merchant TE, Thelissen GR, de Graaf PW, et al. Application of a mixed imaging sequence for MR imaging characterization of human breast disease. Acta Radiol 1993;34:356–61.
6. Heywang SH, Hahn D, Schmid H, et al. MR imaging of the breast using gadolinium-DTPA. J Comput Assist Tomogr 1986;10:199–204.
7. Heywang SH, Wolf A, Pruss E, et al. MR imaging of the breast with Gd-DTPA—preliminary observations. Radiology 1989;71:95–103.
8. Kaiser WA, Zeitler E. MR imaging of the breast: fast imaging sequences with and without Gd-DTPA. Preliminary observations. Radiology 1989;170:681–6.
9. Harms SE, Flamig DP, Hensley KL, et al. MR imaging of the breast with rotating delivery of excitation off-resonance: clinical experience with pathologic correlation. Radiology 1993;187:493–501.
10. Padhani AR. Contrast agent dynamics in breast MRI. In: Warren R, Coulthard A, editors. Breast MRI in practice. London: Martin Dunitz; 2002. p. 43–52.
11. Kriege M, Brekelmans CT, Boetes C, et al. Efficacy of MRI and mammography for breast-cancer screening in women with a familial or genetic predisposition. N Engl J Med 2004;351:427–37.
12. Kuhl CK, Schrading S, Leutner CC, et al. Mammography, breast ultrasound, and magnetic resonance imaging for surveillance of women at high familial risk for breast cancer. J Clin Oncol 2005;23: 8469–76.
13. Tilanus-Linthorst MM, Obdeijn IM, Bartels KC. MARIBS study. Lancet 2005;366:291–2.
14. Stoutjesdijk MJ, Boetes C, Jager GJ, et al. Magnetic resonance imaging and mammography in women with a hereditary risk of breast cancer. J Natl Cancer Inst 2001;93:1095–102.
15. Warner E, Plewes DB, Hill KA, et al. Surveillance of BRCA1 and BRCA2 mutation carriers with magnetic resonance imaging, ultrasound, mammography, and clinical breast examination. JAMA 2004;292:1317–25.
16. Morris EA, Liberman L, Ballon DJ, et al. MRI of occult breast carcinoma in a high-risk population. AJR Am J Roentgenol 2003;181:619–26.
17. Ikeda DM, Hylton NM, Kuhl CK, et al. BI-RADS: Magnetic resonance imaging. In: D'Orsi CJ, Mendelson EB, Ikeda DM, et al, editors. Breast imaging reporting and data system: ACR BI-RADS – Breast imaging atlas. 1st edition. Reston (VA): American College of Radiology; 2003.
18. Edelstein WA, Glover GH, Hardy CJ, et al. The intrinsic signal-to-noise ratio in NMR imaging. Magn Reson Med 1986;3:604–18.
19. Rakow-Penner R, Daniel B, Yu H, et al. Relaxation times of breast tissue at 1.5T and 3T measured using IDEAL. J Magn Reson Imaging 2006;23:87–91.
20. Barth MM, Smith MP, Pedrosa I, et al. Body MR imaging at 3.0 T: understanding the opportunities and challenges. Radiographics 2007;27:1445–62.
21. Kuhl CK, Jost P, Morakkabati N, et al. Contrast-enhanced MR imaging of the breast at 3.0 and 1.5 T in the same patients: initial experience. Radiology 2006;239:666–76.
22. Kuhl CK, Kooijman H. Effect of B1 inhomogeneity on breast MR imaging at 3.0T [letter to the editor]. Radiology 2007;244:929–30.
23. Mountford CE, Stanwell P, Ramadan S. Breast MRI at 3.0 T. Radiology 2008;248:319–20.

24. Friedman PD, Swaminathan PV, Herman K, et al. The importance of bilateral imaging. Am J Roentgenol 2006;187:345–9.

25. Kuhl CK, Kreft BP, Bieling HB, et al. Dynamic breast MRI in premenopausal healthy volunteers: normal values of contrast enhancement and cycle phase dependency. Radiology 1997;203:137–44.

26. Liberman L, Morris EA, Kim CM, et al. MR imaging findings in the contralateral breast of women with recently diagnosed breast cancer. Am J Roentgenol 2003;180:333–41.

27. Lee SG, Orel SG, Woo IJ, et al. MR imaging screening of the contralateral breast in patients with newly diagnosed breast cancer: preliminary results. Radiology 2003;226:773–8.

28. Lehman CD, Blume JD, Thickman D, et al. Added cancer yield of MRI in screening the contralateral breast of women recently diagnosed with breast cancer: results from the International Breast Magnetic Resonance Consortium (IBMC) trial. J Surg Oncol 2005;92:9–15 [discussion 15–6].

29. Slanetz PJ, Edmister WB, Yeh ED, et al. Occult contralateral breast carcinoma incidentally detected by breast magnetic resonance imaging. Breast J 2002;8:145–8.

30. Viehweg P, Rotter K, Laniado M, et al. MR imaging of the contralateral breast in patients after breast-conserving therapy. Eur Radiol 2004;14:402–8.

31. Lehman CD, Gatsonis C, Kuhl CK, et al. MRI evaluation of the contralateral breast in women with recently diagnosed breast cancer. N Engl J Med 2007;356:1295–303.

32. Glockner JF, Houchun HH, Stanley DW, et al. Parallel imaging: a user's guide. Radiographics 2005;25:1279–97.

33. Hendrick RE. Breast MRI: fundamentals and technical aspects. New York: Springer; 2008. p. 156–62.

34. Hendrick RE, Haacke EM. Basic physics of MR contrast agents and maximization of image contrast. J Magn Reson Imaging 1993;3:137–48.

35. Kuhl CK, Schild HH, Morakkabati N. Dynamic bilateral contrast-enhanced MR imaging of the breast: trade-off between spatial and temporal resolution. Radiology 2005;236:789–800.

36. Kuhl C. The current status of breast MR imaging, part I. Choice of technique, image interpretation, diagnostic accuracy, and transfer to clinical practice. Radiology 2007;244:356–78.

37. Kuhl CK, Mielcarek P, Klaschik S, et al. Dynamic breast MR imaging: are signal intensity time course data useful for differential diagnosis of enhancing lesions? Radiology 1999;211:101–10.

38. Gutierrez RL, Strigel RM, Partridge SC, et al. Dynamic breast MRI: does lower temporal resolution negatively affect clinical kinetic analysis? AJR Am J Roentgenol 2012;199:703–8.

39. Schnall MD, Blume J, Bluemke DA, et al. Diagnostic architectural and dynamic features at breast MR imaging: multicenter study. Radiology 2006;238:42–53.

Approach to Breast Magnetic Resonance Imaging Interpretation

Sarah Palestrant, MD, MPhil[a],
Christopher E. Comstock, MD[b], Linda Moy, MD[a],*

KEYWORDS

- Breast cancer • Magnetic resonance imaging • BI-RADS

KEY POINTS

- A systematic and organized approach to the interpretation of breast magnetic resonance (MR) images should be used to improve diagnostic accuracy. Radiologists should develop a consistent viewing protocol and review all images.
- The breast MR imaging reporting should include the clinical history, MR imaging techniques, comparison with prior studies, findings, and the overall Breast Imaging-Reporting and Data System (BI-RADS) assessment.
- Any suspicious morphologic feature should prompt biopsy regardless of the kinetic features.
- The margins of a mass and the type of initial increase of enhancement are two features that strongly predict the likelihood of malignancy.

INTRODUCTION

Dynamic contrast-enhanced (DCE) breast magnetic resonance (MR) imaging is established as an important tool for the detection of mammographically occult cancers and for the evaluation of breast lesions.[1–9] It is used in all aspects of patient management, including preoperative staging for extent of disease, evaluation of treatment response, and continued surveillance for recurrence.[10,11] Breast MR imaging also has emerged as a powerful tool in screening high-risk women, with cancer detection yields of up to double that of mammography and even of mammography and ultrasonography combined.[6,8,12–16] Screening MR imaging has led to the detection of mammographically occult, early stage breast cancers. These breast cancers tend to be small, node-negative tumors with good prognoses.[7,12,14,16]

The success of DCE breast MR imaging interpretation is based, in part, on the reader's ability to correctly detect, assess, and manage suspicious findings. As multiple studies have shown, breast MR imaging is highly sensitive compared with conventional mammography (77%–91% for MR imaging vs 32.6%–50% for mammography), but with lower specificity (81%–97.2% across screening studies for MR imaging vs 93%–99% for mammography).[4,5,7,14,15] Part of the goal of improving interpretation relies on maximizing pretest probability, through patient selection, obtaining all relevant clinical history and reviewing prior imaging and histopathology reports. In addition, interpretation relies significantly on the images, which demand optimal technique. With the images obtained, a systematic and organized approach to interpretation should be used to assess all the

The authors have no financial disclosures.
[a] Department of Radiology, New York University School of Medicine, New York, NY 10016, USA; [b] Department of Radiology, Memorial Sloan-Kettering Cancer Center, New York, NY 10065, USA
* Corresponding author. NYU School of Medicine, NYU Cancer Institute, Breast Imaging Center, 160 East 34th Street, 3rd Floor, New York, NY 10016.
E-mail address: linda.moy@nyumc.org

Radiol Clin N Am 52 (2014) 563–583
http://dx.doi.org/10.1016/j.rcl.2013.12.001
0033-8389/14/$ – see front matter © 2014 Elsevier Inc. All rights reserved.

images. This article discusses practical approaches to breast MR imaging interpretation and reporting.

BEFORE THE EXAMINATION
Current Indications for Breast MR Imaging

The American College of Radiology (ACR) guidelines for the performance of DCE breast MR imaging outline the role the examination plays in breast cancer screening and diagnosis.[17] A common diagnostic indication is preoperative staging to assess the extent of disease in women with invasive carcinoma and ductal carcinoma in situ (DCIS). The sensitivity of MR imaging in detecting in situ and invasive breast cancer is high (between 94% and 100%).[2,3,14] Breast MR imaging is also helpful in the evaluation of residual disease in postlumpectomy women with positive margins and in the detection of a recurrence. Other diagnostic indications include evaluation of treatment response in women undergoing neoadjuvant chemotherapy, detection of an occult primary breast carcinoma in women presenting with a metastatic axillary adenopathy, and lesion characterization when other imaging studies and physical examination are inconclusive. At the authors' institution, breast MR imaging for screening purposes is the most commonly used indication and is summarized briefly here.

In 2007, the American Cancer Society (ACS) issued guidelines for breast cancer screening with MR imaging as an adjunct to mammography.[18] The guidelines stratify asymptomatic women into 3 groups: high, intermediate, and low risk. The ACS recommends annual screening MR imaging for women at high risk for breast cancer. This category includes women who are BReast CAncer genes 1 and 2 (BRCA1 or BRCA2) mutation carriers or who have a first-degree relative with a known BRCA mutation. In addition, first-degree relatives and carriers of the PTEN or TP53 genetic mutations are considered to be at high risk of breast cancer. They include women with Li-Fraumeni syndrome, Cowden syndrome, or Bannayan-Riley-Ruvalcaba syndrome. In addition, women who have undergone radiation therapy to the chest between the ages of 10 and 30 years are also considered high risk. By definition, the high-risk group has a greater than 20% lifetime risk of breast cancer and, as such, should undergo annual screening breast MR imaging and mammography.

The ACS guidelines state that there is insufficient evidence to recommend for or against annual screening MR imaging in women categorized as moderate/intermediate risk for breast cancer.[18]

Women with a lifetime risk of 15% to 20% are placed in this category. They include women with a personal history of lobular carcinoma in situ, atypical lobular hyperplasia, or atypical ductal hyperplasia. Also, women with a personal history of breast cancer, including DCIS, may also benefit from annual screening MR imaging. In addition, women with mammographically dense breasts are considered at moderate risk. It is recommended that the groups of women listed earlier speak with their doctors about the benefits and limitations of supplemental MR imaging screening in addition to mammography. In addition, annual MR imaging screening is not recommended for women whose lifetime risk of breast cancer is less than 15%.

In order to calculate a woman's lifetime risk for breast cancer, various risk models have been proposed. The initial ACS guidelines for screening MR imaging recommended the use of the BRCAPRO (A computer program that uses statistics to predict whether a person has an inherited mutation [change] in the BRCA1 and BRCA2 genes), Claus, or Tyrer-Cuzick models.[18] In 2012 the ACS published a review of current cancer screening guidelines and further discussed the choice of these models.[19] They highlighted the importance of including both maternal and paternal first-degree and second-degree relatives. However, these three models identify different populations deemed eligible for MR imaging screening.[20]

Patient Information Gathering

Once the appropriate patients are selected for breast MR imaging, it is important to obtain the clinical history (ie, the reason for the breast MR imaging). Before the examination, the patient's personal history should be reviewed. It is imperative to learn whether the patient has undergone prior breast procedures, such as biopsies and surgeries, which can help explain imaging findings. The dates and reports for all prior biopsies and surgical excisions should be available. In addition, history of radiation, recent trauma, or certain medications (such as hormonal therapy) lend context to image interpretation. Prior imaging studies should similarly be reviewed at the time of MR imaging interpretation. Often, it is a prior mammogram or ultrasonography result that was the impetus for the MR imaging study. Other times, the prior study may provide additional clues that compliment the patient's history. For instance, a prior mammogram may more readily show a biopsy clip or fat necrosis. The radiologist can then approach the MR images with the knowledge of where to look for a correlate.

In 2 scenarios, namely history of prior procedures or the symptomatic patient, a marker should be placed on the skin, over the site of scar or palpable lump, respectively. The marker of choice is a vitamin E capsule, placed by the radiologist or technologist, as directed by the patient. Placing this landmark superficially on the skin allows radiologists to direct their attention to the area of concern within the breast.

Careful thought should be given to the scheduling of the examination based on the stage of the patient's menstrual cycle. Physiologic enhancement of normal background breast parenchyma may lead to false-positive findings, which in turn may require additional follow-up and/or biopsy. This background parenchymal enhancement (BPE) is influenced by hormonal changes, fluctuating with the menstrual cycle (**Fig. 1**).[21,22] The amount of enhancement is greatest during the first and last weeks of the menstrual cycle, when estrogen, which causes hyperemia, vasodilatation, and capillary leakiness, is at its peak.[22] As such, imaging should take place between days 7 and 14 of the menstrual cycle in order to minimize excessive BPE, which may obscure a suspicious enhancing abnormality.[22] Scheduling staff should ask the patient about the first day of her last menstrual cycle in considering when to appropriately schedule her examination. However, this may only be feasible for screening studies because it may not be desirable to delay imaging in the setting of a patient with recently diagnosed breast cancer referred for local staging before an already-scheduled surgery.

At the authors' institution, before imaging, the patient completes a written questionnaire, conveying her understanding of the examination indication, family history of breast cancer, personal history of biopsy or surgery, first day of last menstrual period, pertinent medication history, and at what facility prior examinations were performed. The technologist also draws a diagram to indicate where the vitamin E capsule has been placed and notes the reason for the marker placement (ie, biopsy or lumpectomy scar vs palpable lump) (**Fig. 2**). The patient must also complete a detailed MR imaging safety questionnaire to ensure that there are no metal implants or other contraindications to undergoing a MR imaging.

EXAMINATION ACQUISITION

There is no standard technique for performing DCE breast MR imaging. Most of the technical parameters including equipment (magnet field strength and type of breast coil), pulse sequences, timing of the dynamic contrast sequences, and postprocessing techniques vary between practice sites. To address these issues, both the ACR and the European Society of Breast Imaging have developed practice guidelines and technical standards for breast MR imaging.[23,24] The ACR also developed a breast MR accreditation program that includes technical requirements for optimizing this examination.[25] Therefore, the MR imaging technique should be included in all breast MR imaging reports. Certain technical issues are summarized later.

Equipment and Positioning

Proper dedicated equipment is necessary to optimize a breast MR imaging examination. The use of

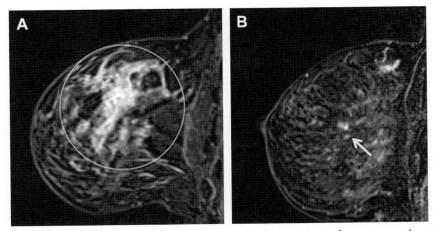

Fig. 1. Sagittal T1-weighted postcontrast subtraction image (*A*) shows 5.3 cm of non–mass enhancement in the right upper, inner breast in this premenopausal woman (*white circle*). The examination took place outside of the recommended window of 7 to 14 days. On the day of biopsy, sagittal T1-weighted postcontrast subtraction image (*B*) shows marked decrease in enhancement. The 8-mm area of enhancement (*white arrow*) was biopsied, pathology yielding benign fibrocystic breast changes.

BREAST MRI QUESTIONNAIRE

Name: _____   AGE: _____   SEX: F or M

Why are you having this study? (**please circle all that apply**)

Abnormal findings Mammogram or Ultrasound   Dense breast
Newly diagnosed breast cancer-pre surgical evaluation   Rule out implant rupture
History of atypia (LCIS, ADH, ALH)   You feel a lump
Post surgical-to check for residual disease   Breast cancer screening
You have tested positive for the BRCA gene
Family member has tested positive for BRCA gene   Other: _____
Strong family history of breast cancer: if yes, who? (mother/grandmother/sister/aunt)
    At what age were they diagnosed?

When was the first day of your last menstrual period? _____
Do you have DCIS? Yes or No
Were you recently diagnosed with breast cancer? Yes or No
Have you ever had breast cancer? Yes or No
    If yes, which breast and when? Right: _____   When? _____
                                    Left: _____   When? _____
    Did the tumor spread elsewhere in your body? Yes or No
    If yes, where did it spread to? _____
        What type of therapy did you receive?
    o Surgery: Right/Left   When? _____
    o Lumpectomy: Right/Left   When? _____
    o Mastectomy: Right/Left   When? _____
    o Chemotherapy: Yes or No   If yes, when? _____
    o Hormonal Therapy: Yes or no   If yes, when? _____
    o Radiation Therapy: Yes or No   If yes, when? _____

Have you had any other breast surgery? Yes or No
    If yes, when and what type?
        o Biopsy: Right: when? _____ Left: when? _____ Results: _____
        o Lumpectomy for *benign* mass: Right: when? _____Left: when? _____
        o Breast implants: Right: when? _____ Left: when? _____
           What type of implants do you have (saline/silicone or a mixture of both?)
        o Breast reduction: Right: when? _____ Left: when? _____

Have you had any other diagnostic breast exams? Yes or No
    If yes, what type of exam?
MRI: When? _____ Where? _____ Results: _____

Mammogram: When? _____ Where? _____ Results: _____

Ultrasound: When? _____ Where? _____ Results: _____

Do you feel a breast lump or mass? Yes or No   If yes, for how long? _____

Additional Tech Notes:

Fig. 2. Sample of patient questionnaire that all patients must complete before the imaging study, in addition to answering questions regarding MR imaging safety. The technologist draws a schematic representation of the breasts in the bottom box, indicating whether a vitamin E capsule was placed. If so, they then also note whether it was placed to indicate an area of palpable concern and/or site of biopsy or surgical scar.

dedicated bilateral breast coils and high-field magnets are essential components to obtain high a signal/noise ratio.[22–28] Breast MR imaging examinations should be performed on at least 1.5-T systems. Good patient positioning is another essential factor for a high-quality study. The patient is placed in the prone position, and both breasts should be symmetrically centered within the coil, placed as deeply in the coil as possible with the nipples pointing downward. More breast coverage may be obtained by placing both arms at the side of the body and not above the patient's head. Also, we have found that mild compression of both breasts decreases motion artifact (**Box 1**).[28]

Imaging Parameters

The pulse sequence parameters (eg, gradient echo or spin echo and whether a two-dimensional or three-dimensional [3D] format was used) should be included in the report. In addition, the scan orientation (axial, sagittal, or coronal), the use of T1-weighted or T2-weighted images, and method of fat suppression should also be reported. Localizer images are initially performed to evaluate for optimal positioning and to ensure full coverage of both breasts and axillae (**Fig. 3**). After these scout images have been reviewed, the noncontrast images can be obtained.

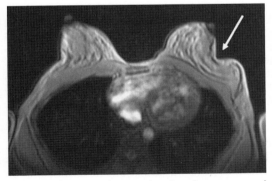

Fig. 3. Axial scout image showing improper positioning of the left breast with the outer breast not well drawn out into the coil (*white arrow*). This improper positioning may result in poor enhancement of the compressed tissue.

A noncontrast T1-weighted gradient-echo sequence without fat saturation is the first sequence that we perform after the scout images. This sequence is particularly helpful to identify fat in benign lymph nodes or hamartomas, to identify fat in scar tissue, and to aid in the diagnosis of benign fat necrosis (**Fig. 4**A, B).[28] Metallic clip signal void may be better delineated on this non–fat-saturated sequence.[29]

A noncontrast T2-weighted gradient-echo fat-saturated sequence is also included to help identify fluid-containing structures, which are usually benign, such as cysts (**Fig. 5**) or seromas (**Fig. 6**A, B). Lymph nodes, fibroadenomas, and occasionally hemorrhage may also be confirmed via their high signal intensity on this sequence.[30] Cancers usually have low to moderate signal intensities, with the rare exception of mucinous cancer and neoplastic necrosis producing T2 hyperintensity.

A precontrast T1-weighted gradient-echo sequence with fat saturation is obtained next. This sequence allows the technologist to see that good fat suppression has been obtained before contrast injection. This sequence is immediately followed by a contrast-enhanced, multiphase T1-weighted gradient-echo fat-saturated series. At present, there are 5 gadolinium contrast agents approved by the US Food and Drug Administration, none of which are labeled specifically for the detection of breast cancer. The labeled dose for all 5 contrast agents is the same: 0.1 mmol/kg at 2 mL/s. Gadolinium is administered via an intravenous injection followed by a 20-mL to 30-mL saline flush. Although there is no consensus for the number of time points or the time intervals to image, the ACR Breast MRI Accreditation Program recommends that the time per sequential acquisition should be less than 2 minutes.[25] At our institution, we perform continuous imaging for 6 to 7 minutes after injection; each acquisition is at less than 2-minute intervals. At least 3 acquisition points are needed, 1 precontrast and 2 postcontrast scans; at the authors' institution, 1 precontrast sequence and 3 postcontrast sequences are performed.[28] Postcontrast sequences are then subtracted from the precontrast T1 series in order to identify true enhancement as opposed to high T1 signal from hemorrhage or proteinaceous material.

Postprocessing

Use of image postprocessing, such as subtraction, maximum intensity projections (MIPs), 3D reconstruction, region of interest analysis, and computer-aided detection software generating automatic color mapping, should also be included in the breast MR imaging report.

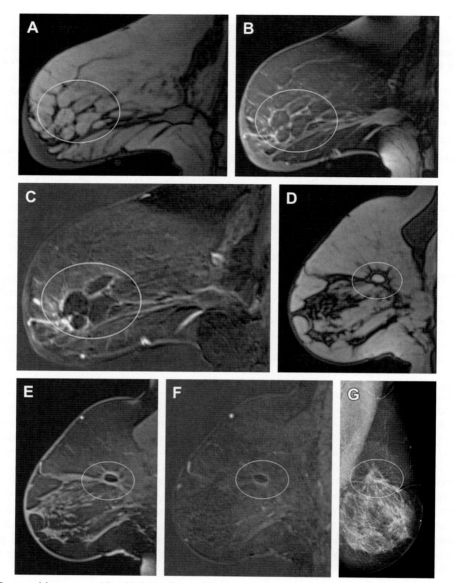

Fig. 4. A 73-year-old woman with a history of right breast cancer status post lumpectomy and radiation. Sagittal non–fat-saturated T1-weighted image (*A*) shows multiple adjacent oval masses of internal fat signal in the lumpectomy bed, measuring up to 6.3 cm in length (*white circle*). Sagittal fat-saturated postcontrast nonsubtracted (*B*) and subtracted (*C*) images show smooth, contiguous rim enhancement with central nonenhancement, consistent with fat necrosis (*white circle*). Companion case: a 57-year-old woman with left breast cancer status post lumpectomy 2 years prior. Sagittal non–fat-saturated T1-weighted image (*D*) shows a 1.6-cm oval, circumscribed, hyperintense mass (*white circle*). Sagittal fat-saturated postcontrast nonsubtracted (*E*) and subtracted (*F*) images show smooth surrounding enhancement, consistent with fat necrosis (*white circle*). Left mediolateral oblique (*G*) 6 months before the MR imaging correlates with MR imaging findings (*white circle*).

INTERPRETATION PROCESS

A systematic and organized approach is recommended when interpreting the breast MR imaging examination. It is important to develop a consistent viewing protocol to ensure that all the images have been reviewed. A global then focused assessment should be used, with inclusion of morphology and kinetics assessment if an abnormality is identified. The language used in conveying this information is also important. For lesion characterization, in an effort to standardize reporting, clinicians should use the ACR MR imaging Breast Imaging-Reporting and Data System (BI-RADS) lexicon classification. In 2003, the first edition of the MR

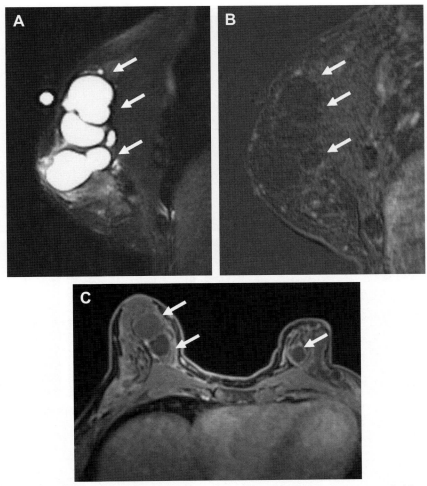

Fig. 5. Sagittal fat-saturated T2-weighted image (*A*) shows multiple, large, adjacent cysts (*white arrows*) in the central/superior right breast. Note the overlying vitamin E marker indicating the area of palpable concern as guided by the patient. Sagittal fat-saturated postcontrast T1-weighted image (*B*) shows no evidence of enhancement in the area of known cysts (*white arrows*). Axial fat-saturated postcontrast nonsubtracted T1-weighted image (*C*) shows 2 of the larger cysts as isointense round masses in the right breast as well as showing additional cysts in the left breast (*white arrows*).

imaging BI-RADS lexicon classification was published in the ACR BI-RADS Breast Imaging Atlas, with an updated version anticipated shortly.[31] These descriptor terms provide a standardized classification for breast imaging studies and show good correlation with the likelihood of breast malignancy. The BI-RADS system informs the referring physicians and radiologists about key findings and identifies appropriate follow-up and management.

Global Approach: Fibroglandular Volume and BPE

In the upcoming ACR BI-RADS – MRI lexicon, the background breast tissue composition will be included in the evaluation of mammograms, breast ultrasonography, and breast MR imaging. Therefore, the first assessment of breast MR imaging should be a global evaluation, in terms of characterizing background fibroglandular tissue (FGT) volume, an anatomic feature, and BPE, a physiologic feature. To evaluate FGT, clinicians must visually assess the amount of nonfatty, noncystic breast parenchyma in relation to the total breast volume on all images of both breasts.[32,33] The volume of fat can be measured by reviewing the non–fat-suppressed and fat-suppressed T1-weighted images, whereas the number and size of cysts can be assessed by evaluating T2-weighted images. With this knowledge of overall fat and cystic components, the amount of FGT can then be

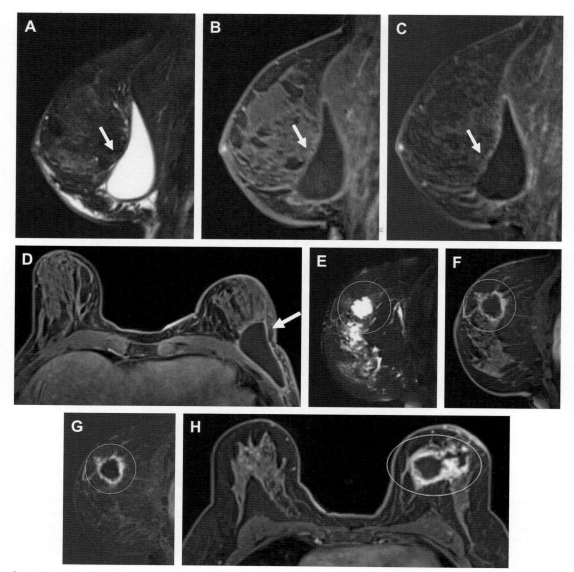

Fig. 6. A 42-year-old woman status post left breast lumpectomy 6 months prior. Sagittal fat-saturated T2-weighted image (*A*) shows a 6-cm homogeneously hyperintense collection (*white arrow*) in the inferior, posterior breast. Sagittal fat-saturated postcontrast nonsubtracted (*B*) and subtracted (*C*) as well as axial fat-saturated post-contrast (*D*) T1-weighted images show smooth, contiguous rim enhancement, consistent with a simple seroma (*white arrow*). Companion case: a 58-year-old woman with history of newly diagnosed left breast cancer, status post surgical excision 3 weeks prior. Sagittal fat-saturated T2-weighted image (*E*) shows a 4.5-cm hyperintense collection (*white circle*) in the upper, central breast. Sagittal fat-saturated postcontrast nonsubtracted (*F*) and subtracted (*G*), as well as axial fat-saturated postcontrast (*H*) T1-weighted images show asymmetric clumped rim enhancement, suspicious for residual disease (*white circle*). Patient underwent reexcision for positive margins, consistent with pathology findings.

calculated in conjunction with the postcontrast subtraction images. The MR imaging assessment of FGT is classified using a 4-point scale, similar to that recommended by the ACR to classify mammographic density, and in accordance with the anticipated BI-RADS MR imaging lexicon classification. A score of 1 is used to describe fatty breasts (<25% glandular); 2, scattered fibroglandular densities (25%–50% glandular); 3, heterogeneously dense breasts (51%–75% glandular); and 4, dense breasts (>75% glandular).[32,33]

With FGT established, clinicians must then assess for BPE. The BPE is enhancement of normal FGT, often in a stippled pattern (tiny dots, separated by normal tissue, sometimes confluent), assessed on the first postcontrast breast MR imaging sequence. In recent studies BPE was visually assessed by examining the breast parenchyma, using a combination of precontrast and postcontrast fat-suppressed T1-weighted and subtraction images. Both the volume and the intensity of enhancement were considered in this global assessment.[32–34] The MIPs are particularly useful to get an overview. The degree of enhancement is categorized into the following descriptive modifiers: minimal (<25% volumetric enhancement), mild (25%–50% volumetric enhancement), moderate (51%–75% volumetric enhancement), or marked (>75% volumetric enhancement) (**Fig. 7**).[32–34] Similar to increased mammographic breast density, moderate and marked BPE can obscure invasive and noninvasive cancer,

and decrease the sensitivity of MR imaging.[34,35] In addition, BPE does not necessarily correlate with FGT; even if the patient has a large volume of FGT, the tissue may not necessarily enhance.

For reasons already discussed, BPE reflects vascularity of the FGT. BPE depends on timing of the menstrual cycle and has been shown to change with hormonal fluctuations.[21,22,35] Recent studies have reported increased BPE as a result of hormone replacement therapy and decreased BPE as a result of antiestrogen medications including tamoxifen,[36] raloxifene,[37] toremifene,[38] and aromatase inhibitors.[39,40] Therefore, information regarding the date of the last menstrual cycle and/or the use of hormone replacement therapy or antiestrogen medications should be documented in the breast MR imaging report.

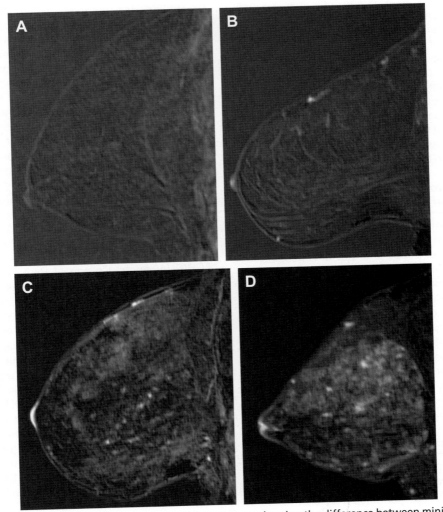

Fig. 7. Sagittal fat-saturated postcontrast T1-weighted images showing the difference between minimal (*A*), mild (*B*), moderate (*C*), and marked (*D*) BPE.

Although BPE has been shown not to correlate with breast density,[41] BPE is similar to breast density in that it is a characteristic of normal breast tissue. Breast tissue that is mammographically dense has been shown to negatively affect accuracy[42,43] and is considered to be an independent risk factor for breast cancer.[44–47] Increased mammographic density, a reflection of both stromal and epithelial tissues, as opposed to fat, is associated with a nearly 5-fold increased risk of developing breast cancer.[44–47] This strong association between breast cancer risk and the amount of fibroglandular tissue as measured by mammograms has been extended to the FGT as measured by MR imaging.[32] Several recent studies suggest that increased BPE may similarly affect both interpretation of breast MR imaging and risk for breast cancer. A positive correlation between follow-up recommendations,[33,34] biopsy rate,[33] and BPE has been shown. However, cancer yield as a function of BPE is an emerging topic that has been reported variably. Hambly and colleagues[34] and DeMartini and colleagues[33] showed no increased incidence of cancer with increase BPE, but King and colleagues[32] suggested a relationship between BPE and breast cancer risk. These recent studies point to potentially important roles of accurately assessing BPE for both examination specificity and patient risk assessment. As such, the ACR BI-RADS committee will likely include FGT and BPE assessments in the upcoming ACR BI-RADS MR imaging lexicon.

Focal Approach: Morphology and Kinetic Assessment

The ability of breast MR imaging to detect cancer depends on differences in vascularity between normal breast tissue and that of a neoplasm. A neoplasm, in order to be detected, needs to be visualized, which is done by the use of contrast enhancement. The most important feature in assessing for cancer is the presence of enhancement of any type[48]; similarly, nonenhancement has a negative predictive value of 100%.[49] As such, if a lesion is identified, a shift to a focused approach is necessary, with first morphologic then kinetic assessment. The first T1-weighted fat-saturation postcontrast images are particularly useful to assess any abnormal enhancement.

Morphologic Assessment

The first step in evaluating lesion morphology on breast MR imaging is to classify the lesion as a focus, mass, or nonmass enhancement.[31] An enhancing lesion that is less than 5 mm is classified as a focus. A focus is a tiny spot or dot of enhancement, which is generally round and smooth and without mass effect. It is usually too small to be characterized further morphologically in terms of margins and pattern of internal enhancement. There is no correlative finding on precontrast imaging.

In contrast, a mass is defined as a 3D, space-occupying lesion. The mass has definable margins and a separable, distinct edge from the surrounding tissue. Once detected, a mass should be described in terms of its shape, margin, and internal enhancement pattern. In the first edition of the BI-RADS – MRI lexicon, the shape of a mass may be classified as round, oval, lobular, or irregular.[31] Its margin may be assessed as smooth, irregular, or spiculated. In addition to shape and margin, the internal enhancement, which describes the pattern of enhancement, should also be assessed. This enhancement may be described as homogeneous, heterogeneous, central, peripheral (ie, rim enhancement), enhancing septations or dark internal septations.

As stated earlier, the descriptor terms show good correlation with the likelihood of breast malignancy. Nunes and colleagues[48] reported that certain MR findings predict benign disease; smooth or lobulated margins had a negative predictive value (NPV) for malignancy of 97% to 100%, absence of lesion enhancement had an NPV of 100%, and enhancement less than surrounding breast stroma had an NPV of 93% to 100%. The presence of dark internal septations in a smooth or lobulated mass is highly specific for a fibroadenoma, with a specificity of 93% to 97%.[26,28] Certain morphologic features strongly suggest malignancy, such as spiculated margins with a positive predictive value (PPV) of 76% to 88% and rim enhancement with a PPV of 79% to 92%.[48,49] Analysis of the cancers detected in the ACRIN (American College of Radiology Imaging Network) 6667 trial found that masses with irregular shapes and irregular or spiculated margins had the highest likelihood of malignancy.[50]

In the upcoming second edition of the ACR BI-RADS – MRI lexicon, it is anticipated that descriptor term lobular will be incorporated into oval shape. The term irregular will be used collectively to describe both shape and margin. The terminology smooth and circumscribed will be used to describe the margins of a mass that has clearly delineated borders. Similar to masses described on mammography and ultrasonography, the term indistinct will be used to describe the margins of a mass that is not sharply outlined from the adjacent breast parenchyma. Two descriptor terms, central enhancement and enhancing internal septations, will likely be excluded from the upcoming ACR BI-RADS – MRI lexicon because they are underused.

The third, and final, category for a lesion is non-mass enhancement (NME), which is an area that does not fulfill the definition of a mass but is larger than a focus. This type of lesion is also further categorized by its distribution and internal enhancement pattern. The standard terminology to describe the distribution of NME includes focal, linear, ductal, segmental, regional, multiregional, or diffuse. Focal refers to NME in a confined area (less than 25% of a quadrant of the breast). Linear enhancement is enhancement in a line that may not have a ductal orientation.[31] Enhancement in a line that may branch or conform to a duct is called ductal enhancement. Segmental enhancement is a triangular region of enhancement with its apex pointing toward the nipple, suggesting a duct or its branches. Regional enhancement is in a large volume of tissue not conforming to a ductal distribution, and may be thought of as a geographic enhancement. Multiple regional enhancement is enhancement in at least 2 large, separate volumes of tissue not conforming to a ductal distribution. Diffuse enhancement is enhancement distributed uniformly throughout the breast. In terms of internal enhancement pattern for NME, it may be homogeneous, heterogeneous, stippled/punctuate, clumped, reticular, or dendritic. The stippled or punctate internal enhancement is similar-appearing, dotlike, enhancing foci. Clumped enhancement is cobblestonelike enhancement, with occasional confluent areas.[31] When NME is detected, assessment of the contralateral breast for symmetric enhancement can be particularly helpful in assessing the level of suspicion for the lesion (Fig. 8).

Although the breast imaging vocabulary for NME has only recently been introduced, studies show that certain descriptor terms show good correlation with the likelihood of breast malignancy. Liberman and colleagues[51] found that the highest rate of subsequent malignancy is seen in lesions classified as ductal enhancement. Ductal enhancement accounted for 21% of MR imaging–detected lesions that had biopsy and had a PPV of 26%. The differential diagnosis of ductal enhancement included carcinoma (usually DCIS), atypical ductal hyperplasia, lobular carcinoma in situ, and benign findings such as fibrocystic change, ductal hyperplasia, and fibrosis. Stippled enhancement is associated with a low incidence of malignancy (25%), whereas clumped, heterogeneous, and homogeneous enhancement are associated with a 60%, 53%, and 67% likelihood of cancer, respectively.[48,52] Segmental distribution of enhancement was associated with a 78% likelihood of cancer, whereas a regional distribution was associated with a 21% likelihood of cancer.

Therefore, mild stippled enhancement with a regional distribution indicates benignity, whereas segmental, clumped enhancement is more likely to indicate malignancy.[48,52] Baltzer and colleagues[53] recently noted that a stippled pattern of enhancement was able to differentiate between benign and malignant NME. Also a new descriptor, a clustered ring appearance, was coined by Tozaki and colleagues[54] to describe heterogeneous enhancement inside clusters of minute ring enhancement. The presence of clustered ring enhancement was found in 63% of malignant lesions and only 4% of benign lesions.

In the upcoming edition of the ACR BI-RADS – MRI lexicon, it is anticipated that the terminology ductal will be incorporated into linear. Linear distribution will also be described as linear branching. A stippled/punctate internal enhancement will likely be removed because the terminology does not indicate abnormality and will be incorporate into BPE. Two additional descriptor terms for internal enhancement, reticular and dendritic, will likely be excluded from the latest ACR BI-RADS – MRI lexicon because they are underused.

When assessing the morphology of a lesion, it is important to review all the source images (ie, the T1-weighted postcontrast fat-saturated images), especially if the patient has moved between sequences. Motion artifact often degrades evaluation of the morphologic features, especially for margin assessment. False enhancement or perceived nonenhancement may occur because of motion artifact. As such, the radiologist must review the postcontrast and subtraction images for discrepancies (Fig. 9).

Kinetic Assessment

Once a lesion has been evaluated morphologically, the next step is to perform the kinetics assessment. This assessment evaluates the change in signal intensity values of an enhancing lesion over time after contrast material injection. Kuhl and colleagues[55] found that many cancers show a rapid wash-in and washout pattern of enhancement compared with benign breast tissue with peak enhancement within the first 2 minutes after injection of contrast (Fig. 10). Therefore, it is important to assess images at early time points after contrast injection, typically less than 2 minutes. In order to perform kinetic analysis, multiple MR imaging acquisitions are conducted after the intravenous contrast bolus injection, hence it is called DCE MR imaging. At present, there is no uniform consensus on what the optimal time frame for each acquisition should be to capture dynamic data for the best diagnostic accuracy. The ACR

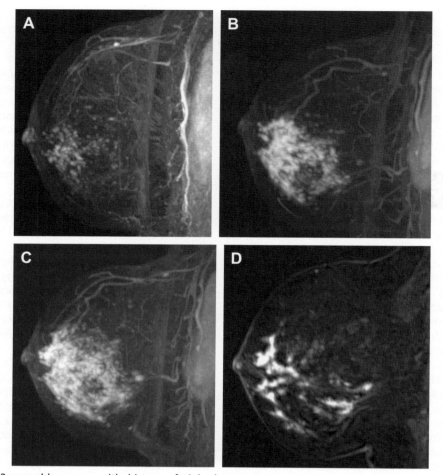

Fig. 8. A 62-year-old woman with history of right breast cancer status post mastectomy presenting with increasing asymmetric, segmental, nonmass enhancement in the left breast. Sagittal fat-saturated postcontrast T1-weighted MIP images of the left breast from baseline (*A*) to first follow-up at the 14-month interval (*B*) to the next follow-up at the 8-month interval (*C*) showing progressively increasing clumped, segmental, nonmass enhancement in the lower, inner left breast, concerning for malignancy. Sagittal fat-saturated postcontrast subtracted T1-weighted (*D*) image is also included for reference. MR-guided biopsy confirmed DCIS.

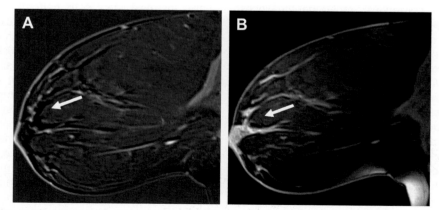

Fig. 9. Motion artifact. Subtracted postcontrast fat-saturated T1-weighted image (*A*) shows a curvilinear black line superior to the nipple, anterior depth (*white arrow*). In conjunction with the nonsubtracted image of the same slice and time sequence (*B*), this line represents misregistration from patient motion between the precontrast and postcontrast sequences.

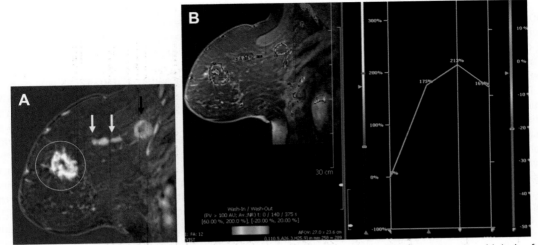

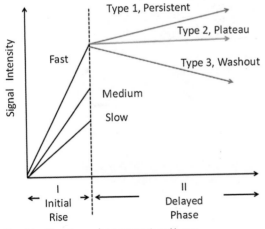

Fig. 10. A 58-year-old woman with biopsy-proven left breast invasive cancer with mixed ductal and lobular features. Sagittal fat-saturated postcontrast subtracted T1-weighted image (*A*) shows the 3.3-cm index lesion at 2:00 (*white circle*) with satellite lesions extending superior and posterior from the dominant mass up to 5.0 cm in extent (*white arrows*), nearing a biopsy-proven malignant axillary node (*black arrow*). All lesions show mixed kinetics, including type III (washout) kinetics (*B*).

Breast MRI Accreditation Program recommends that the time per sequential acquisition should be less than 2 minutes.[25]

Lesion enhancement is quantitatively assessed by obtaining the enhancement kinetics curves, which plot the change in signal intensity values over time. The kinetic curves are divided into the initial increase of enhancement (from the baseline value to the peak enhancement) and the delayed phase (the subsequent changes in signal intensity) (**Fig. 11**). The initial increase calculates the amount of inflow enhancement within the breast from the precontrast T1 sequence to the first-pass postcontrast T1 sequence. There are 3 patterns of initial increase: slow, medium, or rapid. A slow increase is less than or equal to 60% total

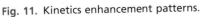

Fig. 11. Kinetics enhancement patterns.

enhancement at 2 minutes; medium is 60% to 100% in 2 minutes; rapid is greater than or equal to 100% increase in 2 minutes. The quantitative characteristic that most strongly indicates a malignancy is rapid initial enhancement.[49,50]

The delayed phase is categorized into 3 enhancement patterns based on the signal intensity–time curve: type I, type II, or type III. Type I is a pattern of persistent (formerly known as progressive) enhancement, with a continuous increase in signal intensity on each successive contrast-enhanced image. Type II is a plateau pattern, in which an initial increase in signal intensity is followed by a flattening of the enhancement curve. Type III, a washout enhancement pattern, involves an initial increase and subsequent decrease in signal intensity.

Kuhl and colleagues[55] reported that the likelihood of malignancy was 6% in lesions with a type I curve, 64% in lesions with a type II enhancement curve, and 87% in lesions with a type III enhancement curve. Type I curves are usually associated with a benign finding (83% benign, 9% malignant).[55] However, there is overlap between these curve types, and cancers may show all 3 patterns of enhancement. Bluemke and colleagues[9] reported that the sensitivity and specificity for a type I curve to be associated with a benign lesion was 52.2% and 71%, respectively. Schnall and colleagues[49] reported that 45% of lesions with a persistent enhancement kinetics proved to be cancers. A type II curve has a sensitivity of 42.6% and specificity of 75% for the detection of malignancy.[9] A type III curve is rarely seen in patients with benign lesions (90.4%), but it has a low sensitivity of 20.5%.[9] Schnall and colleagues[49] noted that 76% of type III curves were associated with cancer. In summary, both type II and type III curves suggest malignancy.

The sensitivity and specificity of breast MR imaging is improved when both morphologic and kinetic features are used to evaluate enhancing lesions. However, interpretation dilemma arises from the overlapping morphologic and kinetic characteristics between benign and malignant lesions. At present, the assessment of the morphologic characteristics is more strongly predict malignancy than the kinetic features.[49,50] The exclusion of cancer solely because of persistent enhancement would lead to increased false-negative results.[49] We find the kinetics assessment to be helpful if the lesion has benign morphologic features. If a lesion has suspicious morphologic features and a benign kinetic curve, a biopsy should be recommended. Although the margin of a mass is the most predictive feature of breast MR imaging interpretation,[52] this analysis depends on the spatial resolution. The spatial resolution of conventional breast MR imaging is lower than that of mammography. Therefore, the irregular borders of a small carcinoma may appear to be circumscribed. In assessing an enhancing circumscribed mass, the enhancement characteristics may help decide whether biopsy is required or whether it is safe to recommend follow-up of the lesion.

Additional Findings

Bilaterality and symmetry of enhancement can help classify the enhancement pattern as normal BPE, and help exclude an underlying abnormality. The BI-RADS lexicon defines symmetric as mirror-image enhancement. Several patterns of normal BPE include a peripheral, posterior, and symmetric pattern of enhancement, also known as picture-framing pattern[56] (Fig. 12) as well as stippled, scattered foci of enhancement in both breasts (Fig. 13).[53] The picture-framing pattern of enhancement is based on the vascular supply to the breast, predominantly supplied by the perforating branches of the internal mammary and the lateral thoracic arteries. This vascular supply leads to a centripetal pattern of enhancement involving all sides with the retroareolar area as the last region to enhance.[53] Because focal areas of BPE may be regional or multiregional, we have found that the addition of a delayed axial postcontrast fat-saturated image is particularly useful to compare the physiologic enhancement in both breasts.[28]

Asymmetric enhancement, defined as enhancement more in one breast than in the other, may be a cause for concern. Common causes for asymmetric BPE include lumpectomy or radiation therapy changes. In these scenarios, a short-term follow-up breast MR imaging may be useful. If there is no relevant clinical history, then the asymmetric BPE should be viewed with suspicion (Fig. 14A, B). The kinetic assessment is particularly helpful in this scenario. In our experience, if washout kinetics are seen, these findings may indicate a high-grade DCIS or an invasive lobular carcinoma.

Aside from the morphologic and kinetic characteristics of a lesion, the size of the lesion may be helpful in assessing the likelihood of malignancy. Liberman and colleagues[57] reported that the PPV

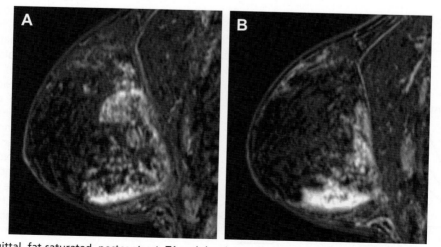

Fig. 12. Sagittal fat-saturated postcontrast T1-weighted images show peripheral, posterior, and symmetric pattern of enhancement in the right (A) and left (B) breasts, also known as picture framing, considered a benign finding.

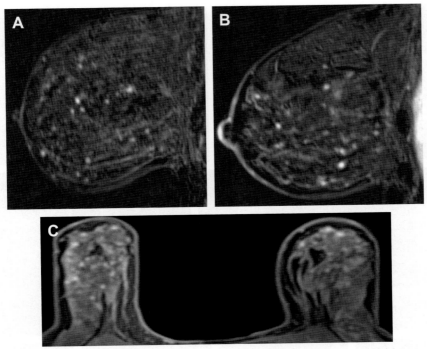

Fig. 13. Sagittal fat-saturated postcontrast T1-weighted images of the right (*A*) and left (*B*) breasts and axial fat-saturated postcontrast T1-weighted image of both breasts (*C*) show stippled, scattered foci of enhancement bilaterally and symmetrically, consistent with a benign cause.

of biopsy for lesions identified at breast MR imaging significantly increased with increasing lesion size. Biopsy is rarely necessary for lesions smaller than 5 mm because of their low (3%) likelihood of cancer. The evaluation of foci was limited because no kinetic analysis was performed. Furthermore, Raza and colleagues[58] reported that foci that were 3 to 4 mm in size were malignant if they were new findings, and had spiculated margins or washout kinetics. They reported that the PPV for malignancy of foci less than or equal to 5 mm was 20.6%. The highest prevalence of cancers was in the same quadrant as the newly diagnosed breast cancer.[58] More recently, Gutierrez and colleagues[59] found that, among all lesions, those greater than 1 cm were more likely to be malignant (34% vs 20%).

Other findings, distinct from the index lesion, may be helpful when deciding the management of the index lesion. These findings include nipple retraction and/or invasion, precontrast high ductal signal, skin thickening (either focal or diffuse) skin invasion, edema (**Fig. 15**), lymphadenopathy (axillary and internal mammary lymph nodes), pectoralis muscle invasion (**Fig. 16**), chest wall invasion (**Fig. 17**), hematoma/blood products, cysts, and abnormal signal void. Abnormal signal void is vague but can be caused by clip artifact (**Fig. 18**), coarse calcifications as from

fat necrosis, or a large vessel. In addition, non-breast findings in the mediastinum or abdomen should be reported.

REPORTING

The breast MR imaging report should include all of the following information: clinical history, MR imaging techniques (magnet and dedicated breast coil, T1-weighted and/or T2-weighted images, dose and type of contrast media, postprocessing techniques), comparison with prior films, the findings, and the final BI-RADS assessment and recommendations. The report should include important information about the findings, including the location of the lesion and its morphologic and kinetic features. Any associated findings (ie, chest wall, skin, or nipple involvement) should be included.

In an effort to standardize reporting, an associated recommendation and management are assigned to the report when the radiologist issues a final BI-RADS assessment. Similar to mammography and ultrasonography, the final assessment is categorized as BI-RADS 0 to 6. A BI-RADS 0 assessment implies that further imaging, usually comparison with prior imaging is recommended. A BI-RADS 1 assessment represents a normal examination with no findings, whereas a BI-RADS

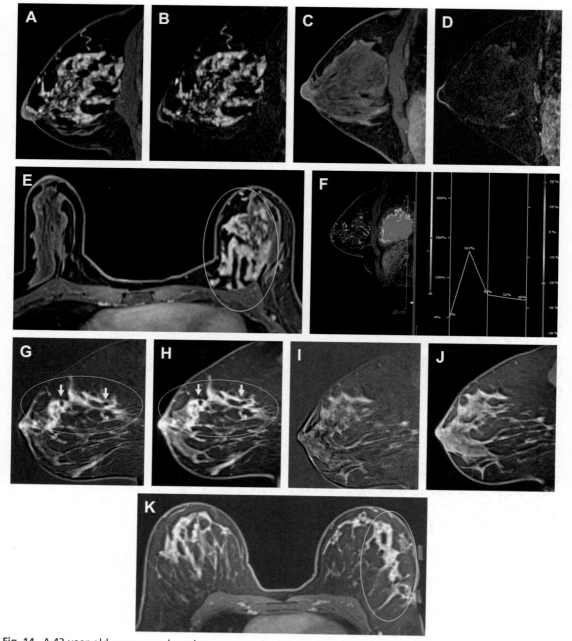

Fig. 14. A 43-year-old woman undergoing preoperative MR imaging staging for known left breast invasive ductal carcinoma proved by ultrasonography-guided core biopsy. Left breast sagittal fat-saturated postcontrast nonsubtracted (*A*) and subtracted (*B*) T1-weighted images show extensive linear, clumped, nonmass enhancement in the left medial breast. Right breast sagittal fat-saturated postcontrast nonsubtracted (*C*) and subtracted (*D*) T1-weighted images show normal BPE. Axial fat-saturated postcontrast nonsubtracted T1-weighted image of both breasts (*E*) shows the asymmetric enhancement in the medial left breast (*white circle*). Color-overlay images show mixed-type kinetics, including washout (type III) kinetics (*F*). Companion case: a 40-year-old woman undergoing preoperative MR imaging staging for known left breast invasive ductal carcinoma proved by stereotactic core biopsy. Left breast sagittal fat-saturated postcontrast nonsubtracted (*G*) and subtracted (*H*) T1-weighted images show a large region of asymmetric enhancement involving the upper, outer left breast (*white circle*); note the round signal voids consistent with the biopsy clips (*white arrows*). Right breast sagittal fat-saturated postcontrast nonsubtracted (*I*) and subtracted (*J*) T1-weighted images show normal BPE. Axial fat-saturated postcontrast nonsubtracted T1-weighted image of both breasts (*K*) shows the asymmetric enhancement in the outer left breast (*white circle*). Note the 2 vitamin E markers overlying the lateral left breast at the site of prior biopsy scars.

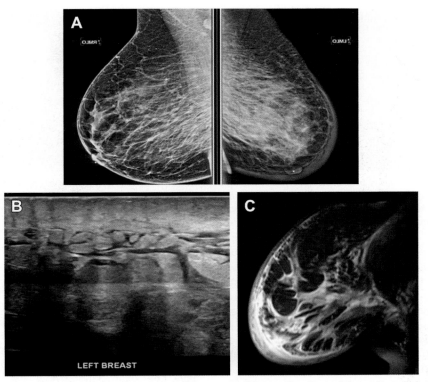

Fig. 15. A 59-year-old woman presenting with left breast swelling and redness. Bilateral mediolateral oblique mammograms (*A*) show the left breast with diffuse skin thickening and increased trabecular pattern of breast parenchyma. Gray-scale sonographic image of the left breast (*B*) shows diffuse skin thickening and subcutaneous edema. Sagittal fat-saturated T2-weighted image of the left breast (*C*) shows diffuse skin and parenchymal edema consistent with inflammatory state. The patient underwent core biopsy of the left breast yielding invasive ductal carcinoma.

2 assessment indicates a normal examination with benign findings. A BI-RADS 3 assessment indicates that a lesion is probably benign and follow-up imaging is recommended, usually at 6 months. At present, there is no clear consensus for how long a probably benign lesion should be followed to confer benignity on MR imaging. A BI-RADS 4 assessment indicates that there is a suspicious abnormality and that biopsy should be considered, with a wide probability of malignancy (2%–95%). For intrainstitutional or interdepartmental audit purposes (ie, to inform the pathologist about the degree of suspicion), the BI-RADS 4 assessment can be subcategorized into BI-RADS 4A, 4B, and 4C. A BI-RADS 4A assessment indicates a low suspicion for cancer (2%–10%), BI-RADS 4B indicates an intermediate suspicion for cancer (11%–50%), and BI-RADS 4C indicates a moderate suspicion for cancer (50%–95%). A BI-RADS 5 assessment indicates a very strong suspicion of malignancy (>95%), whereas a BI-RADS 6 assessment indicates a biopsy-proven cancer.[31]

The management of a suspicious lesion should be clearly stated in the breast MR imaging report. If targeted ultrasonography is recommended to further evaluate an indeterminate lesion, the next steps in the management of the lesion should be outlined, regardless of whether a correlate is seen on ultrasonography. For example, if the

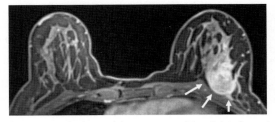

Fig. 16. A 51-year-old woman with right breast palpable cancer in the upper, central left breast (*white arrows*) proved by biopsy to be invasive ductal carcinoma. Although the mass drapes over the pectoralis major muscle, there are no signs of invasion, namely enhancement of the musculature.

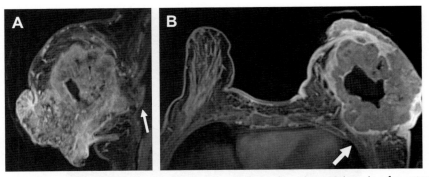

Fig. 17. A 55-year-old woman with left breast metaplastic cancer undergoing MR imaging for extent of disease. Left breast sagittal fat-saturated postcontrast subtracted (*A*) and axial fat-saturated postcontrast nonsubtracted (*B*) T1-weighted images show a 13-cm heterogeneous mass with central necrosis, extending posteriorly to the chest wall and invading the serratus anterior muscle (*white arrow*).

lesion is sonographically occult, 6-month follow-up breast MR imaging is recommended. As an alternative, if no abnormality is detected on ultrasonography, an MR imaging–guided biopsy is recommended. This clear plan of action, from diagnostic MR imaging to diagnostic ultrasonography to MR imaging–guided biopsy, should be set out in the report.

If the radiologist cannot choose between 2 BI-RADS assessments based on 2 separately identified lesions, then the most actionable category should be used. For instance, if a patient with known breast cancer is undergoing the MR imaging examination for extent of disease and is found to have findings suspicious for multifocal, multicentric, or contralateral disease, then a BI-RADS 4 should be given. BI-RADS 6 should not be used, even though the patient already has cancer, because it does not call for further imaging action.

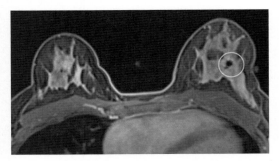

Fig. 18. Axial postcontrast three-dimensional T1-weighted image shows susceptibility artifact from a biopsy clip in the left breast (*white circle*). Such artifact may be useful for identifying the presence and location of a marker clip, but may also interfere with evaluation of the adjacent breast parenchyma.

SUMMARY

Breast MR imaging is becoming increasingly mainstream in the imaging arsenal in the detection of breast cancer and for the evaluation of breast lesions. As such, it is imperative that the radiologist be familiar with which patients should undergo imaging, when these patients should have the examination, how the examination should be performed, and how to interpret and manage the examination results. The clinical indication for the breast MR imaging, prior imaging studies, and pathology reports should be available for review. It is important to have a systematic and organized approach to interpreting breast MR imaging. The radiologist should develop a consistent viewing protocol to ensure that all the images have been examined. The postcontrast and subtraction images should be used to identify enhancement. The T1-weighted images may be used to evaluate for the presence of fat. The T2-weighted images may be used to evaluate for the presence of cysts and other benign high-signal lesions. The ACR BI-RADS lexicon provides standardized terminology to describe the morphologic and kinetic features of enhancing lesion. A final BI-RADS category and recommendation should be included in every breast MR imaging report.

REFERENCES

1. Kuhl CK, Schmutzler RK, Leutner CC, et al. Breast MR imaging screening in 192 women proved or suspected to be carriers of a breast cancer susceptibility gene: preliminary results. Radiology 2000;215:267–79.
2. Orel SG, Schnall MD. MR imaging of the breast for the detection, diagnosis, and staging of breast cancer. Radiology 2001;220:13–30.

3. Morris EA, Liberman L, Ballon DJ, et al. MRI of occult breast carcinoma in a high-risk population. AJR Am J Roentgenol 2003;181:619–26.

4. Kriege M, Brekelmans CT, Boetes C, et al. Efficacy of MRI and mammography for breast-cancer screening in women with a familial or genetic predisposition. N Engl J Med 2004;351:427–37.

5. Leach MO, Boggis CR, Dixon AK, et al. Screening with magnetic resonance imaging and mammography of a UK population at high familial risk of breast cancer: a prospective multicentre cohort study (MARIBS). Lancet 2005;365:1769–78.

6. Trecate G, Vergnaghi D, Manoukian S, et al. MRI in the early detection of breast cancer in women with high genetic risk. Tumori 2006;92(6):517–23.

7. Hagen AI, Kvistad KA, Maehle L, et al. Sensitivity of MRI versus conventional screening in the diagnosis of BRCA-associated breast cancer in a national prospective series. Breast 2007;16: 367–74.

8. Kuhl C, Weigel S, Schrading S, et al. Prospective multicenter cohort study to refine management recommendations for women at elevated familial risk of breast cancer: the EVA trial. J Clin Oncol 2010; 28(9):1450–7.

9. Bluemke DA, Gatsonis CA, Chen MH, et al. Magnetic resonance imaging of the breast prior to biopsy. JAMA 2004;292:2735–42.

10. Lee SG, Orel SG, Woo IJ, et al. MR imaging screening of the contralateral breast in patients with newly diagnosed breast cancer: preliminary results. Radiology 2003;226:773–8.

11. Lehman CD, DeMartini W, Anderson BO, et al. Indications for breast MRI in the patient with newly diagnosed breast cancer. J Natl Compr Canc Netw 2009;7:193–201.

12. Warner E, Plewes DB, Shumak RS, et al. Comparison of breast magnetic resonance imaging, mammography, and ultrasound for surveillance of women at high risk for hereditary breast cancer. J Clin Oncol 2001;19(15):3524–31.

13. Warner E, Plewes DB, Hill KA, et al. Surveillance of BRCA1 and BRCA2 mutation carriers with magnetic resonance imaging, ultrasound, mammography, and clinical breast examination. JAMA 2004;292(11):1317–25.

14. Kuhl CK, Schrading S, Leutner CC, et al. Mammography, breast ultrasound, and magnetic resonance imaging for surveillance of women at high familial risk for breast cancer. J Clin Oncol 2005;23(33): 8469–76.

15. Sardanelli F, Podo F, Santoro F, et al. Multicenter surveillance of women at high genetic breast cancer risk using mammography, ultrasonography, and contrast-enhanced magnetic resonance imaging (the High Breast Cancer Risk Italian 1 study): final results. Invest Radiol 2011;46:94–105.

16. Berg WA, Zhang Z, Lehrer D, et al. ACRIN 6666 investigators. Detection of breast cancer with addition of annual screening ultrasound or a single screening MRI to mammography in women with elevated breast cancer risk. JAMA 2012;307(13): 1394–404.

17. Mainiero MB, Lourenco A, Mahoney MC, et al. ACR appropriateness criteria breast cancer screening. J Am Coll Radiol 2013;10(1):11–4.

18. Saslow D, Boetes C, Burke W, et al. American Cancer Society Breast Cancer Advisory Group. American Cancer Society guidelines for breast screening with MRI as an adjunct to mammography. CA Cancer J Clin 2007;57(2):75–89.

19. Smith RA, Brooks D, Cokkinides V, et al. Cancer screening in the United States, 2013: a review of current American Cancer Society guidelines, current issues in cancer screening, and new guidance on cervical cancer screening and lung cancer screening. CA Cancer J Clin 2013;63(2):87–105.

20. Ozanne EM, Drohan B, Bosinoff P, et al. Which risk model to use? Clinical implications of the ACS MRI screening guidelines. Cancer Epidemiol Biomarkers Prev 2013;22(1):146–9.

21. Kuhl CK, Bieling HB, Giseke J, et al. Healthy premenopausal breast parenchyma in dynamic contrast-enhanced MR imaging of the breast: normal contrast medium enhancement and cyclical-phase dependency. Radiology 1997; 203(1):137–44.

22. Delille JP, Slanetz PJ, Yeh ED, et al. Physiologic changes in breast magnetic resonance imaging during the menstrual cycle: perfusion imaging, signal enhancement, and influence of the T1 relaxation time of breast tissue. Breast J 2005; 11:236–41.

23. American College of Radiology. Available at: www.acr.org. Accessed December 30, 2013.

24. Mann RM, Kuhl CK, Kinkel K, et al. Breast MRI: guidelines from the European Society of Breast Imaging. Eur Radiol 2008;18(7):1307–18.

25. Reference as: American College of Radiology. Available at: www.acr.org. Accessed December 30, 2013.

26. Hendrick RE. Breast MRI: fundamentals and technical aspects. Springer; 2007. ISBN: 978-0-387-73506-1.

27. Rausch DR, Hendrick RE. How to optimize clinical breast MR imaging practices and techniques on your 1.5-T system. Radiographics 2006;26: 1469–84.

28. Chatterji M, Mercado CL, Moy L. Optimizing 1.5-Tesla and 3-Tesla dynamic contrast-enhanced magnetic resonance imaging of the breasts. Magn Reson Imaging Clin N Am 2010;18:207–24, viii.

29. Genson CC, Blane CE, Helvie MA, et al. Effects on breast MRI of artifacts caused by metallic tissue

marker clips. AJR Am J Roentgenol 2007;188:372–6.

30. Kuhl CK, Klaschik S, Mielcarek P, et al. Do T2-weighted pulse sequences help with the differential diagnosis of enhancing lesions in dynamic breast MRI? J Magn Reson Imaging 1999;9:187–96.

31. ACR breast imaging reporting and data system, breast imaging atlas. Reston (VA): American College of Radiology; 2003.

32. King V, Brooks JD, Bernstein JL, et al. Background parenchymal enhancement at breast MR imaging and breast cancer risk. Radiology 2011;260:50–60.

33. DeMartini WB, Liu F, Peacock S, et al. Background parenchymal enhancement on breast MRI: impact on diagnostic performance. AJR Am J Roentgenol 2012;198:W373–80.

34. Hambly NM, Liberman L, Dershaw DD, et al. Background parenchymal enhancement on baseline screening breast MRI: impact on biopsy rate and short-interval follow-up. AJR Am J Roentgenol 2011;196:218–24.

35. Baltzer PA, Dietzel M, Vag T, et al. Clinical MR mammography: impact of hormonal status on background enhancement and diagnostic accuracy. Rofo 2011;183(5):441–7.

36. King V, Kaplan JB, Pike MC, et al. Impact of tamoxifen on fibroglandular tissue, background parenchymal enhancement, and cysts on breast magnetic resonance imaging. Breast J 2012;18(6):527–34.

37. Eng-Wong J, Orzano-Birgani J, Chow CK, et al. Effect of raloxifene on mammographic density and breast magnetic resonance imaging in premenopausal women at increased risk for breast cancer. Cancer Epidemiol Biomarkers Prev 2008;17(7):1696–701.

38. Oksa S, Parkkola R, Luukkaala T, et al. Breast magnetic resonance imaging findings in women treated with toremifene for premenstrual mastalgia. Acta Radiol 2009;50(9):984–9.

39. Mousa NA, Eiada R, Crystal P, et al. The effect of acute aromatase inhibition on breast parenchymal enhancement in magnetic resonance imaging: a prospective pilot clinical trial. Menopause 2012;19(4):420–5.

40. King V, Goldfarb SB, Brooks JD, et al. Effect of aromatase inhibitors on background parenchymal enhancement and amount of fibroglandular tissue at breast MR imaging. Radiology 2012;264(3):670–8.

41. Cubuk R, Tasali N, Narin B, et al. Correlation between breast density in mammography and background enhancement in MR mammography. Radiol Med 2010;115(3):434–41.

42. Carney PA, Miglioretti DL, Yankaskas BC, et al. Individual and combined effects of age, breast density, and hormone replacement therapy use on the accuracy of screening mammography. Ann Intern Med 2003;138:168–75.

43. Kerlikowske K, Grady D, Barclay J, et al. Effect of age, breast density, and family history on the sensitivity of first screening mammography. JAMA 1996;276:33–8.

44. Wolfe JN. Risk for breast cancer development determined by mammographic parenchymal pattern. Cancer 1976;37:2486–92.

45. Wolfe JN. Breast patterns as an index of risk for developing breast cancer. AJR Am J Roentgenol 1976;126(6):1130–7.

46. Byrne C, Schairer C, Wolfe J, et al. Mammographic features and breast cancer risk: effects with time, age, and menopause status. J Natl Cancer Inst 1995;87:1622–9.

47. Boyd NF, Dite GS, Stone J, et al. Heritability of mammographic density, as risk for breast cancer. N Engl J Med 2002;347:886–94.

48. Nunes LW, Schnall MD, Siegelman ES, et al. Diagnostic performance of characteristics of architectural features revealed by high spatial-resolution MR imaging of the breast. AJR Am J Roentgenol 1997;169(2):409–15.

49. Schnall MD, Blume J, Bluernke DA, et al. Diagnostic architectural and dynamic features at breast MR imaging: multicenter study. Radiology 2006;238(1):42–53.

50. Mahoney MC, Gatsonic C, Hanna L, et al. Positive predictive value of BI-RADS MR imaging. Radiology 2012;264(1):51–8.

51. Liberman L, Morris EA, Dershaw DD, et al. Ductal enhancement on MR imaging of the breast. AJR Am J Roentgenol 2003;181(2):519–25.

52. Macura KJ, Ouwerkerk R, Jacobs MA, et al. Patterns of enhancement on breast MR images: interpretation and imaging pitfalls. Radiographics 2006;26(6):1719–34.

53. Baltzer PA, Benndorf M, Dietzel M, et al. False-positive findings at contrast-enhanced breast MRI: a BI-RADS descriptor study. AJR Am J Roentgenol 2010;194(6):1658–63.

54. Tozaki M, Igarashi T, Fukuda K. Breast MRI using the VIBE sequence: clustered ring enhancement in the differential diagnosis of lesions showing non-masslike enhancement. AJR Am J Roentgenol 2006;187(2):313–21.

55. Kuhl CK, Mielcareck P, Klaschik S, et al. Dynamic breast MR imaging: are signal intensity time course data useful for differential diagnosis of enhancing lesions? Radiology 1999;211:101–10.

56. Birdwell RL, Raza S, Odulate AS. Breast MRI: a comprehensive imaging guide. 1st edition. Salt Lake City, Utah: Amirsys; 2010. 11-3-84 to 11-3-99.

57. Liberman L, Mason G, Morris EA, et al. Does size matter? Positive predictive value of MRI-detected

breast lesions as a function of lesion size. AJR Am J Roentgenol 2006;186(2):426–30.

58. Raza S, Sekar M, Ong EM, et al. Small masses on breast MR: is biopsy necessary? Acad Radiol 2012;19(4):412–9.

59. Gutierrez RL, DeMartini WB, Eby PR, et al. BI-RADS lesion characteristics predict likelihood of malignancy in breast MRI for masses but not for nonmasslike enhancement. AJR Am J Roentgenol 2009;193(4):994–1000.

Breast Magnetic Resonance Imaging
Management of an Enhancing Focus

Richard Ha, MD[a],*, Christopher E. Comstock, MD[b]

KEYWORDS

- Breast magnetic resonance imaging • Focus • Kinetics

KEY POINTS

- Managing a small enhancing lesion defined as a focus on breast magnetic resonance (MR) imaging remains a challenge because of lack of clear established guidelines.
- As the spatial resolution of breast MR imaging continues to improve, small lesions measuring 4 to 5 mm can be considered small masses and managed accordingly relying on morphologic characteristics.
- T2 signal intensity and interval change are potential important characteristics of an enhancing focus with predictive value for malignancy and warrant further investigation in a larger study.
- Kinetic analysis is likely not specific for malignancy and should not be used solely to guide management of an enhancing focus.

INTRODUCTION

The American College of Radiology (ACR) Breast Imaging Reporting and Data System (BI-RADS) breast magnetic resonance (MR) imaging lexicon defines a focus as a small isolated dot of enhancement, generally less than 5 mm, that is too small to apply definitive morphologic descriptors or region of interest (ROI) dynamic data.[1] No set criteria for appropriate management are available in the most recent MR imaging BI-RADS lexicon, which promotes the standardization of lesion descriptors and assessment categories based on the results of the ACR BI-RADS Committee.[2,3]

Published studies regarding an enhancing focus identified on breast MR imaging are reviewed to develop a possible management strategy.

CLINICAL SIGNIFICANCE OF AN ENHANCING FOCUS

Although a focus commonly represents a benign cause, such as an intramammary lymph node, papilloma, small fibroadenoma, or fibrocystic change, malignancy has been reported.[4–10] Published literature regarding the malignancy rate of an enhancing focus is variable, ranging from 0.6% to 23%.[4–10]

A study by Liberman and colleagues in 2006[4] retrospectively studied 666 consecutive nonpalpable, mammographically occult lesions detected by MR imaging in 429 women who had diagnostic MR imaging–guided needle localization and surgical biopsy at Memorial Sloan Kettering Cancer Center during a 35-month period. Of the lesions,

No grants.
No disclosures.
[a] Columbia University Medical Center, Herbert Irving Pavilion, 161 Fort Washington Avenue, 10th Floor, New York, NY 10032, USA; [b] Department of Radiology, Memorial Sloan Kettering Cancer Center, 300 East 66th Street, New York, NY 10065, USA
* Corresponding author.
E-mail address: rh2616@columbia.edu

11.1% (74/666) measured 5 mm or less and could have been categorized as enhancing foci. Of these small lesions, 9.5% (7/74) yielded malignancy on subsequent MR imaging–guided biopsy (pathology of the 7 malignant lesions: 5 ductal carcinoma in situ [DCIS] and 2 invasive ductal carcinoma [IDC]). Excluding the 5-mm lesions, the malignancy rate of lesions measuring 4 mm or less was 2.7% (1/37, pathology: DCIS).

Weinstein and colleagues in 2010[5] published an ACR Imaging Network–conducted, prospective multi-institutional MR imaging screening trial of the contralateral breast in women with recent diagnosis of breast cancer. There were 145 BI-RADS 3 lesions in 106 patients. Of 145 BI-RADS 3 lesions, there were 47 foci of enhancement (32.4%). The 1 patient who developed breast malignancy (DCIS) initially had an enhancing focus that was characterized as probably benign and recommended for short-term follow-up. The overall malignancy rate of foci was 2.1% (1/47).

Eby and colleagues in 2009[6] evaluated lesions assessed as BI-RADS 3. Three hundred sixty-two lesions were assessed in 236 patients. The 362 lesions included 168 (46%) foci. Of 168 foci, a single focus of enhancement initially measuring 5 mm and characterized as probably benign showed enlargement on subsequent MR imaging examinations with MR imaging–guided vacuum-assisted biopsy yielding low-grade DCIS. The overall cancer yield of foci was very low, at 0.6% (1/168).

Higher malignancy rates were observed in more recent studies by Abe and colleagues in 2010,[8] Jansen and colleagues in 2011,[9] and Raza and colleagues in 2012.[10] Their malignancy rates in foci ranged from 15% to 20.6%.[7] In combining results of these and the previously mentioned 3 studies, the overall malignancy rate of an enhancing focus is 8.4% (39/467), with 21 invasive cancers and 14 DCIS (Table 1).

Based on published literature, it is clear that malignancy can present as an enhancing focus on breast MR imaging measuring 5 mm or less with most being clinically significant invasive cancers (see Table 1). To develop a strategy of managing these lesions, characteristics of an enhancing focus associated with malignancy from those associated with benignity are further evaluated.

CHARACTERISTICS OF FOCI: EXAMINATION INDICATION

Raza and colleagues in 2012[10] retrospectively reviewed 565 lesions that underwent biopsy with MR guidance and identified 68 lesions measuring 5 mm or less in 61 patients. The malignancy rate of lesions measuring 5 mm or less was 20.6%. The highest prevalence of cancers was in the same quadrant as the newly diagnosed breast cancer, emphasizing the importance of the context in which breast lesions are identified and supporting management of additional indeterminate findings in patients with known cancer with a definitive tissue diagnosis rather than short-term follow-up.

CHARACTERISTICS OF FOCI: KINETIC ANALYSIS

Kinetic analysis was reviewed for its potential role in evaluating an enhancing focus. Specifically, the delayed enhancement pattern was analyzed, which has been reported to have high specificity and high positive predictive value for malignancy.[11]

A study by Eby and colleagues in 2009[6] investigated breast MR imaging BI-RADS 3 lesions. The 362 BI-RADS 3 lesions included 168 (46%) foci. Of those with kinetic analysis (275 of 362 lesions), 60% showed persistent enhancement, 17%

Table 1
Malignancy rates of an enhancing focus

Study	Number of Foci (≤5 mm)	Malignancy Rate, n/N (%)	DCIS	IDC	ILC	IDC/ILC Mixed
Liberman et al,[4] 2006	74	7/74 (9.5)	5	2		
Han et al,[7] 2008	21	4/21 (19)	NS	NS	NS	NS
Eby et al,[6] 2009	168	1/168 (0.6)	1			
Abe et al,[8] 2010	50	3/50 (15)	1	2		
Weinstein et al,[5] 2010	47	1/47 (2.1)	1	0	0	0
Jansen et al,[9] 2011	39	9/39 (23)	5	3		1
Raza et al,[10] 2012	68	14/68 (20.6)	1	9	2	2
Total	467	39/467 (8.4)	14	16	2	3

Abbreviation: NS, Not specified.

plateau enhancement, and 23% washout enhancement. All 69 foci (in 54 patients) with persistent enhancement pattern were benign. The 1 malignant focus showed washout enhancement pattern. The investigators concluded that assigning foci with 100% persistent enhancement to the BI-RADS 2 category would have decreased the frequency of BI-RADS 3 assessment and maintained a likelihood of malignancy in less than 2% of cases.

However, since 2009, several studies have emerged showing significant malignancy potential of persistently enhancing foci, ranging from 11.1% to 18.7%.[8–10] One of the studies by Jansen and colleagues in 2011[9] performed kinetic analysis, yielding a malignancy rate of 18.7% for persistently enhancing foci, 20% for plateau enhancement, and 33.3% for washout enhancement. The delayed enhancement pattern was not specific for malignancy. All 5 studies that investigated the role of kinetic analysis in evaluating an enhancing focus showed no statistical difference between groups of foci with persistent enhancement compared with foci with washout enhancement (Table 2). Additional evaluation comparing groups of foci with persistent enhancement compared with foci with washout enhancement and plateau enhancement also showed no statistical difference (see Table 2).

Similarly, kinetic analysis was not specific in our preliminary study performed at Memorial Sloan Kettering Cancer Center (Ha and colleagues, Radiological Society of North America [RSNA] 2011). We identified 2 malignant foci with persistent enhancement pattern and 2 malignant foci with washout enhancement pattern. The 2 groups were not statistically different. In addition, as the 2

malignant foci with the benign appearing enhancement pattern increased in size on follow-up MR imaging examination, the enhancement pattern changed to the expected washout pattern of malignancy. These results suggest that small malignant lesions do not always show expected enhancement pattern related to increased tumor angiogenesis but instead can have a benign appearing enhancement pattern. Until more definitive, larger studies are performed, kinetic analysis is likely not specific for malignancy and should not be used solely to guide management.

CHARACTERISTICS OF FOCI: T2-WEIGHTED SIGNAL INTENSITY

Kuhl and colleagues in 1999[12] performed one of the first studies to investigate the possible role of using T2 signal intensity to improve diagnostic accuracy of lesions identified on breast MR imaging. In this study, 2 independent radiologists rated the lesions (101 malignant, 104 benign) as having either a low or a high T2 signal with respect to the adjacent glandular tissue. Breast cancers were isointense or hypointense with respect to breast parenchyma in 87% of cases and fibroadenomas were hyperintense in 71%. T2 signal intensity was determined to be helpful in distinguishing between fibroadenomas and breast cancers. Malich and colleagues in 2004[13] also evaluated the potential role of T2-weighted signal intensity in lesion assessment. The study yielded similar results, with most (74%, 313/426) of malignant lesions showing T2 hypointensity and less than 2% (8/426) of malignant lesions showing T2 hyperintensity. These results suggest inherent

Study	Type I Curve with Cancer, n/N (%)	Type II Curve with Cancer, n/N (%)	Type III Curve with Cancer, n/N (%)	Type I Curve vs Type III Curve[a]	Type I Curve vs Type II + III Curve[a]
Han et al,[7] 2008	0/6 (0)	2/9 (22.2)	0/1 (0)	$P = 1.0$	$P = .500$
Eby et al,[6] 2009	0/69 (0)	0/21 (0)	1/30 (3.3)	$P = .30$	$P = .4250$
Abe et al,[8] 2010	1/7 (14.3)	0/29 (0)	2/14 (14.3)	$P = 1.0$	$P = .3704$
Jansen et al,[9] 2011	3/16 (18.7)	2/10 (20)	2/6 (33.3)	$P = .5853$	$P = 1.0$
Raza et al,[10] 2012	5/27 (18.5)	2/21 (9.5)	7/20 (35)	$P = .3111$	$P = 1.0$

Table 2
Kinetic analysis (delayed enhancement pattern)

Type I curve, persistent enhancement pattern; type II curve, plateau enhancement pattern; type III curve, washout enhancement pattern.
[a] Statistical analysis (Fisher exact test, significant if 2-tailed P value ≤.05).

differences in internal composition of malignant lesions that lack signal intensity on T2-weighted images and support categorizing an enhancing focus with T2 hyperintensity as benign.

There are reported cases of breast cancers that can show areas of high T2 signal intensity, including triple-negative tumors, mucinous tumors, and papillary carcinomas.[14–16] However, the lesions in these studies were not foci but larger masses, and in triple-negative cancers, the large irregular areas of high T2 signal intensity pathologically correlated with internal necrosis and not necessarily the lesion itself.

More studies are needed to determine if an enhancing focus with a corresponding T2 hyperintensity can be managed as a benign finding, which could decrease unnecessary follow-up studies, whereas an enhancing focus with T2 hypointensity may warrant at least short-term follow-up if not managed by a biopsy.

CHARACTERISTICS OF FOCI: SIZE

Since the introduction of the term focus defined as "a small isolated dot of enhancement, generally less than 5 mm in size, that is too small to apply definitive morphologic descriptors or ROI dynamic data" in the MR imaging lexicon in 2003, there have been ongoing technical advances in breast MR imaging, resulting in improved spatial resolution.[17–19] As a result, morphologic features can sometimes be evaluated in small lesions measuring 5 mm or less. A study by Raza and colleagues[10] showed that margin could be defined as irregular or spiculated in 60.3% (41/68) of malignant foci that were identified in their study. With expected continued improvement in resolution, lesions measuring 4 to 5 mm could be defined as small masses and lesions measuring 3 mm or less as foci. This development would be in keeping with the intended definition of a focus, which is an enhancing lesion that is too small to characterize with low malignancy potential.

CHARACTERISTICS OF FOCI: INTERVAL CHANGE AND NUMBER

Interval change is another characteristic to consider, especially in patients undergoing breast MR imaging for high-risk screening. Our preliminary study (Ha and colleagues, RSNA 2011) performed at Memorial Sloan Kettering Cancer Center shows significant malignant potential of an enhancing focus that is either new or enlarging. When combined with T2 hypointensity, the malignancy rate was as high as 27.2%, indicating the need for biopsy rather than short-term follow-up.

Also in our preliminary study, malignancy was identified only when 1 or 2 discrete foci were followed. No malignancy was present when 3 or more similar appearing foci were present on the initial breast MR imaging. As more foci are present, these are probably no longer unique and are often described as being part of the normal background parenchymal enhancement, previously described as a stippled pattern, with low likelihood of malignancy. In the new updated lexicon, the enhancing focus will be described as a unique finding, separate from background parenchymal enhancement (Morris MD, updated breast MR imaging lexicon, personal communication, 2013).

SUMMARY

Managing a small enhancing lesion defined as a focus on breast MR imaging remains a challenge because of lack of clear established guidelines. More studies are needed that distinguish specific characteristics of an enhancing focus associated with malignancy from those associated with benignity to determine appropriate management criteria.

As the spatial resolution of breast MR imaging continues to improve, small lesions measuring 4 to 5 mm may be considered small masses and managed accordingly, relying on morphologic characteristics. Otherwise, T2 signal intensity and interval change are potential important characteristics with predictive value for malignancy and warrant further investigation in a larger sample size. Kinetic analysis is likely not specific for malignancy and should not be used solely to guide management of an enhancing focus.

REFERENCES

1. American College of Radiology. Breast imaging reporting and data system (BI-RADS). 4th edition. Reston (VA): American College of Radiology; 2003.
2. Ikeda DM, Baker DR, Daniel BL. Magnetic resonance imaging of breast cancer: clinical indications and breast MRI reporting system [review]. J Magn Reson Imaging 2000;12(6):975–83.
3. Ikeda DM, Hylton NM, Kinkel K, et al. Development, standardization, and testing of a lexicon for reporting contrast-enhanced breast magnetic resonance imaging studies. J Magn Reson Imaging 2001;13: 889–95.
4. Liberman L, Mason G, Morris EA, et al. Does size matter? Positive predictive value of MRI-detected breast lesions as a function of lesion size. AJR Am J Roentgenol 2006;186:426–30.
5. Weinstein SP, Hanna LG, Gatsonis C, et al. Frequency of malignancy seen in probably benign lesions at

contrast-enhanced breast MR imaging: findings from ACRIN 6667. Radiology 2010;255(3):731–7.

6. Eby PR, DeMartini WB, Gutierrez RL, et al. Characteristics of probably benign breast MRI lesions. AJR Am J Roentgenol 2009;193(3):861–7.

7. Han BK, Schnall MD, Orel SG, et al. Outcome of MRI-guided breast biopsy. AJR Am J Roentgenol 2008;191(6):1798–804.

8. Abe H, Schmidt RA, Shah RN, et al. MR-directed ("second-look") ultrasound examination for breast lesions detected initially on MRI: MR and sonographic findings. AJR Am J Roentgenol 2010;194(2):370–7.

9. Jansen SA, Shimauchi A, Zak L, et al. The diverse pathology and kinetics of mass, nonmass, and focus enhancement on MR imaging of the breast. J Magn Reson Imaging 2011;33(6):1382–9.

10. Raza S, Sekar M, Ong EM, et al. Small masses on breast MR: is biopsy necessary? Acad Radiol 2012;19(4):412–9.

11. Kuhl CK, Schild HH, Morakkabati N. Dynamic bilateral contrast-enhanced MR imaging of the breast: trade-off between spatial and temporal resolution. Radiology 2005;236(3):789–800.

12. Kuhl CK, Klaschik S, Mielcarek P, et al. Do T2-weighted pulse sequences help with the differential diagnosis of enhancing lesions in dynamic breast MRI? J Magn Reson Imaging 1999;9(2):187–96.

13. Malich A, Fischer DR, Wurdinger S, et al. Potential MRI interpretation model: differentiation of benign from malignant breast masses. AJR Am J Roentgenol 2005;185(4):964–70.

14. Uematsu T, Kasami M, Yuen S. Triple-negative breast cancer: correlation between MR imaging and pathologic findings. Radiology 2009;250(3):638–47.

15. Günhan-Bilgen I, Zekioglu O, Ustün EE, et al. Invasive micropapillary carcinoma of the breast: clinical, mammographic, and sonographic findings with histopathologic correlation. AJR Am J Roentgenol 2002;179(4):927–31.

16. Monzawa S, Yokokawa M, Sakuma T, et al. Mucinous carcinoma of the breast: MRI features of pure and mixed forms with histopathologic correlation. AJR Am J Roentgenol 2009;192(3):W125–31.

17. Kuhl CK. Breast MR imaging at 3T. Magn Reson Imaging Clin N Am 2007;15(3):315–20.

18. Nnewihe AN, Grafendorfer T, Daniel BL, et al. Custom-fitted 16-channel bilateral breast coil for bidirectional parallel imaging. Magn Reson Med 2011;66(1):281–9.

19. Elsamaloty H, Elzawawi MS, Mohammad S, et al. Increasing accuracy of detection of breast cancer with 3-T MRI. AJR Am J Roentgenol 2009;192(4):1142–8, J Magn Reson Imaging 1999;9(2):187–96.

MR Evaluation of Breast Implants

Michael S. Middleton, MD, PhD

KEYWORDS

- Breast • MR • Implant • Silicone • Saline • Prosthesis • Rupture • Deflation

KEY POINTS

- Addition of breast implant–related magnetic resonance (MR) imaging to breast cancer–related MR imaging examinations is helpful.
- T2-weighted, fat-nulled, water-suppressed MR imaging is useful to evaluate breast implants and soft tissue silicone.
- Intracapsular rupture can be categorized on MR imaging as being uncollapsed, minimally collapsed, partially collapsed, or fully collapsed.

INTRODUCTION

Breast implant magnetic resonance (MR) imaging is useful to evaluate the integrity of breast implants and to determine the relationship of breast implants to any breast lesions that may be present. Additional uses are to evaluate the amount and distribution of soft-tissue silicone, to estimate implant volume, and to determine breast implant type and manufacturer. Soft-tissue silicone may be present as either a result of silicone gel–filled implant rupture or a direct injection of silicone fluid. Plastic surgeons occasionally need to know the volume of implants currently in place so that the correct size can be ordered for replacement. Knowing the implant type, style, and manufacturer can in some cases help evaluate implant integrity and occasionally can provide device failure information to manufacturers or regulatory agencies, and evidence for class action, personal injury, or patent lawsuits.

Evaluation of Implant Integrity

There is an ongoing need to evaluate breast implant integrity. About 10 times as many implants are placed annually now in the United States as were placed in 1992, when the Food and Drug Administration (FDA) breast implant moratorium was instituted (more than 300,000 sets of implants are currently placed annually in the United States, compared with about 32,000 sets/year in 1992 before the FDA moratorium).[1,2] That moratorium was lifted in 2006, and silicone gel–filled breast implants have been available with FDA approval in the United States since then.[3] Recent investigations of implant integrity have shown that implants placed since 1992 have considerably longer lifetimes than earlier implants.[4–10] However, any device can fail, including currently available breast implants. It has been said that breast implants do not last a lifetime; they have a lifetime, but that expected lifetime is now longer than it used to be.[11] Some women will have implants that remain soft and symptom-free forever, but there is a risk for problems such as pain, change of breast size or shape, capsular contracture, implant rupture, extrusion of soft-tissue silicone from a ruptured implant into breast and possibly surrounding soft tissue, and development of silicone granuloma. Patients now considering breast implants are informed that implant rupture can occur, that implants are not considered lifetime devices, and that reoperation may be necessary.[12,13] Furthermore, women with implants are advised to have

Disclosure: Consultant to Allergan.
Department of Radiology, UCSD School of Medicine, 410 West Dickinson Street, San Diego, CA 92103-8749, USA
E-mail address: msm@ucsd.edu

Radiol Clin N Am 52 (2014) 591–608
http://dx.doi.org/10.1016/j.rcl.2014.02.013

an MR imaging examination to check for implant rupture 3 years after placement and then every 2 years thereafter, even if they are not having symptoms, as well as to check whether any new symptoms might be due to rupture, whenever that may be needed.[12,13] It is the author's opinion that checking asymptomatic breast implants with MR imaging every 2 years is too frequent, and that the above-noted advice for biennial MR imaging is based, at least in part, on published high-rupture prevalences of older, less durable implants.[10] Putting aside the question of how frequently MR imaging to check for silent implant rupture is necessary, current FDA-approved manufacturer recommendations support the use of MR imaging to check breast implants for rupture.

There is no definitive proof that silicone implants cause other disease (including cancer), or that implant rupture (in addition to just implant presence) is a factor in that process, despite claims (and lawsuits) since the 1970s to that effect. Studies have not shown a strong association of breast implants with cancer or severe autoimmune disease.[14–16] Patients considering breast implants are informed that current infection, existing cancer or precancer that has not been adequately treated, current pregnancy, and nursing are contraindications to breast implants, and also that safety and effectiveness have not been established in patients with autoimmune disease such as lupus or scleroderma, conditions or medications that interfere with wound healing or blood clotting, reduced blood supply to breast or overlying tissue, ongoing radiation therapy, and certain mental health problems.[12,13]

Relationship to Breast Lesions

In addition to evaluating breast implant integrity, there is also an ongoing need to evaluate the relationship of breast implants and their complications to any breast lesions that may be present.

For patients who are having a contrast-enhanced MR imaging examination for any breast cancer–related reason, addition of breast implant–related imaging should be considered for two reasons. First, breast implant–related complications can mimic breast cancer, just as breast cancer can mimic breast implant–related complications. Second, on a breast cancer–related MR imaging examination, breast surgeons want to be aware of implant-related problems to help avoid complications at surgery and also to have the option to take care of both problems at the same time. Examples of problems that could complicate surgery are capsular contracture, old hematoma, implant rupture, soft-tissue silicone gel or silicone

granuloma, proximity of a lesion to be biopsied or removed surgically to a breast implant, and actual cancer involvement of the fibrous capsule.

For patients who are having a noncontrast breast implant–related MR imaging examination, the possible addition of contrast-enhanced MR imaging sequences to look for breast cancer should be considered. Miglioretti and colleagues[17] found that the presence of breast implants increases the likelihood that breast cancer will not be evident on mammography and therefore the presence of breast implants should be taken into account in decisions of whether to add contrast-enhanced sequences to look for breast cancer, because the presence of implants makes it more likely that breast cancer, if present, will not be detected in mammography.

Soft-Tissue (Extracapsular) Silicone

When silicone gel–filled breast implants rupture, silicone gel can extrude outside the implant fibrous capsule into surrounding soft tissues; when that happens, it is often referred to as "extracapsular" silicone. (The term "intracapsular silicone" refers to silicone gel that is contained within the implant fibrous capsule.)

Silicone fluid was injected directly into breast tissues before and for several years after breast implants became commercially available in the United States in 1964.[18] Occasionally this procedure is still performed in other countries and also rarely in the United States by nonphysician practitioners. These patients' breasts harden over time, and many have undergone subcutaneous mastectomy with implant replacement. Infiltrated silicone (which is not firm and is usually undetectable to palpation) is virtually always present in these cases, even though operation reports often will state that all of it has been removed. The only way to remove all infiltrated silicone fluid would be to remove the tissues in which it resides, which would often require extensive surgery that in practice is not done; only the portion that has become firm or hard (ie, silicone granuloma) is removed. Hence, when these patients present for MR imaging evaluation, infiltrated silicone fluid remaining from prior injections is seen in the breast and often also in other nearby soft tissues including the pectoralis muscles, along with any implants that have been placed. Typically, silicone in soft tissues completely blocks ultrasound transmission and results in extensive overlying density on mammography, which interferes with lesion detection. Although injected silicone is not thought to cause breast cancer, it can prevent early detection, and so sometimes these patients' only hope of early detection is contrast-enhanced breast MR imaging. Because silicone granuloma can enhance, knowing where the silicone is becomes important in detecting breast cancer, for which breast implant–related additional imaging is necessary. For more examples and discussion of these topics, please see Middleton and McNamara.[18]

Implant Volume

Plastic surgeons occasionally request that radiologists provide an estimate of implant volume from MR imaging scans, usually to help in ordering replacement implants. The author has used the Slice-o-Matic software package to do this (Tomovision; Magog, Quebec, Canada; www.tomovision.com), and others have reported that this is also possible with other software packages.[19,20]

Determination of Implant Type and Manufacturer

Patients and their physicians, including radiologists, sometimes would like to know not only what size the implants are, but also the type and style of the implants. This information can help the plastic surgeon advise the patient as to their options and can help the radiologist to know whether the MR imaging appearance seen is normal, or not, for that particular style and manufacturer. Many types and styles of implants are no longer commonly seen and so will not be described here; for more discussion and examples of those more infrequently encountered implants, please see the online paper by Middleton and McNamara[21] and their book.[18]

When the breast implant class action lawsuits in the United States were most active, in the mid 1990s and early 2000s, there were numerous requests from attorneys as well as from patients and physicians to identify breast implant types, styles, and manufacturers. Information from materials discovered in those legal proceedings, as well as medical records, MR imaging scans, computed tomographic (CT) scans, mammograms, and actual physical implant examinations conducted and photographs taken during and after explantation surgery, was used to compile a catalog and an atlas of implant photographs and imaging findings, to which the reader is referred for details on the styles and types of breast implants that have been used for breast reconstruction and augmentation since the late 1940s.[18]

Breast MR imaging also can be useful for research and surveillance regarding device failure incidence, prevalence, complications, and mechanism of failure. Breast MR imaging was the study procedure used in the FDA breast implant study[10,22] and in clinical trials conducted by breast implant manufacturers[4–9] and has been used most recently to investigate problems with the French PIP implants for which removal is being recommended in many countries.[11,23–25]

NORMAL BREAST MR IMAGING APPEARANCES AND IMAGING TECHNIQUE

Fourteen types of breast implants have been described,[18,21,26] only a few of which are frequently seen at this time (**Table 1**). The two main types are the *saline-filled* and *single-lumen silicone gel–filled* types. Each of these consists of a silicone elastomer implant shell (sometimes called the envelope, or the bag) and fill material (saline, or silicone gel). Saline-filled implants

Table 1
Common breast implant types currently in use

	Inner Lumen Fill	Outer Lumen Fill	Valve
Saline filled	Saline	n/a	Usually diaphragm type, occasionally leaflet type for some older implants
Single-lumen, silicone gel-filled	Silicone gel	n/a	None
Standard double-lumen	Silicone gel	Saline	Leaflet type
Gel-gel double-lumen	Silicone gel	Silicone gel	None
Reverse double-lumen expander-implant	Saline	Silicone gel	A thin tube leading to a subcutaneous fill port is threaded through outer-lumen and inner-lumen leaflet valves for inner-lumen sequential filling. That tube is intended to be pulled after that inner-lumen filling is complete.

most commonly have a diaphragm valve anteriorly that has a characteristic appearance on MR imaging and mammography (**Fig. 1**). Silicone gel–filled implants also have a characteristic appearance on MR imaging (**Fig. 2**), but can be difficult to distinguish from standard double-lumen implants if saline is absent from their outer lumen. Both will show so-called implant shell folds, which are in-foldings of implant shell. These folds are expected and are part of the normal appearance of breast implants. Rarely, very large or very over-filled implants will show no folds, in any plane, but that is the exception.

Mammography, Ultrasound, and CT Imaging

Mammography will show extracapsular silicone from ruptured silicone gel–filled implants well, unless it is too far posterior in the breast or off the film. However, with rare exceptions, it will not show intracapsular rupture, of any stage, at all. Hence, as might be expected, early estimates of rupture prevalence (about 5%) were grossly underestimated when only mammography was used for its detection.[27] Another pitfall of mammography is that contour abnormalities and calcification of the fibrous capsule are sometimes overinterpreted as being evidence of rupture. These appearances are not useful indicators of implant rupture, because they often are present for older implants even when the implants are not ruptured. On the other hand, mammography will show silicone fluid breast injections, deflated saline-filled implants, the plane in which implants are placed (subglandular or submuscular), the outer saline-containing lumen of standard double-lumen implants, and the characteristic appearance and the type of saline-filled breast implants. This information can be useful. For example, knowing that an implant is saline-filled from mammography can obviate breast MR imaging to look for silicone gel–filled implant rupture, because mammography can definitively show that an implant is saline-filled. With regard to implant identification, a case was seen where a lawsuit was averted when a woman was sure her plastic surgeon placed silicone gel–filled implants against her wishes and switched her medical records to show that she had saline-filled implants, which she had asked for and which indeed she did have, as shown definitively on old mammograms.

Ultrasound can reliably detect extracapsular silicone granuloma (and silicone, and probably polyurethane in lymph nodes), perhaps better than MR imaging, using the so-called "snowstorm" sign.[28] It can also detect intracapsular rupture quite well if the operator is sufficiently experienced and knows what to look for.[29,30] However, the level of required experience is not common, and so it is probably best, unless an individual has sufficient expertise, to limit conclusions based on ultrasound to extracapsular findings.

CT scans can show many implant abnormalities, but usually not as well as MR imaging. Hence, given that CT scans use ionizing radiation, evaluation of implants with CT should be limited to evaluating incidental findings on CT scans obtained for other purposes.

MR Imaging

MR imaging has limitations, which are later discussed, but nevertheless is still the most accurate method available to noninvasively evaluate silicone gel–filled breast implants. Breast implant imaging currently can be performed well on essentially all types of 1.5-T and 3-T MR imaging scanners from all major manufacturers, using

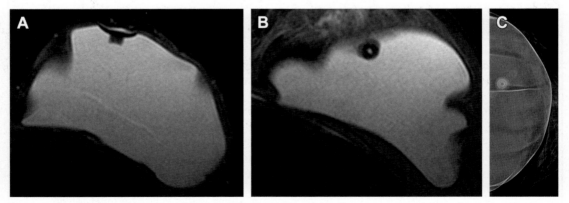

Fig. 1. Saline-filled breast implant: (*A*) T2-weighted MR image showing cross-section view of anterior diaphragm valve; (*B*) T2-weighted MR image showing en-face view of anterior diaphragm valve; (*C*) mammogram of same patient shown in (*B*), showing en-face view of diaphragm valve and its two side-straps, low-density fill material (saline), and clearly identifiable higher density implant shell.

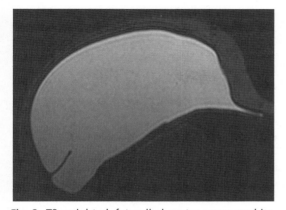

Fig. 2. T2-weighted, fat-nulled, water-suppressed image of single-lumen silicone gel–filled implant, showing a normal implant shell fold, and the slightly thickened posterior implant shell elastomer patch.

off-the-shelf standard sequences. Despite that statement, there are imaging acquisition pitfalls and choices that can compromise image usefulness, so provided here is a practical discussion of silicone gel and implant basics, and acquisition technique.

Silicone molecular structure

Silicon is a tetravalent atom (atomic number 14, atomic weight 28.085), and like carbon (which is also tetravalent), can form long-chain molecules. Those long-chain molecules typically consist of several hundred backbone siloxane ($-Si-O-$) subunits. The class of long-chain molecules that contain backbone siloxane subunits are generically referred to as silicones. Methyl groups ($-CH_3$) are attached to most of the silicon (Si) atoms on that backbone (**Fig. 3**), and methyl groups are also attached at the ends. Hence, silicone is also called polydimethylsiloxane. In this form, silicone is a viscous liquid, like honey; it is not a gel that can hold its shape. To formulate a gel that can hold its shape from silicone fluid, some of the long chains of silicone need to be chemically cross-linked to each other. If cross-linked silicone chains are mixed in an appropriate

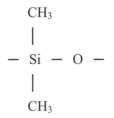

Fig. 3. Schematic structure of one subunit of a long-chain silicone molecule.

way in appropriate amounts, a silicone gel results (like a matrix of cross-linked long silicone chains, immersed in a bath of more silicone long chains that are not cross-linked, in about a 1:4 ratio). That gel is what silicone gel–filled implants are filled with. Implant shells are made of the same components, but under appropriate conditions of heat and pressure an elastomer forms (essentially a silicone rubber). That is what the shells of breast implants are made of.

During manufacture, the outer surface of breast implant shells is commonly made textured because it is thought that texture reduces the likelihood of capsular contracture. Textured implants often develop a layer of waterlike fluid around the implant, within the fibrous capsule (see Ref.[21] for an example).

The inner surface of implant shells is typically coated with a substance to help reduce silicone fluid bleed out of the implants, because so-called low-bleed implants are thought to be less prone to capsular contracture. If a new implant were to be placed, out of the box, on a sheet of paper for a week, there would be a slippery stain on that paper—that is silicone fluid bleed. All silicone gel–filled breast implants do that; it is not by itself a sign of rupture.

When the implant shell of a silicone gel–containing implant develops defects, holes, or tears, silicone gel escapes, and that is called rupture.

Some older implants from the 1960s and 1970s, which are now only occasionally seen, have so-called fixation patches of various numbers and kinds attached to their posterior surface that are meant to engender tissue ingrowth, and hence, fixation of the implant to surrounding tissues, to prevent rotation. The idea was that some of the resultant shape of the breast after implant placement is due to the shape of the implant itself, and so fixation was thought to be a good idea. The ingrowth ends up involving the inner surface of the fibrous capsules surrounding these implants.

Anatomy

Breast implants can be placed in the subglandular (or prepectoral) plane, under breast glandular tissue and over pectoralis major; or the submuscular (or retropectoral) plane, under pectoralis major. Muscle coverage for submuscular implants can be variable, and implants can even be placed under pectoralis minor. For reconstruction, implants can be placed under a latissimus dorsi flap that has been brought forward from the back. For MR imaging, it is usually sufficient to specify the plane in which the implants have been placed. Two studies of older implants have reported that submuscular implants have a higher risk of rupture than subglandular implants.[10,26]

Incisions to place implants can be axillary, infra-mammary, or peri-areolar.

Parameter settings in breast implant MR imaging

Extracapsular silicone Silicone is similar to water in that it has a longer T2 value than fat. Hence, if implants are imaged with standard off-the-shelf MR imaging T2-weighted sequences, silicone will be brighter than fat, as will water, but water will be brighter than silicone because water has a longer value of T2 than silicone. **Fig. 4**, for example, shows a T2-weighted image in which there is no suppression or fat nulling of any kind: water is brighter than silicone, and silicone is brighter than fat. This image is not optimal, however, to look for silicone outside the fibrous capsule. Ideally, the radiologist wants an image in which silicone is bright and everything else (ie, both water and fat) is dark, so that it is possible to say, "my confidence is high that none of the silicone gel from inside the implant, which is bright, is outside of the fibrous capsule where effectively the only other signal intensities are from water and fat, and if (bright) extracapsular silicone were present in any significant amount, I would see it." To accomplish that, water and fat both have to be dark. One sure way to do that is to apply water suppression and fat nulling to a T2-weighted sequence. An example of this kind of sequence

is shown in **Fig. 5**, in which the silicone is bright, and both fat and water are dark. This sequence will allow the radiologist to detect any significant extracapsular silicone outside the fibrous capsule that may be present, or to exclude it with high confidence.

Intracapsular silicone The technical goal in detecting intracapsular rupture of silicone gel–filled breast implants is to determine whether silicone gel is present outside the implant shell, or not. If (bright) silicone gel on T2-weighted sequences is definitively seen outside the implant shell, inside the fibrous capsule, then implant rupture is inferred; an actual break, disruption, or tear in the silicone elastomer shell is almost never directly seen. The technical image acquisition problem to be overcome is that silicone elastomer shells of breast implants are sometimes very thin (~0.05 mm) and are most often, even on modern implants with thicker shells, well under a millimeter thick. This statement means that on standard 2D T2-weighted images with 3- to 4-mm slice thickness, implant shells (dark on T2-weighted sequences) are almost always volume averaged with adjacent silicone gel (bright on T2-weighted sequences). This can be managed to some extent because even though implant shells are volume averaged with surrounding silicone gel, the shells are so much darker than the silicone gel that they can still be seen if implant resolution is sufficiently high. How high? On unilateral 20-cm field-of-view (FOV) images, most implant shells can be seen over most of their surface if the acquisition matrix is 256 × 192, slice thickness is 4 mm, and one image acquisition is acquired (ie, one signal

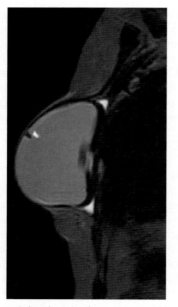

Fig. 4. T2-weighted sagittal unsuppressed image of a single-lumen silicone gel–filled breast implant, unsuppressed, showing bright intracapsular water-like fluid, gray silicone gel, and darker breast fatty tissue.

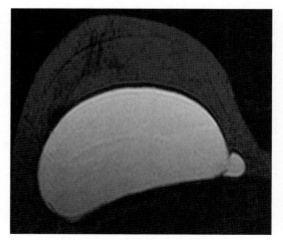

Fig. 5. T2-weighted, fat-nulled, water-suppressed image of a ruptured single-lumen silicone gel–filled breast implant with a small medial collection of extruded extracapsular silicone gel.

average). Sensitivity for rupture will be noticeably decreased if slice thickness is increased to 5 mm and/or the acquisition matrix is decreased to 256 × 128.

To recognize normal shell fold patterns reliably, slice gaps of 0 mm are usually required. If only one imaging plane can be acquired, the axial plane is preferred because, for some reason, the way implants settle in breasts and the patterns of folds that result are more likely to show implant rupture in the axial plane than imaging in the sagittal plane.

Breast implant MR imaging pulse sequences

Useful MR imaging pulse sequences are summarized in **Table 2**. There are also other ways to image breast implants using both off-the-shelf standard sequences and proprietary sequences. Evident rupture and larger amounts of extracapsular silicone may be easily detected on almost any sequence that offers some contrast between water, fat, and silicone. The author prefers using the sequences described here because they can detect both intracapsular rupture and extracapsular silicone; they are robust and implementable across sites and scanner manufacturers using standard MR imaging scanner software and hardware, and they have been used on several thousand patients with breast implants at the author's site and elsewhere. They do require some care to acquire, as is discussed later, but the level of expertise required is not more than MR imaging technologists are typically used to. Also, the basic

principles and goals of breast implant MR imaging using these sequences apply also to other methods of breast implant imaging:

1. Bilateral 2D sagittal T2-weighted, unsuppressed: Acquiring one sequence that uses no suppression or nulling of any kind can be helpful to resolve problems of implant-fill material identification that may result from failure of water suppression, failure of silicone suppression, or failure of fat nulling (see **Fig. 4**). It can act as a "truth-teller" sequence in that signal from water will always be greater than silicone signal, and silicone signal will always be greater than fat signal. It can also serve as a localizer sequence to help plan other sequences, and to spot superior and very rarely inferior spread of extracapsular silicone that may not be included on other (axial) sequences.

2. Unilateral 2D axial T2-weighted, fast spin-echo, fat-nulled, water-suppressed: As noted above, a good sequence to image silicone gel–filled breast implants is unilateral axial 2D T2-weighted, fast spin-echo imaging with inversion-recovery fat nulling and water suppression, 4-mm slice thickness, 0-mm slice gaps, and 256 × 192 acquisition matrix (see **Fig. 5**). Inversion times of 140 to 180 ms are used to accomplish fat nulling. To reduce imaging time, echo train lengths of about 15 are used; these result in higher fat signal, but that is effectively reduced by the fat nulling. These

Table 2
Useful breast implant MR imaging sequences

	Description	Main Parameters	Uses
1	Bilateral 2D sagittal T2-weighted, unsuppressed, body coil	Fast spin-echo, ETL = 8–10, 8-mm slice thickness, 4-mm gaps, TR >3000 ms, 256 × 192 matrix, 1 average	Scout sequence that allows differentiation of water from silicone in cases of failure of nulling or suppression
2	Unilateral 2D axial T2-weighted, fast spin-echo, fat-nulled, water-suppressed, breast coil	Fast spin-echo, ETL = 15, 4-mm slice thickness, 0 mm gaps, TR >3000 ms, 256 × 192 matrix, 1 average	Main sequence to detect extracapsular soft-tissue silicone; also useful for most intracapsular implant rupture
3	Unilateral 2D axial T2-weighted, fast spin-echo, silicone-suppressed, breast coil	Fast spin-echo, ETL = 15, 4-mm slice thickness, 0 mm gaps, TR >3000 ms, 256 × 192 matrix, 1 average	Auxiliary sequence to increase confidence in extracapsular soft-tissue silicone
4	Unilateral high-resolution 2D axial T2-weighted, fast spin-echo, water-suppressed, breast coil	Fast spin-echo, ETL = 15, 3-mm slice thickness, 0 mm gaps, TR >3000 msec, 256 × 256 matrix, 2 averages	High-resolution increased at expense of soft-tissue silicone detection capability, useful for thin shell and some standard double-lumen implants where early rupture determination is difficult

Abbreviation: ETL, echo train length.

sequences typically take 2 to 4 minutes to acquire, per breast. Sensitivity for intracapsular rupture detection can be increased by acquiring images with 256 × 256 matrix.

3. Unilateral 2D axial T2-weighted, fast spin-echo, silicone-suppressed: Improved confidence in detecting extracapsular silicone can be achieved if silicone instead of water suppression is used and no fat nulling is applied, resulting in images in which water is very bright, fat is medium gray, and silicone is dark. If silicone is present in soft tissues, it will show up as bright against a dark background on the fat-nulled, water-suppressed images (see **Fig. 5**), and dark against a medium-gray background on silicone-suppressed images (**Fig. 6**). This sequence is not good to detect intracapsular rupture because dark implant shell folds are not well seen against a background of dark silicone gel.

4. Unilateral high-resolution 2D axial T2-weighted, fast spin-echo, water-suppressed: Higher resolution settings (256 × 256 acquisition matrix, 3-mm slice thickness, 0-mm slice gaps) may be necessary to detect rupture for older, thin shell implants from the mid-1970s to the mid-1980s, and some standard double-lumen implants where saline is absent from the outer lumen. In those cases, to attain adequate signal-to-noise, 2 signal averages are required. Because the purpose of this sequence is specifically to detect implant shell folds, there is less need for fat nulling and it can be omitted to save time. **Figs. 8**, **10** and **13A** were obtained with this sequence.

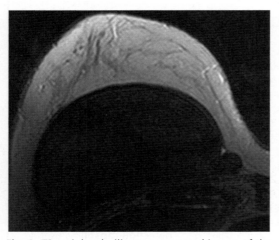

Fig. 6. T2-weighted, silicone-suppressed image of the same implant showed in **Fig. 5**, showing the small medial collection of extruded extracapsular silicone gel now imaging with sharply defined dark signal against the surrounding (unsuppressed) breast fatty tissue.

MR image acquisition hints and pitfalls

This section is intended mainly for MR imaging technologists, although radiologists may also be interested. The discussion is provided in some depth, which is often needed to provide practical assistance in acquiring these pulse sequences. Several common errors that can occur in breast implant imaging follow:

1. MR imaging indications for imaging saline-filled breast implants: Saline-filled breast implants do not benefit from MR imaging evaluation, unless there is an interest in possible soft-tissue silicone from a prior implant, evaluation of previous silicone fluid injections, or there is uncertainty whether the implant is saline-filled. Also, some tissue expanders that contain an integral magnet are MR imaging contraindicated. Keeping these factors in mind will help avoid unnecessary, or even risky, MR imaging scanning.

2. Recognizing saline-filled implants: Knowing whether an implant is saline-filled or silicone gel–filled can help with MR imaging. Not infrequently, patient history is incorrect or misleading. If definitive documentation of implant type is not available (such as implant manufacturer's labels), there are at least a dozen ways to tell from imaging alone whether implants are saline-filled. Ways to recognize or suggest that an implant is saline-filled include

   • Implant fill material is less dense than implant shell on mammography (**Fig. 1**C)
   • Implant fill material is less dense than silicone gel on CT
   • There is no posterior displacement of posterior implant surface on ultrasound[29,30]
   • Large water peak on sequence setup MR spectrum (Typically, most MR scanner manufacturers offer an option during prescanning to check the MR spectrum. This check is usually sufficient to identify the main water, fat, and silicone peaks and to determine the frequency of any peak by placing a vertical cursor over that peak.)
   • Marked chemical shift of implant fill material compared with fat on unsuppressed MR images
   • Same signal intensity on unsuppressed T2-weighted images as waterlike fluid elsewhere in the body
   • Darker signal than silicone gel on T1-weighted MR images
   • Dark signal on water suppression MR imaging T2-weighted sequences
   • Bright signal on silicone suppression MR imaging T2-weighted sequences

- Bright signal on fat suppression MR imaging T2-weighted sequences
- Presence of diaphragm valve on mammography, CT, or MR imaging (Diaphragm valves are small cylinder-shaped elastomer structures, typically 5 to 10 mm in diameter and up to 10 mm in depth, usually mounted anteriorly on saline-filled implants to permit filling at time of placement [see Ref.[21] for illustrations].)
- Presence of leaflet valve on mammography, CT, or MR imaging (Leaflet valves are 7- to 10-mm-wide elastomer strips, usually 3 to 4 cm in length, usually mounted posteriorly on standard double-lumen and some other types of implants, to permit filling of the saline-containing lumen at the time of placement [see Ref.[21] for illustrations].)

3. Choice of acquisition frequency: To choose the correct operating frequency for any particular breast implant MR imaging sequence involving chemical suppression requires familiarity with the basic spectrum of water, fat, and silicone (**Fig. 7**). The water, fat, and silicone spectral peaks shown in **Fig. 7** are schematically represented as single peaks, whereas in reality each is much more complex. For example, fat has 7 major spectral peaks.[31] However, fat and silicone suppression in breast implant imaging require only qualitative interpretation, and so acting as if the spectrum consists only of the single water peak, the major methylene ($-CH_2-$) peak of fat, and the major methyl group ($-CH_3$) peak of silicone is not inappropriate for this application.

Choosing the operating frequency correctly is a 2-step process. In step 1, we must find a reference frequency—this can be either water, fat, or silicone. Suppose a breast contains a large implant that is saline filled (based on clearly seeing a diaphragm valve, for example),

with very little overlying fatty or other tissue. We then know that there will be one spectral peak and it will be the water peak. Place the MR pre-scanning spectrum cursor over the water peak and write down its frequency (for example, suppose it is 63,500,000 Hz). At 1.5 T, knowing just that one number, we then also know that the fat frequency is about 220 Hz lower than that (63,499,780 Hz), and the silicone frequency is about 300 Hz lower than water (63,499,700 Hz). The second step is scanner-dependent and software-dependent, and so it will vary, but it is often known by the MR imaging technologists for your scanner, or the applications group for your scanner manufacturer may be able to help. Suppose we are setting up a water suppression sequence, and for that sequence on your scanner you know you have to scan at the fat frequency. From step 1, we know the fat frequency, so we can plug in the correct number and run the scan. Suppose the scenario is changed: the patient has a large silicone gel–filled implant and no overlying tissue. In step 1, you can place a cursor on that spectral peak—it will be the only peak present—and we also know it has to be the silicone peak from the appearance of the images. It will be approximately 63,499,700 Hz, and so we will again know that to suppress water, we can plug in the frequency of fat, which is 643,499,780 Hz, and then we are ready to scan. This method works for any single peak, any combination of 2 peaks, or for all 3 peaks, which can occur for, possibly, a standard double-lumen implant in a fatty breast where water, fat, and silicone are all present.

4. Choice of where to place the spectrum box for step 1, above: To see a prescanning spectrum on most or all scanners for step 1 (above) before you scan, you need to specify or accept a default location for where that setup spectrum will be obtained, or you might need to actively specify that location yourself. This location is scanner-dependent and may require some practice that is specific to your site and scanner. In general, if you place a spectral region of interest (ROI) over whatever you want to suppress, the frequency you see of the (usually one) peak in your spectrum should correspond to where you chose to place the ROI. If you placed the ROI over a saline-filled implant, the frequency of that peak (and there should be only the one peak) should be that of the water peak, and similarly also for fat or silicone if you place the ROI over those areas. If you or the scanner automatically places the ROI over both breasts, there often will be more than

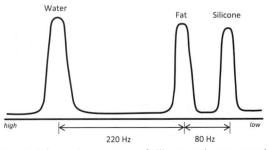

Fig. 7. Schematic spectrum of silicone gel, water, and fat. Silicone and fat are separated by about 80 Hz, and fat and water are separated by about 220 Hz at 1.5 T. (These differences are doubled at 3 T.)

one peak, but using the method described above, you should be able to proceed to step 2 to choose an operating frequency and then scan. When you have done this once and it works, it should be correct for future scans using that placement protocol.

5. Choice of imaging volume: For the sagittal unsuppressed/localizer sequence, the body coil should be used; the selected FOV should be approximately 32 cm centered on the breasts, and imaging should be performed from axilla to axilla. For the fat-nulled, water-suppressed axial sequence and the silicone-suppressed axial sequence, the whole breast should be selected (usually 20 cm FOV is adequate, 22 cm for large breasts); the breast surface coil should be used in unilateral mode, and the maximal number of slices that can obtain signal from the surface coil should be selected (at our site, that is 41 contiguous slices of 4-mm-thickness). For the high-resolution axial images, the image volume should be coned tightly to the implant and the breast surface coil used in unilateral mode.

Normal MR imaging appearance and variants of silicone gel–filled breast implants

Single lumen Single-lumen silicone gel–filled breast implants, which are the most common type at this time, show several normal-variant appearances of implant folds; no folds (rare), floppy folds (**Fig. 8**), volume-averaged folds (**Fig. 9**), folds that bisect or trisect the implant (**Fig. 10**), and complex folds (**Fig. 11**). These folds are all cross-

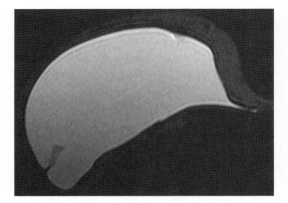

Fig. 9. T2-weighted, fat-nulled, water-suppressed image of a single-lumen silicone gel–filled breast implant, showing a volume-averaged fold in the lower left corner of the image. This appearance results from the fold being directed in a slightly different angle at the top, compared with the bottom of the voxels in this slice.

sectional appearances of the same phenomenon: when an underfilled bag (the implant) is placed into a confined space, it conforms to the space and in-folds on itself as needed to fit into that space. Those in-foldings are the folds seen on MR imaging. The complex fold pattern is the one that most closely mimics the appearance of implant rupture. However, these appearances are different, and if one scrolls up and down

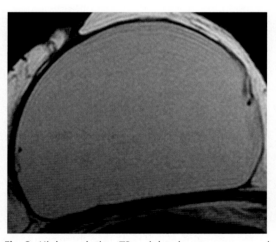

Fig. 8. High-resolution, T2-weighted, water-suppressed image of an intact single-lumen silicone gel–filled breast implant, showing a floppy fold along the left edge of the implant. The fold appears completely dark, with no evidence of silicone within the fold, outside the implant appears whole.

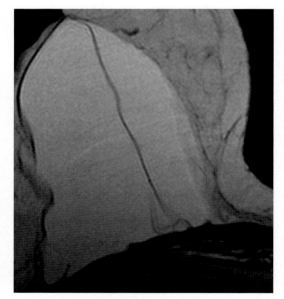

Fig. 10. High-resolution, T2-weighted, water-suppressed image of an intact single-lumen silicone gel–filled breast implant, showing a fold apparently bisecting the implant. This is just an in-folding from slices above and below this slice. This appearance is a pitfall for rupture, but is not a sign of rupture.

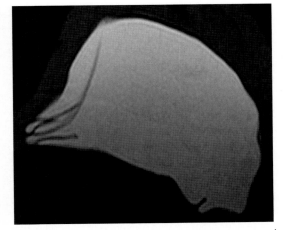

Fig. 11. T2-weighted, fat-nulled, water-suppressed image of a single-lumen silicone gel–filled breast implant, showing a series of complex-appearing shell folds in the left part of the image. This is a pitfall for rupture and is not a sign of rupture. The key is to notice that the shell folds extend all the way to the edge of the implant, and so not present as a series of folds with rounded edges completely surrounded by silicone gel, which would then indicate rupture.

through the slices of a series showing complex folds, it will be clear that they are only in-foldings, and that there is no evident silicone outside the implant as a whole, along the inner surface of the fibrous capsule, or within the folds themselves.

A normal variant appearance of submuscular single-lumen silicone gel–filled breast implants is bunched folds medially under the pectoralis major muscle (**Fig. 12**). This variant is a consequence of these implants having thin pliable shells and of

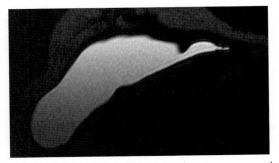

Fig. 12. High-resolution, T2-weighted, water-suppressed image of an intact single-lumen silicone gel–filled breast implant, showing a bunched or pinched appearance medially. This example is a common pitfall for rupture, but is not a sign of rupture. The implant is just conforming to the structures and pressures around it, and the presence of pectoralis major just medial to the implant often results in this appearance.

being underfilled objects placed into a confined space, under muscle.

Numerous additional examples of these normal imaging variants are illustrated in Ref.[18]

Standard double-lumen Standard double-lumen implants have silicone gel in the inner lumen and saline in the outer lumen. Some older versions have a single posterior thicker silicone elastomer shell patch to which both the inner and the outer shells are attached; on some of those implants a leaflet valve mounted on that central patch is used to fill the outer lumen, and in others a posterior leaflet valve mounted separately on its outer shell (not the central shell patch) is used for that task. This design is referred to as the "shared-patch" design. More recent standard double-lumen implants consist of a true bag-in-a-bag design, each with its own posterior shell patch; in this type of implant, the leaflet values are mounted on the outer, posterior implant shell. References[18,21,26] contain illustrations of several examples of this kind of implant.

Gel-gel double lumen The gel-gel double-lumen implant is a high-profile device intended for breast reconstruction; that is, it is intended to provide form and profile in addition to bulk to take the place of tissue that has been removed. It has a different but recognizable normal appearance that should not be mistaken for intracapsular rupture. Reference[18] contains illustrations of this kind of implant.

Reverse double-lumen expander-implant The reverse double-lumen expander-implant is intended for reconstruction, but is also used for augmentation. When used for reconstruction, where overlying tissue is minimal, the idea is that softer, more natural feeling silicone gel in the outer lumen is closer to the skin, and saline is placed in the inner lumen to permit expansion and sizing. If used as an expander-implant, it is placed in the breast with the fill point piece at the distal end of the fill tube placed subcutaneously in the axilla for serial filling over time. When the breast skin has been appropriately expanded, the fill tube is pulled, effectively converting the device to a permanent implant. References[18,21,26] contain illustrations of this kind of implant.

ABNORMAL IMAGING FINDINGS
Diagnosis of Rupture

Fibrous capsules can form around implants within days of placement.[32,33] They can vary from thin and translucent to tough but flexible, and then later in some patients they can contract, assume a more spherical shape, become painful, calcify, and even ossify.[34] Capsular contracture is at least partly a foreign body reaction that may be related to silicone fluid bleed, implant rupture, physical contact of tissue with the implant surface, other silicone specific factors (because silicone chemistry varies), chronic infection, implantation surgery factors, or patient factors; in other words, it is not known what causes it, but it is known that it occurs and is not uncommon.

Breast implant rupture usually is due to small defects or worn areas of implant shell that eventually begin to ooze silicone gel into the intracapsular space, within the fibrous capsule. Occasionally implant shells tear *in vivo*, but that might happen after an earlier smaller defect develops. Capsular contracture is not by itself a clear indication that an implant is ruptured, but there may be an association with rupture because both capsular contracture and rupture are more likely as implants age.

Breast implant intracapsular rupture can be staged, from early to advanced (**Table 3**): the stages are uncollapsed, minimally collapsed, moderately collapsed, and fully collapsed rupture (**Fig. 13**).[18,26] Any of these stages can be accompanied by extracapsular silicone, either from the implant itself or from a prior implant. The presence of definite extracapsular soft-tissue silicone does not imply that the implant is in a state of partially or fully collapsed rupture; many implants that are in states of uncollapsed and minimally collapsed rupture develop capsule defects through which silicone escapes to extracapsular soft tissues. Describing intracapsular rupture by stage, using common terminology, can be helpful to surgeons

and patients to help them decide what to do and when to do it, and can help inform the surgeon of the condition of patients' implants preoperatively.

Fig. 13 shows some of the various signs of implant rupture. For further examples, see Ref.[18,26]

Uncollapsed (ie, very early) rupture is characterized by silicone gel (bright signal on water-suppressed images) present in folds—that is, outside the implant as a whole, inside the fibrous capsule, but not (yet) between stretches of implant shell and fibrous capsule. This appearance is referred to by a variety of names: keyhole sign, teardrop sign, inverted teardrop sign, and noose sign.[18,26] All of these signs refer to variants of the same phenomenon: the presence of silicone within in-foldings of implant shell, outside the implant as a whole. The inference is that if enough silicone is present in those locations to be seen on MR imaging, the implant must be (at least) in a state of uncollapsed rupture. That is not entirely true, as is discussed later, but in most cases if any of these appearances is seen, the implant is probably ruptured.

Minimally collapsed rupture refers to the second stage of intracapsular rupture where silicone gel not only is present within shell in-foldings, but also is present between stretches of implant shell and fibrous capsule. This appearance is referred to by two names: the back-patch sign, and the subcapsular line sign.[18,26] The back-patch, or shell patch, of an implant is a silicone elastomer disc of variable diameter (as small as ~25 mm, as large as ~105 mm) placed on the posterior surface of implants. It is often readily identifiable on MR imaging and rarely if ever is included in an in-folding of implant shell because it is thicker and

Table 3		
MR imaging stages of breast implant intracapsular rupture		
Stage	**Category**	**Description**
I	Uncollapsed	Silicone gel is seen on MR imaging within shell folds, outside the implant shell, inside the fibrous capsule, but not adjacent to stretches of implant shell/fibrous capsule
II	Minimally collapsed	Silicone gel is seen on MR imaging not only within shell folds, but also along stretches of implant shell/fibrous capsule boundary, or behind the implant posterior elastomer patch
III	Partially collapsed	Implant shell partially collapsed on itself on MR imaging, but with some semblance of still being an implant containing silicone gel; large amounts of silicone gel are outside the implant proper, within the fibrous capsule
IV	Fully collapsed	Implant shell is seen on MR imaging to be collapsed on itself in layers and folds, centrally or peripherally, within the fibrous capsule; the silicone gel is no longer in the implant shell, and the implant shell is now collapsed and mostly emptied of silicone gel, which surrounds it within the fibrous capsule

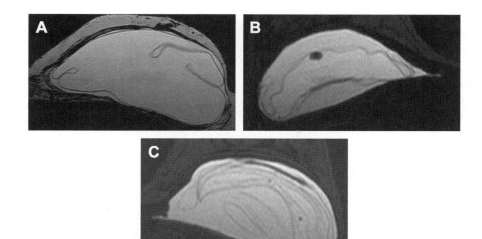

Fig. 13. Three examples of implant rupture are shown here. The first example is a high-resolution image with water suppression, and the other 2 examples are fat-nulled and water-suppressed. (*A*) An example of minimally collapsed rupture. The keyhole and subcapsular line signs are seen here. If only the keyhole sign was seen, this would have been called uncollapsed rupture. (*B*) A standard double-lumen implant in a state of partially collapsed rupture. Note that the 2 leaves of implant shell can just be seen, attached to each side of the shared posterior shell patch. Partially collapsed rupture is probably more common for standard double-lumen implants than for single-lumen silicone gel–filled breast implants, for implants in these advanced stages of rupture. (*C*) The appearance of a double-lumen implant (again, with a shared posterior shell patch) in a state of fully collapsed rupture. Note that there appear to be too many lines; this has been called the double wavy-line sign. (*From* Middleton MS, McNamara MP. Breast implant imaging. Philadelphia: Lippincott Williams and Wilkins; 2003; and Middleton MS. Magnetic resonance evaluation of breast implants and soft-tissue silicone [review]. Top Magn Reson Imaging 1998;9:92–137.)

stiffer than implant shell, so silicone seen outside of it not only indicates rupture, it indicates that more silicone gel is outside the implant than is seen in uncollapsed rupture.

Partially collapsed rupture refers to implants that have more silicone gel outside the shell than those in a state of minimally collapsed rupture, but have not yet fully progressed to being in a state of fully collapsed rupture. One sign has been described that occurs in this, and in the final (fully collapsed) stage, called the C-sign.[18,26] It refers to some early implants from Heyer Schulte (early versions of Styles 2000, 2100, and 2200, from the late 1960s and early 1970s) whose shell patches (~40–60 mm diameter) were notably thick and tended to curl when the implant shell collapsed to the point that there is not enough silicone gel remaining within the implant to keep the shell patches flat. When viewed cross-sectionally, the shell-patches look like the letter C. Because these implants are now quite old, they will only rarely (if ever) be encountered at this time.

Fully collapsed rupture refers to the final stage of intracapsular rupture when the implant shell is fully collapsed within the silicone gel that it used to contain. This appearance is referred to by 2 names: the wavy-line sign, and the linguini sign.[18,26] Both refer to the above-described appearance of implant shell, fully folded in on itself, perhaps torn into pieces.

The term herniation has been used to describe those situations whereby parts of the actual implant shell are extruding through a defect in the implant fibrous capsule. Herniated implants may or may not be ruptured.

Diagnosis of Deflation

Saline-filled implants are usually said to deflate, not to rupture. Once there is a defect in the shell or the valve of a saline-filled implant, it usually empties in a day to a week. No imaging of any kind is needed for these diagnoses—the patient herself, and her plastic surgeon, know what has happened, and there are often symptoms such as pain, burning, and perceived loss of profile and size. However, if an imaging examination is done for another reason when there is a deflated saline-filled implant in place, the appearance is characteristic. Examples are shown in Refs.[18,26]

Diagnosis of Soft Tissue Silicone

Extracapsular silicone can be seen in 4 forms: diffusely infiltrated silicone fluid or gel, silicone gel collections with or without their own fibrous capsules, silicone granuloma (which can be thought of as a silicone-infiltrated scar/fibrous tissue), and silicone adenopathy.

The first two forms have the same T2-weighted signal intensity as silicone gel within breast implants. The third and fourth forms can have foci of the same T2-weighted signal as silicone gel in implants, but much or all of the remainder will have less signal intensity than silicone gel in implants and typically will have an inhomogeneous appearance. The reason relates to how silicone granuloma and silicone adenopathy forms. Silicone granulomas start as silicone gel, but tissue ingrowth occurs (of tissue with scarlike or waterlike signal intensity), resulting in a final lower signal on water-suppressed T2-weighted sequences compared with silicone gel. Silicone adenopathy develops slightly differently. On water-suppressed images, most nodes, which are T2-bright, will be dark. As silicone enters nodes, they can enlarge and eventually will show increased signal on water-suppressed images. The threshold of silicone that can be detected depends on the signal intensity of nodes without silicone, which depends on sequence parameters like the degree of water suppression. Hence, the very smallest amounts of silicone in nodes are not evident on fat-nulled, water-suppressed MR imaging, and the levels above that can be detected are sequence-dependent.

Implant rupture and extrusion into extracapsular tissues can be caused or exacerbated by closed capsulotomy, a procedure that is currently discouraged in a warning from breast implant manufacturers.[12,13] Rarely, migration of silicone gel following extrusion from ruptured implants can extend into the brachial plexus and the arms.[18,26,35–38]

Differential Diagnosis

Most diagnoses of advanced implant rupture and extracapsular silicone are definitive, with no differential alternatives. Depending on the imaging method and resolution used, uncollapsed and even minimally collapsed rupture may not be evident due to volume averaging resulting in false negatives; they are usually not false negative missed diagnoses; however, they are false negative diagnoses that are beyond the capability of

the imaging as obtained. Even with the best imaging available and the most experienced readers, there is slight overlap between the upper limits of normal silicone fluid bleed from intact implants that can be seen outside the implant shell in folds, and the lower limits of the earliest uncollapsed rupture than can be diagnosed from MR imaging from seeing small amounts of silicone outside the implant shell in folds. The problem is that silicone fluid and silicone gel are not distinguishable by MR imaging; they are both brighter than fat and less bright than water on T2-weighted sequences. With the MR imaging signs of rupture that are present, it is assumed that silicone definitively seen outside the implant shell means rupture, but that assumption breaks down for the very smallest amounts of silicone that can be seen on MR imaging. Hence, there is a threshold below which it cannot be determined whether an implant is ruptured or not, and there is a range above that whereby imaging quality and reader experience factors come into play, so that some implant rupture might not be definitively recognizable, even to experts.

The most common interpretation pitfall in breast MR imaging is distinguishing complex folds (see **Fig. 11**) from collapsed rupture (**Fig. 13C**). Several additional examples are shown in Ref.[18] The key to distinguishing these entities is to scroll through the images and question whether the folds go all the way to the inner surface of the fibrous capsule surface, which mitigates strongly toward complex folds, or whether they are rounded everywhere and always separated from the fibrous capsule by clearly identified silicone gel.

The same kinds of arguments hold for extracapsular soft-tissue silicone. For clearly evident silicone fluid collections and silicone granulomas, there is no differential; it is known that they are silicone gel collections and granulomas, respectively (**Fig. 14**). It is not known whether they do not also contain cancer, but in our limited experience to date, we have never seen that, so it is rare or does not occur. The situation is somewhat complicated because cancer is diagnosed partly from enhancement, and silicone granulomas can enhance, but they usually enhance with benign characteristics.

If implant-related imaging is not done during a breast cancer–related MR imaging, or is not done adequately, it may not be possible to tell whether a mass is a silicone granuloma or a cancer. Implant-related sequences described here and elsewhere can usually help resolve these dilemmas. An example of the use of implant-related imaging to help sort out the granuloma-versus-cancer question is included in Ref.[18]

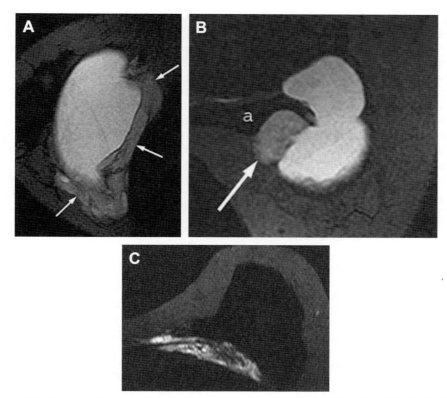

Fig. 14. T2-weighted images showing 3 silicone granulomas (*arrows* in *A* and *B*) adjacent to the implant fibrous capsules. The first example is fat-nulled (*A*), and the other 2 examples (*B,C*) were obtained instead with a long TE (more than 200 ms), which was how fat was darkened before inversion-recovery was available for fast spin-echo sequences. All 3 images are water-suppressed. The first 2 examples (*A,B*) show ruptured silicone gel–filled implants, and the third example (*C*) shows an intact (subglandular) saline-filled implant (dark because it is water suppressed). The silicone granuloma for the third case (*C*) came from a previously ruptured submuscular silicone gel–filled implant.

Additional Pearls, Pitfalls, and Variants

It can sometimes be difficult to distinguish uncollapsed and minimally collapsed rupture of single-lumen silicone gel–filled implants, from silicone gel that has escaped from the inner lumen into the outer lumen of standard double-lumen implants, where no saline was ever placed in the outer lumen or where the outer lumen saline escaped previously. Old mammograms are probably the most helpful here—the older the better—because saline in the outer lumen of a standard double-lumen implant has a characteristic and recognizable appearance. Medical records can help learn the implant type. High-resolution implant imaging can sometimes identify both the inner and the outer lumen shell, occasionally with small waterlike bubbles between them, and that can help. It may not be possible to tell the difference from MR imaging alone. Usually it can be assumed that a silicone gel–filled implant is a single-lumen design simply because uncollapsed and minimally collapsed rupture of that implant type is common, and the appearance described above of the standard double-lumen implant with the saline gone and silicone in the outer lumen is rare.

Failed water suppression of breast soft tissues can result in a kind of T2 shine-through of T2-bright waterlike structures, like benign lymph nodes, some fibroadenomas, and other T2-bright lesions and structures. If a reader rigorously assumes that all bright objects on fat-nulled, water-suppressed images are silicone gel or granuloma, eventually this situation will be encountered. The solution is to always be vigilant to the possibility of failed water (or silicone, or fat) suppression. A sign that water suppression has failed is that nearby structures that are known to be water-based, like blood vessels, are bright also. This is a reliable rule of thumb. Use of the silicone-suppressed sequence described above also can help.

Large breast seromas and hematomas can mimic the appearance of saline-filled implants. The key here is to think of seromas and hematomas when shell folds or a valve is not seen.

Very rarely, hematomas develop within implant fibrous capsules. These hematomas are likely to have been present since implant placement. Sometimes there is a history of breast enlargement and persistent pain in the postoperative period; however, these are not silicone granulomas, because silicone granulomas do not form within implant fibrous capsules. One should consider this possibility if an inhomogeneous, non-silicone material with a waterlike signal is seen within the fibrous capsule.

What the Referring Physician Needs to Know

Referring physicians should know when to request breast implant–related MR imaging, on its own and in conjunction with breast cancer–related contrast-enhanced MR imaging. Women with suspected rupture, for whom there is no genetic or other concern for breast cancer, can have non-contrast implant-related MR imagings if there is clinical concern for rupture. The author disagrees that screening for silent rupture should be done every 2 years, as mentioned in breast implant product inserts.[12,13] The author contends that the timeframe is too often. Every 10 years would be a comfortable screening timeframe, and even that may be too often. As part of the informed consent process, it would be helpful to inform prospective breast implant recipients that problems can and do occur, that most of those problems can be handled medically or surgically, and that MR imaging screening every 10 years is available as a safety net to detect the small number of silent ruptures that might have developed so that they are caught before more serious local complications develop.

For patients receiving contrast-enhanced breast MR imaging for breast cancer–related reasons, the author would counsel the opposite: some level of breast implant–related imaging should be included for patients with silicone gel–filled implants in place unless there is a good reason not to include it, such as, a previous recent breast MR imaging was done where implants were evaluated, with no intervening change in the feel, shape, or size of the breasts and no concern for implant rupture. The reason for including breast implant–related imaging in these examinations is that any breast cancer–related findings that are found or are being followed should take into account the condition and position of any silicone gel–filled implants that are in place. In these scenarios, probably one sequence per breast (pre-contrast, 2D axial, T2-weighted, fat-nulled, water-suppressed) would be adequate. Saline-filled breast implants are automatically and adequately evaluated by any routine T2 imaging that is done as part of breast cancer–related MR imaging, so no additional imaging needs to be done to evaluate them.

Referring physicians should also know that imaging breast tissue expanders containing integral magnets with MR imaging is contraindicated, that MR imaging evaluation of saline-filled implants is not indicated, and that, in general, unless there are extenuating or additional circumstances, MR imaging to evaluate capsular contracture is not indicated.

After breast implant–related MR imaging examinations are performed, referring physicians would benefit from knowing the following:

- Implant type (saline-filled, silicone gel–filled)
- Plane of placement (submuscular, subglandular)
- Implant condition (no evidence of rupture, uncollapsed rupture, minimally collapsed rupture, partially collapsed rupture, or fully collapsed rupture)
- Amount, location, and state (infiltrated gel, free gel, silicone gel cyst, silicone granuloma) of any extracapsular soft-tissue silicone that might be present, and
- Relation of implants and any soft-tissue silicone that may be present to breast cancer–related findings.

If a new breast implant–related finding is found and the referring physician is not a plastic surgeon, referral should be made to a plastic surgeon.

SUMMARY

Breast implant MR imaging is widely available, although technical challenges prevent successful imaging at some sites. This article covered some of those problems and provided suggested approaches and solutions for MR imaging technologists and radiologists to help overcome those challenges. Current breast implant sequences can be time-consuming, especially when performed in addition to breast cancer–related MR imaging, and so development of more rapid, high-resolution, fat-nulled, water-suppressed imaging, or its equivalent, would be helpful.

Most radiologists are familiar with the appearance of partially and fully collapsed rupture and extensive soft-tissue silicone, but many may not be familiar with the strengths and limitations of MR imaging to detect early implant rupture and small amounts of soft-tissue silicone. Some may not be fully comfortable distinguishing complex folds from fully collapsed rupture. This work discussed those problems and referred readers to more complete publications for further detail.

This article discussed in some detail what the referring physician needs to know, including recommendations for screening. Also, the author expressed disagreement with current recommendations to use MR imaging to screen women with breast implants every 2 years, instead suggesting that perhaps screening every 10 years would be more appropriate. This topic is worthy of further consideration and, if necessary, further research.

REFERENCES

1. American Society of Plastic Surgeons, 2012 Plastic Surgery Statistics Report. Available at: http://www.plasticsurgery.org/Documents/news-resources/statistics/2012-Plastic-Surgery-Statistics/full-plastic-surgery-statistics-report.pdf. Accessed February 6, 2014.
2. Nommsen-Rivers L. Cosmetic breast surgery—is breastfeeding at risk. J Hum Lact 2003;19:7–8.
3. Regulatory History of breast Implants in the U.S. Available at: http://www.fda.gov/MedicalDevices/ProductsandMedicalProcedures/ImplantsandProsthetics/BreastImplants/ucm064461.htm. Accessed February 5, 2014.
4. Hedén P, Nava MB, van Tetering JP, et al. Prevalence of rupture in inamed silicone breast implants. Plast Reconstr Surg 2006;118:303–8.
5. Spear SL, Murphy DK, Slicton A, et al, Inamed Silicone Breast Implant U.S. Study Group. Inamed silicone breast implant core study results at 6 years. Plast Reconstr Surg 2007;120:8S–16S.
6. Cunningham B, McCue J. Safety and effectiveness of Mentor's MemoryGel implants at 6 years. Aesthetic Plast Surg 2009;33:440–4.
7. Hammond DC, Migliori MM, Caplin DA, et al. Mentor Contour Profile Gel implants: clinical outcomes at 6 years. Plast Reconstr Surg 2012;29:1381–91.
8. Maxwell GP, Van Natta BW, Murphy DK, et al. Natrelle style 410 form-stable silicone breast implants: core study results at 6 years. Aesthet Surg J 2012; 32:709–17.
9. Stevens WG, Harrington J, Alizadeh K, et al. Five-year follow-up data from the U.S. clinical trial for Sientra's U.S. Food and Drug Administration-approved Silimed® brand round and shaped implants with high-strength silicone gel. Plast Reconstr Surg 2012;130:973–81.
10. Brown SL, Middleton MS, Berg WA, et al. Prevalence of rupture of silicone gel breast implants revealed on MR imaging in a population of women in Birmingham, Alabama. AJR Am J Roentgenol 2000;175:1057–64.
11. Middleton MS. Invited panel presentation: Long-term problems in the augmentation patient. American Society of Plastic Surgeons (ASPS), 2013 Annual Meeting. San Diego, October 15, 2013, 10:00 to 11:00 AM.
12. Mentor product insert datasheet dated August 2010. Available at: http://www.mentorwwllc.com/Documents/gel-PIDS.pdf. Accessed February 5, 2014.
13. Allergan Directions for Use dated December 2009. Available at: http://www.allergan.com/assets/pdf/L034-03_Silicone_DFU.pdf. Accessed February 5, 2014.
14. Brinton LA, Lubin JH, Burich MC, et al. Breast cancer following augmentation mammoplasty (United States). Cancer Causes Control 2000;9:819–27.
15. Brinton LA, Brown SL. Breast implants and cancer. J Natl Cancer Inst 1997;89:1341–9.
16. Gabriel SE, Woods JE, O'Fallon M, et al. Complications leading to surgery after breast implantation. N Engl J Med 1997;336:677–82.
17. Miglioretti DL, Rutter CM, Geller BM, et al. Effect of breast augmentation on the accuracy of mammography and cancer characteristics. JAMA 2004;291:442–50.
18. Middleton MS, McNamara MP. Breast implant imaging. Philadelphia: Lippincott Williams and Wilkins; 2003.
19. Rudolph R, Forcier N. Calculation of silicone breast implant volumes using breast magnetic resonance imaging. Aesthet Surg J 2009;29:310–3.
20. Herold C, Reichelt A, Stieglitz LH, et al. MRI-based breast volumetry—evaluation of three different software solutions. J Digit Imaging 2010;23:603–10.
21. Middleton MS, McNamara MP Jr. Breast implant classification with MR imaging correlation: (CME available on RSNA link). Radiographics 2000;20:E1. Available at: http://pubs.rsna.org/doi/full/10.1148/radiographics.20.3.g00mae11.
22. Berg WA, Nguyen TK, Middleton MS, et al. MR imaging of extracapsular silicone from breast implants: diagnostic pitfalls. AJR Am J Roentgenol 2002;178:465–72.
23. Helyar V, Burke C, McWilliams S. The ruptured PIP breast implant. Clin Radiol 2013;68:845–50.
24. Chummun S, McLean NR. Poly implant prothèse (PIP) breast implants: our experience. Surgeon 2013;5:241–5.
25. Kolios L, Hirche C, Spiethoff A, et al. Complications of Poly Implant Prothèse breast implants: the current discussion. Expert Rev Med Devices 2013;10:167–70.
26. Middleton MS. Magnetic resonance evaluation of breast implants and soft-tissue silicone. Top Magn Reson Imaging 1998;9:92–137 [review].
27. Destouet JM, Monsees BS, Oser RF, et al. Screening mammography in 350 women with breast implants: prevalence and findings of implant complications. AJR Am J Roentgenol 1992;159:973–8.
28. Harris KM, Ganott MA, Shestak KC, et al. Silicone implant rupture: detection with US. Radiology 1993;187:761–8.

29. Middleton MS, McNamara MP Jr. MR and ultrasound imaging of breast implants and soft-tissue silicone. Imaging 1997;9:201–26.

30. McNamara MP Jr, Middleton MS. Ultrasound of breast implants and soft tissue silicone. In: Whitman GJ, editor. Ultrasound clinics, vol. 6. Philadelphia: Saunders; 2011. p. 345–68 (3).

31. Hamilton G, Yokoo T, Bydder M, et al. In vivo characterization of the liver fat ^{1}H MR spectrum. NMR Biomed 2011;24:784–90.

32. Vistnes LM, Ksander GA, Kosek J. Study of encapsulation of silicone rubber implants in animals. A foreign body reaction. Plast Reconstr Surg 1978;62:580–8.

33. Vistnes LM, Ksander GA. Tissue response to soft tissue silicone prostheses: capsule formation and other sequelae. In: Rubin LR, editor. Biomaterials in reconstructive surgery. St Louis (MO): Mosby; 1983. p. 516–28.

34. Peters WJ. Massive heterotopic ossification in breast implant capsules. Aesthetic Plast Surg 1985;9:43–5.

35. Foster WC, Springfield DS, Brown KL. Pseudotumor of the arm associated with rupture of silicone-gel breast prostheses. Report of two cases. J Bone Joint Surg Am 1983;65:548–51.

36. Sanger JR, Matloub HS, Yousif NJ, et al. Silicone gel infiltration of a peripheral nerve and constrictive neuropathy following rupture of a breast prosthesis. J Bone Joint Surg Am 1983;65:548–51.

37. Persellin ST, Vogler JB 3rd, Brazis PW, et al. Detection of migratory silicone pseudotumor with use of magnetic resonance imaging. Mayo Clin Proc 1992;67:891–5.

38. Teuber SS, Ito LK, Anderson M, et al. Silicone breast implant-associated scarring dystrophy of the arm. Arch Dermatol 1995;131:54–6.

Contrast-Enhanced Digital Mammography

Maxine Jochelson, MD

KEYWORDS

- Digital mammography • Contrast • Neovascularity • MR imaging

KEY POINTS

- Contrast-enhanced mammography can improve the sensitivity of digital mammography.
- Contrast-enhanced mammography is less sensitive but more specific than breast MR imaging.
- Contrast mammography is significantly less expensive than MR imaging and could potentially be used for screening patients who are unable to undergo breast MR imaging.

CONTRAST-ENHANCED MAMMOGRAPHY

Mammography remains the only breast screening examination proved to reduce breast cancer mortality in the general screening population. Multiple randomized studies have demonstrated a 30% to 40% reduction in mortality for women actually screened.[1–3] Mammography is inexpensive and widely available, but its sensitivity is limited: 70% to 85% overall but dropping to 30% to 50% in high-risk women with dense breast tissue.[4–6]

Certain breast cancers are more likely to be associated with false-negative mammograms. Among them are lobular carcinomas, which grow in a linear pattern and, therefore, may not form a discrete mass, and noncalcified ductal carcinoma in situ. Small nonspiculated masses are common sources of false-negative mammograms. Oval-shaped circumscribed masses may be misinterpreted as benign.

Once a cancer is diagnosed, mammography may underestimate the size and/or extent of a primary tumor. As a result, re-excision is necessary in approximately 30% of patients[7,8] undergoing breast conservation. Also, mammography may not identify additional foci of malignancy in other quadrants of the breast.

There is continuing improvement in mammography, most recently due to the conversion from analog to digital mammography. Although digital mammography does not improve the overall sensitivity of mammography, it has been shown to improve sensitivity in women with dense breast tissue.[9] More importantly, digital mammography has provided a template on which to develop more-advanced breast imaging technology. Tomosynthesis was developed as a method to image the breast by removing overlying layers of breast tissue so that lesion characteristics and margins are better seen. This topic has been discussed in an article elsewhere in this issue. As stated by Johns and Yaffe,[10] however, removal of overlying structures may not be sufficient to guarantee lesion detection because the difference in attenuation coefficients between fibroglandular and cancerous tissue ranges from only 4% at 15 keV to 1% at 25 keV.

Contrast-enhanced mammography is the second type of advanced technology stemming from the digital platform. The theory behind contrast mammography is based on the success of breast MR imaging, which is currently the most sensitive of all breast imaging techniques, with sensitivities reported up to 98%.[11,12] MR imaging detects

Department of Radiology, Memorial Sloan-Kettering Cancer Center, Weill Cornell Medical College, 300 East 66th Street #711, New York, NY 10065, USA
E-mail address: jochelsm@mskcc.org

Radiol Clin N Am 52 (2014) 609–616
http://dx.doi.org/10.1016/j.rcl.2013.12.004

occult breast cancers in approximately 4/100 to 5/100 high-risk women. It also detects occult multifocal or multicentric cancers in approximately 16% of all patients with known breast cancer.[13] The exquisite sensitivity of MR imaging is the result of a combination of anatomic and physiologic imaging. The physiologic component of MR imaging is primarily its ability to detect enhancing tumor vascularity after contrast administration. Tumor vascularity may be detected before a discrete mass is present. As a result, MR imaging has been shown to demonstrate cancers at an earlier stage in high-risk women who are screened yearly with MR imaging compared with those screened with mammography alone.[14] In this population, MR imaging has also been shown to improve overall survival (93% vs 74.5% in historical cohorts).[15,16]

MR imaging is expensive and time consuming, however, and cannot be performed on all patients. Additionally, good-quality MR imaging is not universally available. Women who are claustrophobic and women with pacemakers or other implanted metallic materials cannot undergo breast MR imaging. Therefore, there is a need for an alternate method to use both contrast enhancement and anatomy for detection of breast cancer. The performance of mammography using contrast material to diagnose breast cancer has been studied for several decades.

DIGITAL SUBTRACTION ANGIOGRAPHY

In 1985, Ackerman and colleagues[17] reported their experience using digital subtraction angiography (DSA) of the breast in 22 patients in an attempt to differentiate benign from malignant disease without performing a surgical biopsy. They injected 30 mL of contrast at 25 mL/s into the right atrium; 32 to 40 images were obtained. In this initial group there were 7 true positive results, 11 true negative results, 2 false-positive results, 1 false-negative result, and 1 equivocal case. These results must be interpreted, however, with caution. One of the malignant lesions was considered a true negative because the mammogram was negative. Additionally, lesions less than 2 cm were not well seen. This somewhat invasive procedure, therefore, did not perform well enough to continue with its use.

It was observed that the degree of tumor angiogenesis correlates with tumor growth and metastatic potential.[18] Haga and colleagues[19] investigated whether tumor enhancement on DSA correlated with disease-free survival. They performed DSA in 103 women and found all tumors enhanced. They compared maximum densities of enhancement and demonstrated that higher densities of enhancement were associated with decreased disease-free survival.

TEMPORAL TECHNIQUE

More recently, contrast-enhanced mammography has been performed using a temporal technique. A baseline image is obtained in a single view performed just above the K-edge of iodine (33 KeV) with the breast mildly compressed. The same iodinated contrast used for CT scans is injected intravenously after which multiple images of the breast are obtained over a period of 5 to 7 minutes. The noncontrast image is subtracted from the contrast images. This technique is successful in detecting cancers. Jong and colleagues[20] studied 22 women who were to undergo breast biopsies for suspected breast cancers. They demonstrated enhancement in 8/10 (80%) of the cancers in their study. Seven of 12 benign lesions did not enhance, but there were 5/22 (23%) false-positive examinations. These included 3 fibroadenomas and 2 patients with fibrocystic changes.

Diekmann and colleagues[21] performed a multireader study involving 70 patients with 80 lesions and demonstrated that the addition of contrast to digital mammography improved sensitivity from 43% to 62%. Not surprisingly, improvement in sensitivity was more likely to occur in women with dense breasts than women with fatty breasts. Dromain studied 20 women with suspicious mammographic findings. There was enhancement in 16/20 (80%) cancers. The size of 97% of the tumors correlated well with size at histology. In her study, the enhancement curves in the cancers differed from those seen with MR imaging. With contrast-enhanced mammography, most cancers demonstrated gradually increasing enhancement as opposed to the rapid enhancement with washout pattern classically seen with cancers on MR imaging. Rapid enhancement with wash out was only seen in 4 of the patients having contrast mammography. It is uncertain as to whether this difference in enhancement pattern is related to the breast compression performed with the temporal technique or is a characteristic of the difference between gadolinium and the iodinated contrast used for contrast mammography. Additionally, the enhancement patterns in Dromain and colleagues'[22] series did not correlate with the microvessel counts demonstrated on pathology.

Although the technique of temporal contrast-enhanced mammography is able to demonstrate cancers with good sensitivity, there are several disadvantages associated with this technique.

Despite breast compression, patient motion caused artifacts; it is difficult for patients to remain still for 7 minutes. Additionally only 1 view of one breast can be obtained per injection, making it difficult to localize abnormalities. Moreover, the contralateral breast is not imaged at all.

CONTRAST-ENHANCED DUAL-ENERGY DIGITAL MAMMOGRAPHY

Contrast-enhanced dual-energy digital mammography (CEDM) is an alternate attempt at combining contrast enhancement with digital mammography. This technique uses nonionic iodinated contrast at 1.5 mL/kg. Each exposure provides a low-energy image below the K-edge of iodine (33 KeV) and a high-energy image above the K-edge of iodine. The tube voltage used is based on breast thickness and glandularity and ranges from 26 to 30 kV (peak) for low-energy images to between 45 and 49 kV (peak) (**Fig. 1**) for the high-energy images. The 2 images are recombined, the background breast parenchyma is eliminated, and an image with any iodine-enhanced lesions is produced.

Lewin and colleagues[23] first performed mammography with dual-energy technique using a mammography unit that was not designed for use with contrast. Nevertheless, they successfully injected contrast followed by the performance of the low- and high-energy images while the breast was compressed. Subtraction of the 2 images yielded an iodine image; 26 patients with mammographic or clinical findings were imaged. There were 13 invasive cancers; 11 of them enhanced strongly and 2 enhanced weakly, confirming the ability of contrast-enhanced mammography using dual-energy technique to demonstrate breast cancer.[23]

As a result of this promising study, a dedicated unit was developed to perform CEDM. It basically adapted a digital mammography unit (Senographe DS, GE Healthcare, Buc, France) for this purpose. The standard digital mammography unit was modified to allow the use of a specialized filter, which could shape the x-ray spectrum specifically to perform CEDM. The prototype unit used manual technique for breast thickness and density. Newer units allow for automated or manual technique. Iodinated contrast is administrated using a power injector with a high flow rate. Patients are seated during intravenous injection of the contrast material. When injection is complete, they begin what for them seems routine mammography. With the new dual-energy units, compression time is no greater than 15 seconds per view and the entire study can be performed within 5 minutes.

The earliest clinical trials were performed imaging 2 views of a single breast. Dromain and colleagues[24] studied 120 women with either abnormalities detected on screening or with clinical problems not resolved by routine mammography or ultrasound. They reported that 74/80 (92%) of cancers enhanced and 13/50 (26%) of benign lesions enhanced. The addition of contrast-enhanced mammography to mammography had significantly better results than mammography alone. Contrast-enhanced mammography plus mammography trended toward improvement over mammography and ultrasound[24] but this did not reach statistical significance.

With positive results of CEDM in a single breast, the next step was to attempt bilateral

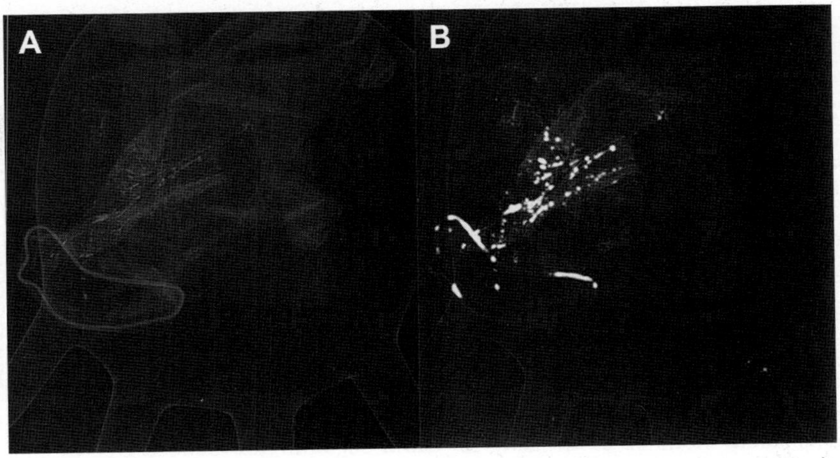

Fig. 1. (*A*) Glove lined with iodinated contrast filmed with keV under 33 shows contrast as water density. (*B*) Same glove with recombination of low-energy and high-energy images demonstrates the iodine. (*Courtesy of* D. David Dershaw, MD, New York, NY.)

contrast-enhanced digital mammography. Jochelson and colleagues[25] performed a 2-phase study. The purpose of the initial phase was to determine the feasibility and if need be optimize the technique of performing bilateral CEDM. The second part of the study was to evaluate the ability of CEDM to detect a known cancer within the breast and compare its sensitivity with digital mammography and breast MR imaging. The ability to detect multifocal/centric disease was also evaluated and compared with mammography and MR imaging for both sensitivity and specificity; 82 patients were enrolled.

The first portion of the trial included 10 patients and demonstrated that bilateral CEDM was feasible and easy to accomplish. The optimal time to begin imaging after contrast enhancement was determined to be approximately 3 minutes. The order in which the images were obtained was varied to determine if it mattered if the side containing the cancer was imaged early or late or whether the *craniocaudal (CC)* or mediolateral oblique *(MLO)* images needed to be performed in a certain order. The study demonstrated that the order did not matter. Tumor enhancement was seen for up to 10 minutes after injection. All patients tolerated the procedure well with no adverse effects.

Fifty-two patients were available for data analysis to determine the accuracy of CEDM compared with digital mammography and MR imaging. CEDM and MR imaging each detected 50/52 (96%) of the index lesions (**Fig. 2**), which was significantly better than mammography, which detected 42/52 (81%). All but 2 of the lesions detected by CEDM were within 5 mm of the actual size of the tumor at pathology. Both invasive and intraductal cancers were detected.

Two additional malignant lesions were present in the ipsilateral breast in this group of patients. CEDM detected 14/25 (56%) whereas MR imaging detected 22/25 (88%) (**Fig. 3**). CEDM demonstrated 2 false-positive lesions and MR imaging found 8 in the ipsilateral breast. In the contralateral breast there was a single cancer, Paget disease, which was not demonstrated by either CEDM or MR imaging. There were 5 false-positive results on MR imaging and none on CEDM in the contralateral breast. The overall lesion detection rate was 64/77 (83%) for CEDM and 72/77 (94%) for MR imaging. Although CEDM was less sensitive, the true positive rate was significantly higher than MR imaging: 64/66 (97%) for CEDM versus 72/85 (85%) for MR imaging.[25]

Entities other than cancer enhance. Just as with MR imaging, the walls of cysts and seroma

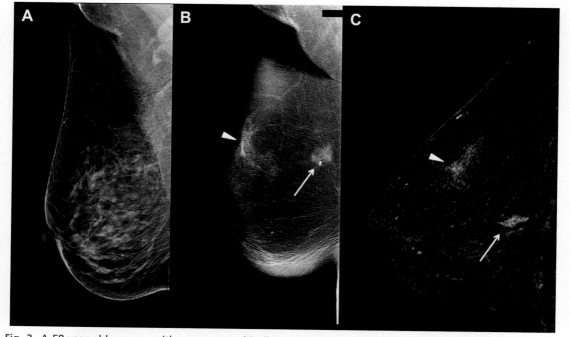

Fig. 2. A 58-year-old woman with mammographically occult invasive ductal carcinoma of the right breast. (*A*) Right MLO mammogram shows no abnormality. (*B*) CEDM demonstrates rounded area of enhancement surrounding a biopsy clip (*arrow*) consistent with known cancer. More anterior area of enhancement due to uptake in seroma after benign biopsy (*arrowhead*). (*C*) Sagittal subtraction image from MR imaging demonstrates the cancer posteriorly (*arrow*) and seroma anteriorly (*arrowhead*).

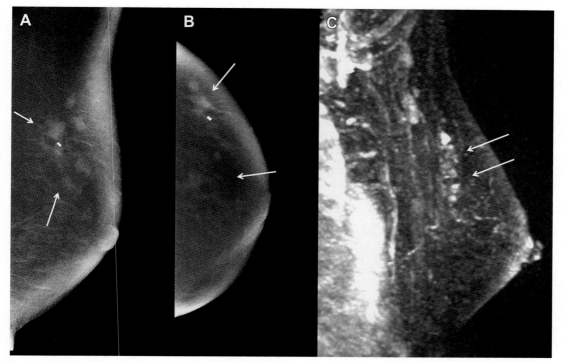

Fig. 3. A 49-year-old woman with a palpable mass left upper outer quadrant biopsy proved to be invasive lobular carcinoma. (*A*) CEDM MLO and (*B*) CEDM CC views show multiple enhancing lesions consistent with multicentric cancer (*arrows*). (*C*) MR imaging, maximum intensity projection image, of the left breast demonstrating multiples lesions (*arrows*).

cavities may enhance (**Fig. 4**). These findings are easy to recognize and do not warrant histologic confirmation. False-positive findings may be seen, however, in benign lesions, such as fibroadenomas, pseudoangiomatous stromal hyperplasia (PASH) (**Fig. 5**), and radial scars that have enhanced on contrast mammography, requiring histologic confirmation. Additionally, just as with MR imaging, there may be background parenchymal enhancement (BPE). At this time, it is uncertain as to whether it is related to timing in regard to menstrual cycle as it is on MR imaging. It is also uncertain as to whether it is a sign of increased cancer risk as has been suggested with BPE on MR imaging.[26]

At this time a method to perform biopsies using CEDM is not available. Abnormalities detected by CEDM are often also seen on MR imaging so that MR imaging–guided core biopsy may be performed. Alternatively, targeted ultrasound may also identify some of these lesions. As with all new modalities, however, a method for performing biopsies is necessary. Work is under way to accomplish this.

Another contrast-enhanced breast imaging technology to consider is contrast-enhanced digital breast tomosynthesis (CE-DBT). Chen and

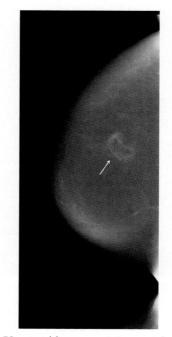

Fig. 4. A 58-year-old woman status post–benign core biopsy right breast with a peripherally enhancing seroma (*arrow*).

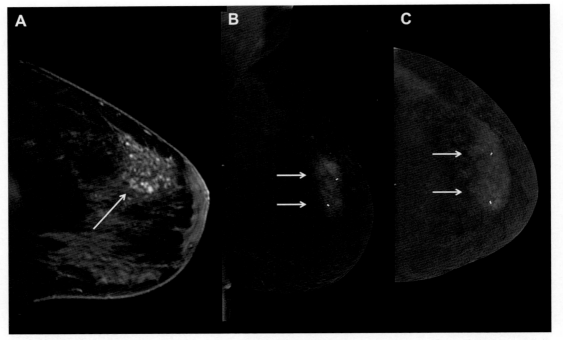

Fig. 5. PASH. (*A*) A 47-year-old high-risk woman who had focal non–mass enhancement (*arrow*) during screening MR imaging. Biopsy showed PASH. (*B*) CEDM MLO and (*C*) CEDM CC views also demonstrate a focal area of enhancement corresponding to the MR imaging finding (*arrows*).

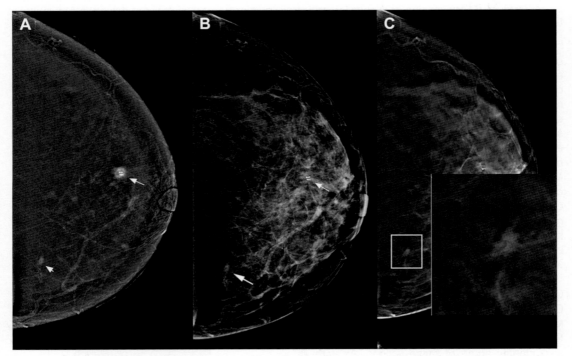

Fig. 6. A 45-year-old woman with biopsy-proved invasive ductal carcinoma. (*A*) Standard mammogram shows biopsy markers (*long arrow*) at the site of the biopsy-proved cancer. The lesion is not visible; a 5-mm lesion is identified in the medial breast (*short arrow*). (*B*) Dual-energy CEDM image shows the known cancer (*long arrow*). A 5-mm enhancing focus in the medial breast (*short arrow*) cannot be characterized. (*C*) Low-energy tomosynthesis image acquired as part of the CEDM study shows the enhancing lesion (*box*) irregularly shaped (*inset*), greatly raising the likelihood of malignancy. The lesion was later proved a second invasive ductal carcinoma. (*Courtesy of John Lewin, MD, Denver, CO.*)

colleagues[27] performed a pilot study in 13 patients with Breast Imaging Reporting and Data System 4 or 5 lesions on mammography and ultrasound. There were 11 cancers of which 10 enhanced. They concluded that CE-DBT could be used as an adjunct to digital mammography for breast lesion characterization. Carton and colleagues[28] performed CE-DBT on a single patient with known breast cancer and compared it with MR imaging. They used both temporal and dual-energy techniques. As in prior studies, there was less motion artifact with dual energy compared with temporal imaging. They were able to demonstrate that the CE-DBT examination compared favorably with MR imaging.[28] Tomosynthesis used after CEDM enables improved lesion and margin analysis so may add to the specificity of CEDM (**Fig. 6**).

At the time this article is being written, CEDM has been studied only in patients with known cancers or in patients with clinical and/or imaging abnormalities so that the results of the data until now cannot be applied to screening. To my knowledge, no prospective trial to evaluate the accuracy of CEDM in the screening setting has been published, although such trials are under way.

SUMMARY

CEDM is a promising new technology that combines anatomic evaluation of the breast with the physiologic characteristic of contrast enhancement of the neovascularity associated with malignant tumors. Early experience suggests that CEDM is more sensitive than digital mammography and more specific than MR imaging. Potential uses may include staging of known breast cancers, additional evaluation of mammographic or clinical abnormalities, evaluation of the post-lumpectomy breast for recurrent tumor, and screening for cancer. It may be an alternative to screening MR imaging and even potentially screening ultrasound. A great deal more prospective research is required to better assess its ability to screen.

REFERENCES

1. Tabar L, Vitak B, Chen TH, et al. Swedish two-county trial: impact of mammographic screening on breast cancer mortality during 3 decades. Radiology 2011;260:658–63.
2. Berry DA, Cronin KA, Plevritis SK, et al. Effect of screening and adjuvant therapy on mortality from breast cancer. N Engl J Med 2005;353:1784–92.
3. Broeders M, Moss S, Nystrom L, et al. The impact of mammographic screening on breast cancer mortality in Europe: a review of observational studies. J Med Screen 2012;19(Suppl 1):14–25.
4. Kerlikowske K, Carney PA, Geller B, et al. Performance of screening mammography among women with and without a first-degree relative with breast cancer. Ann Intern Med 2000;133:855–63.
5. Kuhl CK, Schmutzler RK, Leutner CC, et al. Breast MR imaging screening in 192 women proved or suspected to be carriers of a breast cancer susceptibility gene: preliminary results. Radiology 2000;215:267–79.
6. Leach MO, Boggis CR, Dixon AK, et al. Screening with magnetic resonance imaging and mammography of a UK population at high familial risk of breast cancer: a prospective multicentre cohort study (MARIBS). Lancet 2005;365:1769–78.
7. Morrow M, Jagsi R, Alderman AK, et al. Surgeon recommendations and receipt of mastectomy for treatment of breast cancer. JAMA 2009;302:1551–6.
8. McCahill LE, Single RM, Aiello Bowles EJ, et al. Variability in reexcision following breast conservation surgery. JAMA 2012;307:467–75.
9. Pisano ED, Gatsonis C, Hendrick E, et al. Diagnostic performance of digital versus film mammography for breast-cancer screening. N Engl J Med 2005;353:1773–83.
10. Johns PC, Yaffe MJ. X-ray characterisation of normal and neoplastic breast tissues. Phys Med Biol 1987;32:675–95.
11. Morris EA, Liberman L, Ballon DJ, et al. MRI of occult breast carcinoma in a high-risk population. AJR Am J Roentgenol 2003;181:619–26.
12. Berg WA. Rationale for a trial of screening breast ultrasound: American College of Radiology Imaging Network (ACRIN) 6666. AJR Am J Roentgenol 2003;180:1225–8.
13. Houssami N, Ciatto S, Macaskill P, et al. Accuracy and surgical impact of magnetic resonance imaging in breast cancer staging: systematic review and meta-analysis in detection of multifocal and multicentric cancer. J Clin Oncol 2008;26:3248–58.
14. Warner E, Hill K, Causer P, et al. Prospective study of breast cancer incidence in women with a BRCA1 or BRCA2 mutation under surveillance with and without magnetic resonance imaging. J Clin Oncol 2011;29:1664–9.
15. Rijnsburger AJ, Obdeijn IM, Kaas R, et al. BRCA1-associated breast cancers present differently from BRCA2-associated and familial cases: long-term follow-up of the Dutch MRISC Screening Study. J Clin Oncol 2010;28:5265–73.
16. Heijnsdijk EA, Warner E, Gilbert F, et al. Difference in natural history between breast cancers in BRCA1 and BRCA2 mutation carriers and effects of MRI screening-MRISC, MARIBS, and Canadian studies combined. Cancer Epidemiol Biomarkers Prev 2012;21(9):1458–68.

17. Ackerman LV, Watt AC, Shetty P, et al. Breast lesions examined by digital angiography. Work in progress. Radiology 1985;155:65–8.

18. Weidner N, Semple JP, Welch WR, et al. Tumor angiogenesis and metastasis–correlation in invasive breast carcinoma. N Engl J Med 1991;324:1–8.

19. Haga S, Watanabe O, Shimizu T, et al. Analysis of the tumor staining obtained by preoperative IV-DSA for breast cancer patients: density and metastasis correlation. Breast Cancer Res Treat 1997;43:129–35.

20. Jong RA, Yaffe MJ, Skarpathiotakis M, et al. Contrast-enhanced digital mammography: initial clinical experience. Radiology 2003;228:842–50.

21. Diekmann F, Freyer M, Diekmann S, et al. Evaluation of contrast-enhanced digital mammography. Eur J Radiol 2011;78:112–21.

22. Dromain C, Balleyguier C, Adler G, et al. Contrast-enhanced digital mammography. Eur J Radiol 2009;69:34–42.

23. Lewin JM, Isaacs PK, Vance V, et al. Dual-energy contrast-enhanced digital subtraction mammography: feasibility. Radiology 2003;229:261–8.

24. Dromain C, Thibault F, Muller S, et al. Dual-energy contrast-enhanced digital mammography: initial clinical results. Eur Radiol 2011;21:565–74.

25. Jochelson MS, Dershaw DD, Sung J, et al. Bilateral contrast-enhanced dual-energy digital mammography: feasibility and comparison with conventional digital mammography and MR imaging in women with known breast carcinoma. Radiology 2013; 266(3):743–51.

26. King V, Brooks JD, Bernstein JL, et al. Background parenchymal enhancement at breast MR imaging and breast cancer risk. Radiology 2011; 260:50–60.

27. Chen SC, Carton AK, Albert M, et al. Initial clinical experience with contrast-enhanced digital breast tomosynthesis. Acad Radiol 2007; 14:229–38.

28. Carton AK, Ullberg C, Maidment AD. Optimization of a dual-energy contrast-enhanced technique for a photon-counting digital breast tomosynthesis system: II. An experimental validation. Med Phys 2010; 37:5908–13.

Index

Note: Page numbers of article titles are in **boldface** type.

Radiol Clin N Am 52 (2014) 617–621
http://dx.doi.org/10.1016/S0033-8389(14)00051-7
0033-8389/14/$ – see front matter © 2014 Elsevier Inc. All rights reserved.

radiologic.theclinics.com

Moving?

Make sure your subscription moves with you!

To notify us of your new address, find your **Clinics Account Number** (located on your mailing label above your name), and contact customer service at:

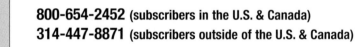

Email: journalscustomerservice-usa@elsevier.com

800-654-2452 (subscribers in the U.S. & Canada)
314-447-8871 (subscribers outside of the U.S. & Canada)

Fax number: 314-447-8029

Elsevier Health Sciences Division
Subscription Customer Service
3251 Riverport Lane
Maryland Heights, MO 63043

*To ensure uninterrupted delivery of your subscription, please notify us at least 4 weeks in advance of move.

ELSEVIER

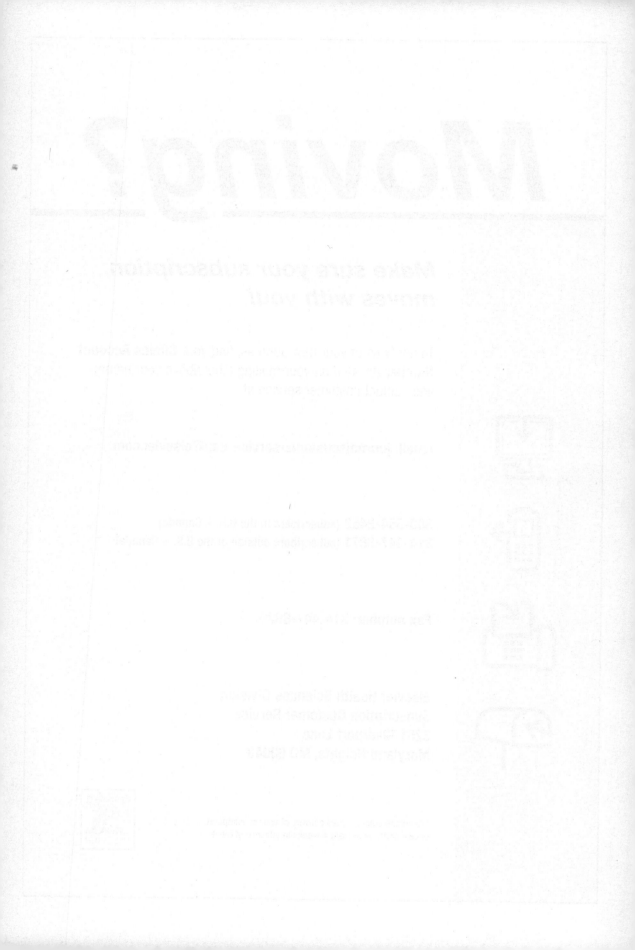